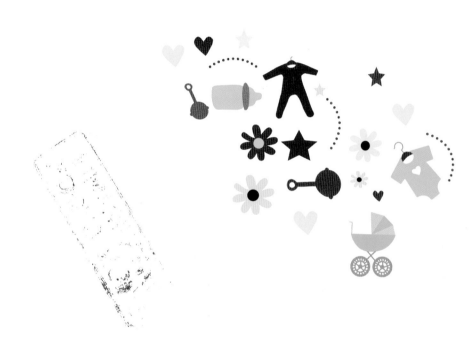

pregnancy
the beginner's guide

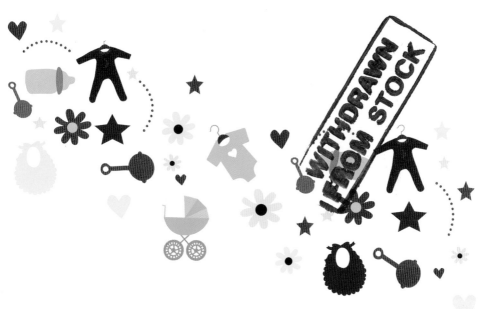

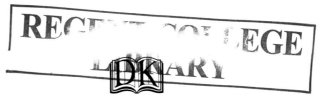

DK

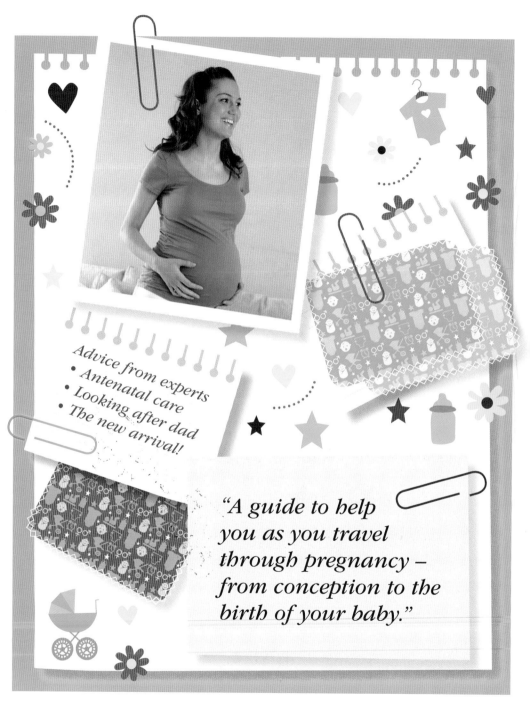

Advice from experts
• Antenatal care
• Looking after dad
• The new arrival!

"A guide to help you as you travel through pregnancy – from conception to the birth of your baby."

pregnancy
the beginner's guide

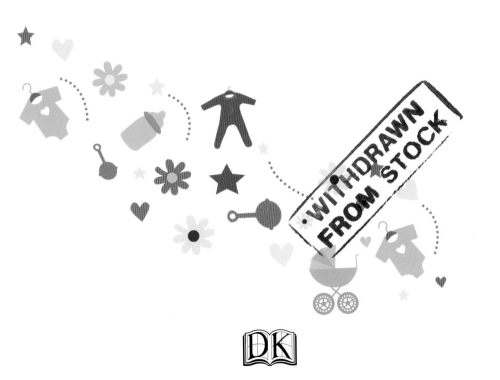

DK

LONDON, NEW YORK, MUNICH, MELBOURNE, AND DELHI

Senior Editors
Christine Stroyan, Katharine Goddard

Senior Art Editors Claire Patané, Jane Ewart

Project Editors
Becky Alexander, Joanna Edwards

Project Art Editors Charlotte Johnson,
Claire Shedden, Elaine Hewson, Ria Holland

Jacket Designer Rosie Levine

Illustrator Bryony Fripp

Producer, Pre-Production
Sarah Isle, Raymond Williams

Senior Producer Alex Bell

Creative Technical Support
Sonia Charbonnier

Managing Editor Penny Smith

Senior Managing Art Editor
Marianne Markham

Publisher Mary Ling

Creative Director Jane Bull

Consultant Judith Barac

Writers Shaoni Bhattacharya, Claire Cross,
Elinor Duffy, Kate Ling, and Susannah Marriott.

Every effort has been made to ensure that
the information in this book is complete
and accurate. However, neither the publisher
nor the authors are engaged in rendering
professional advice or services to the
individual reader.

The contents of this book are not intended
as a substitute for consulting with your
healthcare provider. All matters regarding the
health of you and your baby require medical
supervision. Neither the publisher nor the
authors shall be liable or responsible for any
loss or damage allegedly arising from any
information or suggestions in this book.

First published in Great Britain in 2014 by

Dorling Kindersley Limited

80 Strand, London WC2R 0RL

1 2 3 4 5 6 7 8 9 10

001-196608-Feb14

A CIP catalogue record for this book
is available from the British Library.

ISBN: 978-1-4093-3871-0

Printed and bound in China by
Leo paper products Ltd.

Discover more at **www.dk.com**

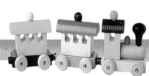

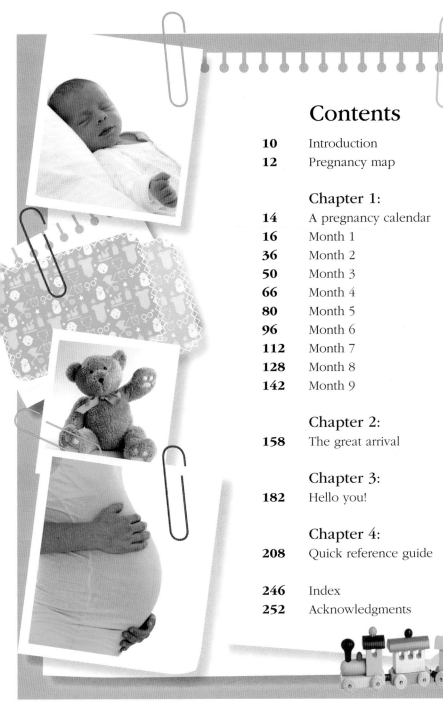

Contents

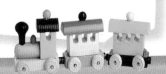

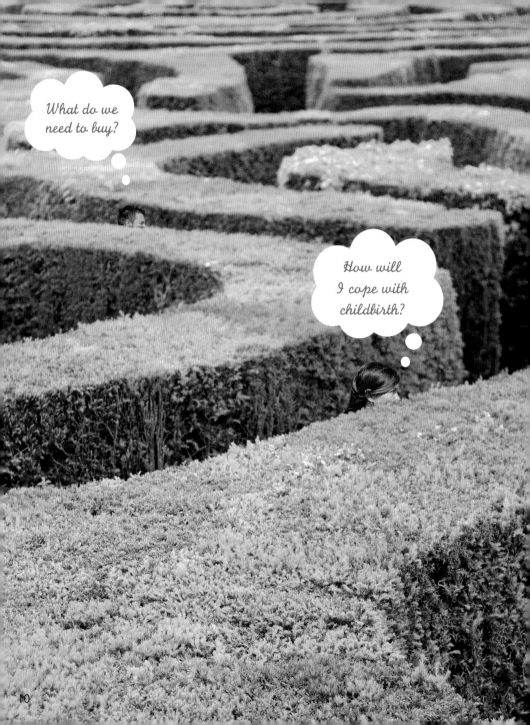

Introduction

FINDING YOUR WAY

WELCOME TO PREGNANCY! This journey begins without you even knowing it, and ends with the happiest day of your life – the day you meet your baby. When you reach your destination one thing is for sure – your path will have changed forever, and in the best way possible.

THIS VOYAGE will take you to strange new places, such as antenatal clinics and birthing classes; you will have to get used to a different style of clothing, a change in diet, and a language you have never come across before. The journey may test your relationship with your loved ones, but will also bring you closer than ever.

PREGNANCY is an emotional rollercoaster, too – your hormones run riot throughout the nine months, your body is no longer your own, and you will bounce from elation to exhaustion and back again as your life gradually shifts to accommodate enormous and unprecedented change. And then, suddenly, you have a tiny person in your care, who relies on you for everything and who will bring you more joy than you could have ever thought imaginable.

DO YOU NEED TO KNOW what to do, what to eat, and where to go? Look no further for all the answers: let *Pregnancy: The beginner's guide* be your constant companion as you make your way through this wonderful new world. This book will be your key to blending in, to understanding what's going on, to knowing what's ahead, and most importantly to making the most out of every minute. You will never do this for the first time again, so don't waste a moment worrying when you could spend it understanding, marvelling, and enjoying the trip of a lifetime.

You're pregnant!

YOUR PREGNANCY JOURNEY

You are about to embark on an epic adventure, with each step taking you closer to meeting your baby. You have 40 weeks to get acquainted with all things baby!

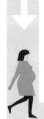

FIRST TRIMESTER

HALFWAY THERE!

FIRST ANTENATAL APPOINTMENT
Yes, you are pregnant! Your hormones are busy getting ready for baby.

Weeks 5–8
FEELING PREGNANT?
Morning sickness may kick in as your body goes through amazing changes. Get plenty of rest, eat well, and look after yourself.

SECOND TRIMESTER

H

H

Weeks 9–12
YOUR FIRST SCAN You get to see and hear your baby for the first time, and he will be checked to see that everything is well. You will also find out the estimated delivery date – when baby is due! You can get an image to take home, and may start telling people.

Weeks 17–21
20-WEEK SCAN
The sonographer will check that baby is growing well, while you get to watch your baby move around. Baby has grown and you may find out if it's a boy or girl!

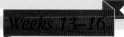

Weeks 13–16
LOOKING PREGNANT You might have a bump by now, and the secret is out! You may need to buy new clothes.

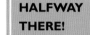

This is a travel guide to your journey from conception to delivery.

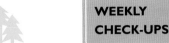
WEEKLY CHECK-UPS

370,000 BABIES ARE BORN EVERY DAY

THIRD TRIMESTER

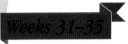
Weeks 31–35

GET ORGANIZED

Enjoy your antenatal classes, and meet lots of parents-to-be. Start packing a hospital bag so you have everything you need, ready for action.

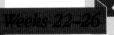
Weeks 22–26

AND RELAX! You are probably feeling great; blooming in fact. Your skin and hair look good, and you have more energy. This could be the perfect time to take a holiday.

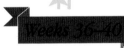
Weeks 36–40

COUNTING DOWN

Baby is nearly ready to be born. Good luck on your new adventure!

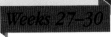
Weeks 27–30

PLANNING THE BIRTH Visit hospitals and birthing centres, and book antenatal classes. Talk to work about maternity leave.

13

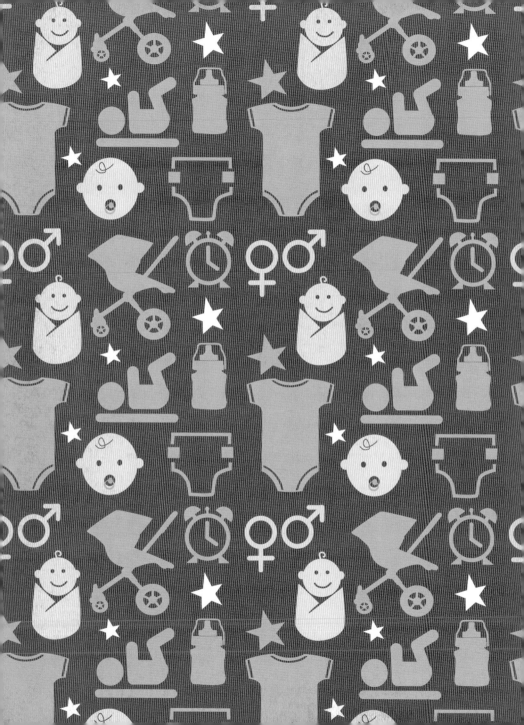

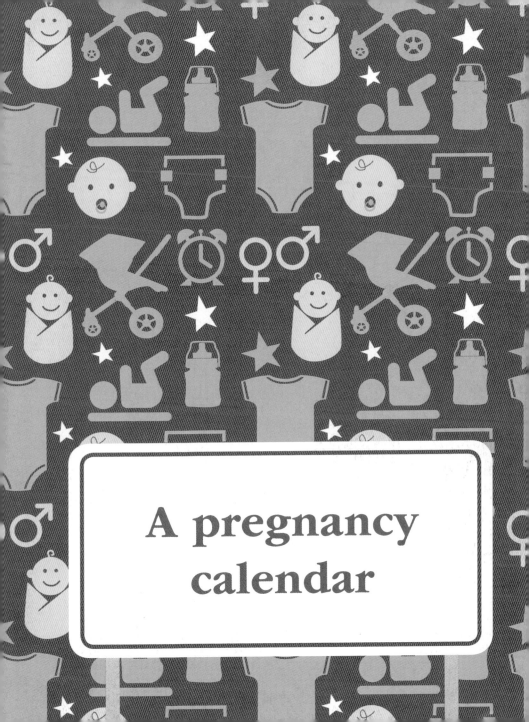

A pregnancy calendar

The journey begins

Get ready for the trip of a lifetime! Even if you don't look or feel any different, your body is busy getting ready for all the new tasks it has to perform.

✳ We have lift-off!

Levels of the female hormone oestrogen, produced by your ovaries, rise rapidly during the first weeks of pregnancy. It increases blood flow to your organs, and thickens the lining of your uterus to create a welcoming environment for the implanting embryo. Working alongside the hormone progesterone, oestrogen also triggers the mammary glands to swell, making your breasts feel unusually tender and heavy or tingly. Your body is getting ready for breastfeeding.

✳ It's like jet-lag

Triggering many of the tell-tale signs and sensations of early pregnancy, progesterone levels also rise after conception. For the next few weeks progesterone is produced in the corpus luteum, the follicles in your ovary that burst to release the egg that was fertilized. Progesterone has a sedative effect, contributing to the unexplained exhaustion you may feel. It also relaxes your muscles and ligaments, allowing your uterus to expand. At such high levels, progesterone slows the muscle contractions that move food through your digestive system, resulting in food taking longer to be processed. This actually benefits your pregnancy – nutrients have longer to be absorbed into

x2

BLOOD FLOW to your uterus has already doubled. Your heart is now working hard to supply both of you!

78%

OF WOMEN suffer from low-to-moderate antenatal psychosocial stress (anxiety).

your bloodstream – but it can also lead to indigestion, heartburn, gas, and constipation. Progesterone thickens your cervical mucus, sealing your baby safely in your uterus. It's all very clever!

✳ Testing positive

Human chorionic gonadotrophin (hCG) starts to be produced by the embryo after it implants, about a week after conception. It surges until the end of the first trimester, when it drops away steadily. This is the hormone that triggers a positive result in a pregnancy test kit. HCG prompts the corpus luteum to produce enough oestrogen and progesterone to keep the embryo safely embedded and nourished until the placenta can take over production.

✳ Over the speed limit

Your metabolism speeds up after conception to support the extra demands of your organs and growing baby. Your heart pumps faster to boost blood flow to every organ, and you start to breathe more rapidly in order to deliver nutrients and oxygen to your baby. No wonder so many expectant mums feel tired!

Think about booking your first antenatal appointment.

Travelling together

Pregnancy can be a nerve-wracking adventure for both partners, even if you have been planning it for ages. Get ready for emotional swings from delight to incredulity – for both of you.

✽ PMS plus

Hormonal changes are at their most dramatic now. In fact, early pregnancy can feel like the worst case of PMS. The surge in hormones can make you moody, bloated, irritable, argumentative, and likely to burst into tears for no reason. Just being aware of this makes it more bearable, and should help your partner empathize. It's your hormones not a personality transplant! When hormone levels even out from week 12, so should your emotions.

✽ Going long-haul

You and your partner have a lot of big subjects to cover – work, money, childcare, but you don't have to cover everything right now. You both have months to get used to the idea of having a baby; if you like, plan to set aside time to talk things through regularly.

✽ Your changing roles

You also don't have to decide what kind of parents to be yet, but it can help to start thinking about your backgrounds and expectations of family life. Think back to your childhoods – what do you

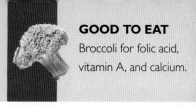
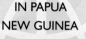

remember fondly, what do you wish had been different, what would you borrow from other parents you think have done a great job.

✳ Be honest

It's best not to bluff your way through the early weeks and pretend that everything is great if it isn't. Some days pregnancy will feel like a bad idea and very few parents feel completely ready for it. The first antenatal appointment, feeling tired, wanting to share the news, worrying about money – talk to your partner if you feel anxious.

IN PAPUA NEW GUINEA
traditionally a woman does not tell her husband she is pregnant; instead she confides in family, who tell neighbours. When the husband finds out, he can't let on until the first in a series of pregnancy feasts.

✳ Expect the unexpected

Are your reactions to pregnancy what you expected? Your partner's reactions may not meet your expectations either. Becoming a parent involves finding out about your partner – like how he or she copes when faced with life changes and responsibility. You both may need to learn empathy, practise patience, and get better at talking things through. It's all good preparation for when your baby is older!

✳ Planning for your first appointment

Write down any questions you have for your first antenatal appointment. You can ask about anything that is worrying you. Your midwife, when you meet her, will be able to answer the questions and hopefully reassure you.

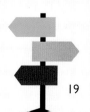

19

The sperm decides the sex of the baby, since it carries either an X or Y chromosome.

A love story

If you thought falling in love with your partner was an incredible adventure, then the romance gets really serious once egg and sperm meet. In just seven days they collide, mingle, and start a whole new person.

✳ Boy meets girl

When egg and sperm meet in your fallopian tube, they fuse to create a new cell, the zygote, in which the genetic material (DNA) they each carry mixes together. Here, your 23 chromosomes join your partner's 23 chromosomes forming a single cell with 46 chromosomes. Your baby's sex, as well as its unique looks and character, are entirely determined by this meeting and mixing of male and female DNA.

✳ The magic happens

For the first 12 hours of life the zygote remains a single cell. It starts to move down your fallopian tube, aided by the movement of tiny, hair-like structures called cilia, which propel it towards your uterus. About 30 hours into its journey, the zygote divides in two. In another 15 hours, these two cells divide to become four. And after about 72 hours have passed since fertilization, those four have divided into

Baby's progress bar: you are now 10% complete

LOADING

| 10% | 20% | 30% | 40% | 50% |

BY DAY FOUR, the embryo contains at least 12 cells. Within a few weeks, it will grow to form a cluster of cells. Your baby already contains 46 chromosomes.

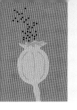

HOW BIG?
Your baby is now the size of a poppy seed.

eight cells, and the initial loose bunch of cells has become a tight ball. This process of cell-division continues, over and over, until there is a cluster of around 100 cells, now called a blastocyst. At this stage, a cavity develops within the blastocyst and its cells separate to form two structures: a shell-like outer layer, and an inner cell mass.

✳ Hello baby

Around five days after conception the blastocyst finally reaches your uterus, where it slows down and rolls along the sticky uterus wall. Then, on about day six, the outer layer of cells starts to burrow into the thickened uterus lining in a process known as implantation. As it implants, the blastocyst secretes the hormone hCG, which tells your body to make enough oestrogen and progesterone to support the first 12 weeks of pregnancy. After about three days implantation is complete. Once safely burrowed into the lining of your uterus, the blastocyst's inner cell mass will change and specialize in order to develop into an embryo, while its outer layer begins to form the placenta.

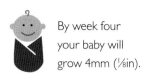

By week four your baby will grow 4mm (⅙in).

Cells at work

Deep inside your uterus an embryo is busy developing from a tiny cluster of cells. By the end of week four it has created its own beating heart.

✳ Secure luggage

After implantation, the amniotic sac starts to form from the outer cells of the blastocyte, building a protective bubble around your growing baby. The sac will fill with amniotic fluid to keep the baby warm and hydrated and act as a shock absorber. It is encircled by another protective layer, called the chorion. Tiny fingerlike "villi" reach out from here and root into the wall of your uterus, tapping into your bloodstream in order to bring nutrients and oxygen to the baby. The chorion will eventually grow into the placenta, but until this is fully formed, the embryo derives nourishment from a yolk sac, attached to it by a stalk.

✳ Ready for action

The implanted blastocyst contains an inner group of cells, each of which is programmed to create one specific aspect of the embryo. In a process called differentiation, which begins in week three, this cell mass divides into three distinct layers: the ectoderm,

DID YOU KNOW?

PREGNANCY STARTS before you have even missed your period! Baby is busy growing for three to four weeks before you know.

10,000

By one month, the embryo is 10,000 times larger than its initial single cell.

mesoderm, and endoderm. The cells in these layers already know whether they will become skin, skeleton, or organs, and are ready to start fulfilling these amazing and unique functions.

IN INDIAN AYURVEDIC MEDICINE, the embryo is said to be formed from the five elements that are the building blocks of all life in the universe: earth, water, fire, air, and ether. The soul enters the embryo once it is formed.

✳ Outer layer

Ectoderm cells now start to form the outer layer of your baby's body, made up of skin and hair, including the skin cells that give us pigment. So your baby's hair and eye colour is being decided right now! They also form the central nervous system and the sensory organs.

✳ Middle layer

Mesoderm cells will develop into your baby's skeleton, muscles, heart, circulatory system, reproductive organs, and kidneys. Your baby's bone marrow and blood are also manufactured in this layer, alongside fat, bone, and cartilage.

✳ Inner layer

Endoderm cells make up the inner layer, and will develop into body systems including the entire digestive tract, the respiratory system, and the urinary tract, along with all the organs these systems will require to function. It's quite a substantial list, including the liver, pancreas, stomach, lungs, intestines, and bladder. There are also cells within this layer that will eventually create eggs and sperm.

Trip of a lifetime

With any long journey to a highly-anticipated destination, it's always good to know roughly when you're going to get there, and pregnancy is definitely no different. You've got a lot of planning to do!

✳ Doing the maths

For the sake of convenience, a baby's estimated date of delivery (EDD) is calculated as 40 weeks from the first day of the mother's last period – the specific time of conception would be far too hard to work out. Most women with regular cycles will ovulate about two weeks after their period, so conception will usually take place around that time. This means that for the first two of the 40 weeks, the pregnancy hasn't even begun – so the baby's real time in the womb is actually only 38 weeks. If the mathematics involved in this calculation seem boggling, help is at hand: there is a host of online calculators that, when given the date of your last period, can do the maths for you. Women with irregular cycles should be aware that for them using this method can be rather hit-and-miss; the measurements taken during ultrasound dating scans are more accurate.

✳ Why is a due date important?

Working out your EDD is important for several reasons. First, it will allow the midwife and

ANYWHERE FROM 38–42 WEEKS
is considered a normal length for a
pregnancy, and 80–90% of women
will give birth within this range.

MORE THAN FOUR BABIES
are born in the world every
second – that's 133 million
births every year!

doctor to accurately monitor your baby's growth. It will also allow
you and your partner to start thinking about future changes in your
lives, in addition to planning for maternity leave, booking scans, and
attending antenatal visits.

✷ Patience is a virtue

The EDD might seem a lifetime away when you first discover you're
pregnant, yet many expectant mums have to wait beyond this date
for baby to arrive. There are many reasons for this – if it is a first
pregnancy, if there is a history of post-term babies, or just if baby
isn't ready to come out yet.

✷ Ready to pop

If you reach 42 weeks, you may feel well overdue on your pregnancy
journey, but actually it's still within normal ranges. Nevertheless, most
doctors would encourage induction of labour or close monitoring
after 40 weeks plus 10 days. This is because amniotic fluid levels may
begin to drop, the placenta becomes less efficient, and the baby will
only get bigger and become more difficult to deliver. Only 5 per cent
of women stay pregnant beyond 42 weeks, and in many cases this is
down to an incorrect due date prediction.

✷ Long time coming

Every day past your due date may feel like an eternity, but spare a
thought for Beulah Hunter who, in 1945, allegedly waited 375 days
for her slow-developing but perfectly healthy baby, Penny, to be
born. This remains the longest viable human pregnancy on record!

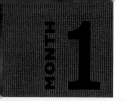

Checking you are OK

Once you tell your doctor that you are pregnant you will be booked in for a number of appointments and scans, with a whole support team to look after you!

❋ What is the lingo?

Antenatal (meaning "before birth") care is the healthcare you receive while pregnant. You will have regular appointments to monitor you and your baby throughout your pregnancy. Don't worry if this is your first time in this new world; you will be given plenty of information to help you.

❋ Who will I see?

First you need to book an appointment with your usual doctor, who will confirm that you are pregnant. You will then be transferred to the midwife team who will guide you safely through this journey. Most likely you will see more than one midwife during your nine months, so always carry your antenatal notes with you. If you need specialist care you may also have appointments with a consultant. At any appointment you have, feel free to ask questions, and write down any that occur to you between appointments. Your midwife will answer your questions and reassure you.

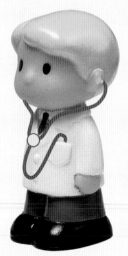

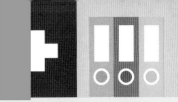

Antenatal care

✳ Check-in time

Your first meeting with a midwife at 8–12 weeks is called the "booking-in appointment". This can take up to two hours and you will be asked questions including the date of your last period, whether you smoke, and if you are eating well, and whether you need to see a doctor for any reason. The aim of this is to establish how best to care for you, and to monitor how your pregnancy is progressing. You may also be given information about local antenatal classes.

✳ Departure lounge checks

You will be asked to provide a blood sample and urine sample so your team can find out if you are in tip-top health. The tests will check your iron levels and blood type, and look for any genetic diseases, urine infections, diabetes, and sexually transmitted diseases. If you have any medical concerns, your doctor will help you to deal with them. Your baby's growth will be monitored at each check by measuring your bump from the top of your womb to your pelvic bone. Your midwife may also listen to baby's heartbeat. You will also have at least two ultrasound scans (see pages 58–59 and 88–89).

✳ Final destination

A midwife will discuss a schedule of care with you. Appointments will probably be monthly until the third trimester when they may be weekly. If there is any cause for concern you may move to a hospital where they have scanning equipment and access to consultants.

Most women only need extra calories during the last trimester – 200 calories each day. That's a banana and a piece of toast.

Fruit juices, herbal teas, smoothies, and of course water make great thirst quenchers when pregnant.

What can I eat?

Forget eating for two – that's been proved wrong (sorry!). Eating a healthy, balanced diet throughout your pregnancy is best for you and your baby.

✳ Looking after you and your baby

Your diet takes on a new significance now you are pregnant. After all, what you eat is what your baby eats, too. Eating regular, nutritious meals and snacks will give you the energy you need for each day, alleviate nausea, and help you sleep better. There are a few foods to avoid, or cut back on (see opposite), to prevent food poisoning and the risk of E. coli, listeria, salmonella, and toxoplasmosis. Any alcohol will pass to your baby, so if you do drink, take advice first.

✳ Folic acid and vitamin D

Your midwife will advise you to take 400 micrograms (mcg) of folic acid throughout your first trimester; this is important as it helps to prevent birth defects. You should also take 10mcg of vitamin D every day throughout your pregnancy, and continue for as long as you are breastfeeding to help your baby's bones develop healthily. If you take a multivitamin, check that it does not contain vitamin A, as this is not advised as a supplement during pregnancy.

Stop!

Pâté Avoid all types, including vegetable pâtés.

Mould-ripened soft cheese This includes Camembert, Brie, soft-rind goat's cheese, Roquefort, Danish blue, and Gorgonzola.

Raw eggs Risk of salmonella.

Raw or undercooked meat Especially minced meat, such as steak tartare or burgers.

Liver products Contain high levels of vitamin A.

Medicinal herbs Check with a midwife or doctor before taking any medicinal herbs.

Deep-sea fish Including shark, marlin, and swordfish.

Raw shellfish Cooked shellfish are usually safe.

Unpasteurized milk Risk of salmonella.

Cold meats Salami, Parma ham, chorizo, pepperoni, and processed ham due to risk of toxoplasmosis.

Caution

Caffeine Pregnant women are advised to cut back on caffeine as it can contribute to low birth weight. 200mg a day is the advised limit, which is the equivalent of two mugs of tea or instant coffee. Chocolate also contains caffeine – dark chocolate contains about 50mg per 50g/2oz bar, as does cola.

Sushi See page 223. If in doubt, choose cooked or vegetable sushi options.

Tuna Two tuna steaks or four medium cans a week is the recommended limit, as tuna contains high levels of mercury.

Vegetables Must be washed to remove all traces of soil.

Commercially prepared foods Can contain listeria. Ready meals should be heated to a high temperature. Re-wash bagged salad leaves.

Safe

Yogurt Made from pasteurized milk, including with probiotics.

Honey All types of honey.

Herbal teas Four cups a day is the recommended limit.

Mayonnaise If made without raw egg.

Many cheeses Hard cheeses and those made from pasteurized milk are safe.

Vegetables that contain vitamin A Spinach, for example, contains a different type of vitamin A to the one in supplements and liver.

Pasteurized cream This is safe because listeria is killed by pasteurization.

Prawns If cooked thoroughly.

Coleslaw As long as the eggs in the mayonnaise are pasteurized, which they are in most shop-bought varieties.

Peanuts Good source of protein but not if your partner has an allergy.

A healthy balance

Whether you like to cook or prefer to buy ready-made meals, making some thoughtful choices will help you to eat well. Mix in delicious superfoods to give you and your baby a nutritional boost.

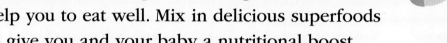

✳ Food for thought

Aim to eat a mix of all the food groups, including a variety of vegetables, fruit, carbohydrates, and proteins. This is not the time for low-carb diets! On an ideal day, your food should contain 50–60 per cent carbohydrates, 25 per cent essential fats, and 20 per cent proteins. Good sources of carbohydrate include wholegrains, such as wholemeal bread, brown rice, pulses, and grains. Protein is found in pulses, nuts, eggs, dairy produce, meat, and fish. Essential fats come from nuts, seeds, oily fish, and eggs. Aim to have carbohydrates, protein, and essential fats in every meal.

✳ Need a little extra

If you eat a varied diet then you will get the range of vitamins and nutrients that you need, but pregnancy can place extra demands on even the most foodie mum-to-be. Iron-rich foods are important during pregnancy to prevent tiredness and anaemia. To help absorb iron, eat plenty of vitamin C-rich foods such as fruit or peppers.

✳ Vegetarian and gluten-free

If you know you cannot, or do not want to, eat certain foods, for example if you are diabetic or vegetarian, and are worried you may be missing essential nutrients, seek advice from a nutritionist. If you need to avoid gluten make sure you get enough energy from carbohydrates, such as sweet potatoes, quinoa, and bananas.

✳ Superfoods

You need a balanced, varied range of foods throughout your pregnancy to keep you and your baby in tip-top condition. The chart below shows a selection of the vitamins and nutrients your body can obtain from eating certain fresh foods. You may also like to refer to pages 216–221 for more information on eating well.

Vitamin A	Broccoli, carrots, sweet potatoes
Vitamin B	Broccoli, eggs, wholegrains
Vitamin C	Broccoli, citrus fruits, berries, avocados
Vitamin D	Yogurt, milk, hard cheeses
Vitamin K	Spinach, dairy produce
Folic acid	Nuts and seeds, green leafy vegetables (such as broccoli, kale, and spinach), pulses, lentils, citrus fruits, fortified cereals, avocados
Iron	Leafy green vegetables, beans and lentils, lean red meats, fortified cereals, tofu
Zinc	Nuts and seeds, beans and lentils, lean red meats
Calcium	Dairy produce, tofu
Omega-3/fatty acids	Oily fish, omega-3-enriched eggs, nuts
Protein	Nuts, eggs, oily fish, dairy produce
Potassium	Banana, avocados, sweet potatoes

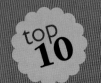

I'm tired of being tired
COMMON COMPLAINTS
IN EARLY PREGNANCY

WHAT TO DO

1 ### Fatigue
You feel exhausted and just can't do as much as you used to.

Cut down on going out in the evenings and have power naps. Listen to your body, eat healthily, and take it easy as much as possible. Tiredness should improve in the next trimester.

2 ### Sickness
You feel sick unless you eat a loaf of bread. You ARE actually sick – a lot. It's a nightmare!

Eat little and often, and snack. Eating ginger products can help. If you can't keep anything down, see a doctor as dehydration can be dangerous in pregnancy.

3 ### Bloating and constipation
You have a tummy full of wind and stools like rabbit droppings.

Eat lots of fibre, drink more water, and exercise daily, as this stimulates the bowel. Don't use laxatives without consulting your doctor first. Try not to strain as this causes haemorrhoids.

4 ### Breast changes
Your breasts are growing alarmingly and your nipples are changing colour.

Get measured for maternity bras (no underwires). These will support your chest and help ease soreness. Rub olive or argan oil into your skin to prevent stretch marks.

5 ### Headaches
You're having lots of irritating minor headaches.

Drink plenty of water to stave off dehydration and avoid becoming too tired. You can take paracetamol safely during pregnancy, but not ibuprofen.

NEW HEALTH NIGGLES You may well experience some, if not all, of these symptoms during your first trimester. If any are extreme, seek medical advice.

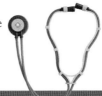

CRAVINGS could be a sign that your body needs extra minerals.

WHAT TO DO

Top 10

6 Weeing all the time
You need to go to the loo more often than usual.

This is caused by hormonal changes and the growth of the baby, and there's not much you can do. It's annoying, because it can disturb your sleep, so try to take a rest in the day.

7 Can't sleep
Tossing and turning, need the loo, weird taste in your mouth, crampy legs… great!

Remind yourself that you WILL be able to manage the next day and try to relax. Develop coping strategies, such as taking an afternoon nap – this is important and not a sign of laziness!

8 Cramp
Agonizing cramp in your thighs, legs, and feet.

Stretch out your leg or foot, or ask your partner to massage the cramped muscles. Some doctors say extra calcium intake can help, so ingest more milk, cheese, or bananas.

9 Food cravings
You can't stop thinking about a nice snack of fried eggs with mint sauce.

You are not alone in wanting favourite comfort foods such as chocolate. If you find you are craving things such as soil, charcoal, or other non-food substances, talk to your doctor.

10 Mood swings
One minute you are laughing, the next crying.

This is normal. Sometimes just knowing that and telling those close to you is all you need to cope. Eating healthily can really help, too.

33

MONTH

1

Weeks 1–4
DAD'S SURVIVAL
GUIDE

DID YOU
KNOW?

The big news!

Congratulations – you're going to be a father. From the moment the thin blue lines appear your life changes; the positive pregnancy test signals a new phase of your life.

✳ Surprise!

It's big news. Huge. So it's hardly surprising if you experience mixed feelings, perhaps elation, pride, relief, trepidation, or downright terror? If the news is a surprise you might even be in total shock. All of this is completely natural – after all, this is probably the biggest thing that has ever happened to you. It is also the biggest thing to happen to your partner, and it is her who will be going through the most changes, so she is going to need your support, and that begins right now. Start as you mean to go on and smile, hug her, give her a kiss, and tell her this is the best news you've ever heard.

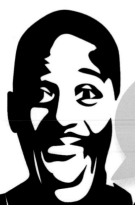

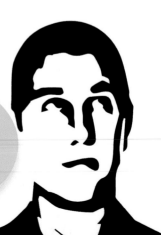

CELEBRATE YOUR amazing news with a good night out and discuss everything that's wonderful and crazy about beginning this new life.

YOUR PARTNER was born with all her eggs; half your baby is as old as her.

THE AVERAGE EJACULATION contains 40–600 million sperm but only about 200 will be hardy enough to make it past the cervix and into the womb.

EACH MONTH the average couple has only a 20% chance of conceiving. It's not easy!

✳ Unreal life

Initially it may all seem a bit unreal; there is no bump, no scan picture, and your partner looks the same. You may decide not to tell anyone for a few more months, which can make it all seem less tangible. You can, however, talk with your partner about the future, practicalities, and fantasize about how much fun the three of you are going to have over the rest of your lives.

✳ From tiny acorns

At this point your baby is only tiny, but she's already firmly fixed into the lining of your partner's womb, and is busy growing. Your partner will be experiencing very few symptoms, but she may start to have a sense that something is different, or have early nausea, and her breasts may grow slightly as the pregnancy hormones start to influence her body. Your partner may feel more tired than usual, or she may not really notice anything different. It is time to simply let the news sink in and start to adjust to this new phase of life.

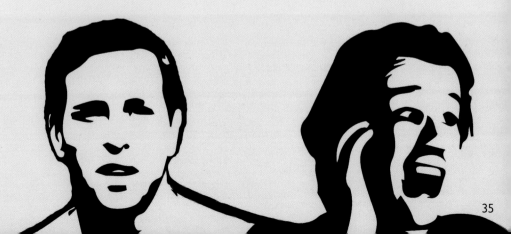

Anytime sickness

Remember how it felt to be travel sick? Well, that's how it feels to have "morning sickness", which is very common during this stage of pregnancy. Sadly, for some women this nausea can occur at anytime.

✱ How are you feeling?

Many women start experiencing pregnancy symptoms around the time they miss their first period; thankfully most ease after week 12. You may experience nausea and vomiting, but other symptoms include a metallic taste in the mouth or an increase in saliva. You may have greater sensitivity to smell or food, and crave bland, filling foods, such as white bread, plain pasta, milk, and potatoes. Combined with the overwhelming exhaustion of early pregnancy, suffering from intense morning sickness can be particularly debilitating. If you can't keep any food or water down (a condition known as hyperemesis gravidarum [HG]) you need to see a doctor or midwife.

✱ What's happening inside

Morning sickness is most often attributed to rising hormones, particularly the effects of high levels of oestrogen. This also contributes to your heightened sense of smell. Increased progesterone is linked to sluggish digestion, and a peak of hCG (see page 17) in month two triggers the nausea. Certain scientists explain it as an evolutionary adaptation; we instinctively choose bland foods to protect us from ingesting potentially toxic plants. Bland foods are also easy to digest and the extra carbohydrates are craved when your body is saying you are tired.

✱ Take it easy

If pregnancy is making you feel tired, then listen to your body. Tiredness has been shown to worsen symptoms of morning sickness, so rest when you need to. Stay in bed a little longer in the morning if you can, rest during breaks at work rather than rushing around, and take a nap at weekends.

✱ Self-help strategies

Eating small, frequent, carbohydrate-rich snacks, such as rice cakes, oat biscuits, or a slice of toast, can help to reduce morning sickness. Ginger can be extremely effective at preventing and alleviating pregnancy nausea. Most research studies recommend taking 250mg (which is ½ tsp) of powdered ginger root four times a day – you can buy this in tablets and capsules. You could also try using fresh ginger in your cooking, such as in a stir-fry, or try nibbling ginger biscuits. Vitamins C and K are also thought to ease symptoms; these can be found in fresh blackcurrants, kiwi fruits, peppers, and spinach. A lack of vitamin B6 has been linked with pregnancy nausea, so eat wholegrains, potatoes, milk, cod, and bananas, which are all good sources.

Going out/staying in

You probably haven't yet told many people you are pregnant, which can make work and social situations tricky. How do you handle tiredness, nausea, and not drinking alcohol without giving the game away?

✳ Make a few changes

Your body is working overtime and you aren't alone if you feel tired at work or on your commute. Many women choose not to make their pregnancy common knowledge at work until the first trimester is safely over, but talking to a sympathetic line manager or personnel manager could help make this stage of pregnancy easier. In the UK you are entitled to paid time-off for antenatal appointments, and your company is obliged to reconsider your workload if it is no longer suitable. You may be able to negotiate flexible hours to avoid the rush hour, and working from home occasionally can be a huge help if you're suffering from morning sickness.

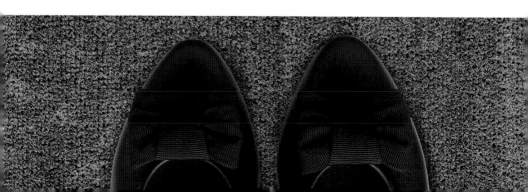

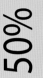

DID YOU KNOW?

MOST TRAIN COMPANIES give pregnant season ticket-holders a free upgrade.

50% OF WOMEN EXPERIENCE NAUSEA AND VOMITING DURING PREGNANCY.

✳ Eating out

Your tastes can change in the early weeks of pregnancy, so you may not fancy your usual favourites. As you need to eat regularly, late suppers might not work for you. Snack beforehand if you have to, but perhaps make arrangements for lunch instead of dinner.

✳ Alcohol-free

If you're known as someone who enjoys a drink in social situations, declining a glass can make heads turn. To keep the secret for a while longer, volunteer to drive when out with friends. You could choose drinks that look similar, such as grape juice instead of red wine.

✳ Change your routine

Why not arrange to meet at the cinema or theatre rather than a crowded bar; you will be guaranteed a seat! Or invite people to your home, where you can lounge with your feet up and serve just the food and drink you fancy (or even order it in). But maybe the best nights, for a while, will be the ones you spend on the sofa with a box set wearing your pyjamas. Relaxation is the new hedonism.

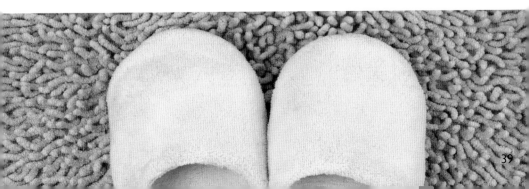

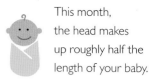

This month, the head makes up roughly half the length of your baby.

Budding and unfurling

By now you can just make out the form of your rapidly developing baby – rounded inwards in a C-shape. Even at this early stage, many key body parts are taking shape and manoeuvring into position.

✳ The little grey cells

By week five, a dark line of cells emerges along the back of the embryo, reflecting the final position of the spinal cord. At the top are two "lobes" that fold and develop into the neural tube. These changes are the start of the central nervous system, including the spinal cord and brain. From around six weeks, brain activity can be detected.

✳ A beating heart

The heart develops this month as no more than a tube, but it is in its final position at the front of the embryo. It begins beating around 21 days after conception and this can be picked up on a scan, though you won't be able to hear it on a Doppler device (heart detector) for a while yet. Shortly afterwards, it will flex into an S-shape so that the parts that will become the organ and atria are in the correct place.

Baby's progress bar: you are now 20% complete

LOADING ...

| 10% | 20% | 30% | 40% | 50% |

DID YOU KNOW?

BABY RESEMBLES a tadpole in shape – at six weeks she has a tail, but this soon withers and by eight weeks has practically gone.

HOW BIG?
Your baby is now the size of a blackberry.

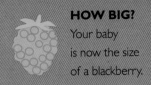

From here, four chambers separate. A precursor to blood starts to circulate through key blood vessels – at this point made up almost entirely of red blood cells.

✳ Early tummy

Another tube makes itself visible from week five – this one extending all the way from your baby's mouth to her tail end, and will eventually become her entire digestive system. All the organs she'll need to process and expel food emerge from this one simple tube.

✳ Budding limbs

Tiny bumps swell at the sides of the embryo from around weeks six and seven, which mark the beginnings of limbs. The arms and legs will lengthen out from these buds, like paddles or flippers, with ridges at the ends that transform into hands and feet. Soon there will be discernible fingers and toes, and by the end of the month the webbing that connects them will have all but vanished.

Take 400mcg of folic acid daily to safeguard development of your baby's neural tube.

Baby's first face

At the beginning of month two, your baby's head is large in proportion to the rest of his body, but by week eight you'll be able to make out a distinctly human-shaped face.

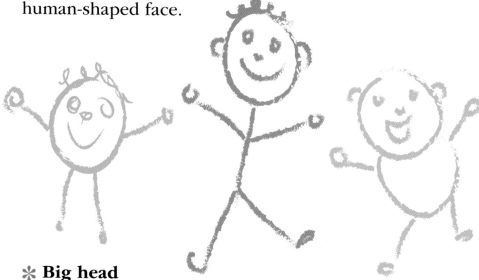

✳ Big head

By week six your baby has gill-like features at the top of his body, which will evolve over the next few weeks into a face. Inside a large head, his brain is developing five distinct sections and nerve cells are connecting up the wiring that will link your baby's brain with every other part of his body via neural pathways. By the end of this month, his neck will have started to stretch out from his head, which becomes more rounded and recognizably human in shape.

DID YOU KNOW?

YOUR BABY IS officially a fetus from eight weeks onwards. This stems from the Latin word for "young one" or "offspring".

150

The number of beats per minute of the fetal heart by week six.

✳ Face building

Bones are starting to replace cartilage and fuse together in the face, and as tissue joins together, recognizable features including the nose, forehead, cheeks, upper lip, and jaw become visible. Teeth buds are beginning to grow inside the jaw, and a rudimentary tongue is evident in his emerging palate. Openings appear for the nostrils, too.

✳ Fresh eyes

A large, dark circle at each side of your baby's face indicates that his eyes are now developing. Pigment is already detectable in the early retina, and, by week eight, the optic nerves connecting each eye to the brain will have developed, and eyelids will have grown over his eyes.

✳ Early ears

The internal structures of the ears start to form around week six, also forging connections to the developing brain. The external parts of the ear form as dips on the surface of the head, spaced wide apart on either side.

✳ Skin layering

At the beginning of week five your baby's skin is composed of one simple layer, but two weeks later it will have developed a top layer, known as the "periderm", and a basal (base) layer. Tiny hair follicles also start to form in the skin at about this stage, but you won't find any actual hair growing until next month.

Being tired is your body's way of telling you to ease up – stress during pregnancy can raise your blood pressure, so take it easy. Luckily, this early fatigue will improve in the second trimester.

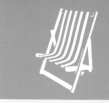

Relax and take it easy

You are pregnant, but the phone still rings, the laundry still piles up, and work deadlines loom as large as life. The key to managing stress when you are pregnant is to look after yourself.

✳ Stress less

It's been proven that for most people a healthy diet, combined with plenty of sleep and relaxation, reduces stress and generally makes life easier. And these things are even more important now that your body is working hard to make a baby. Take a step back, and stay on top. By caring for yourself you are caring for your baby, too.

Eating well

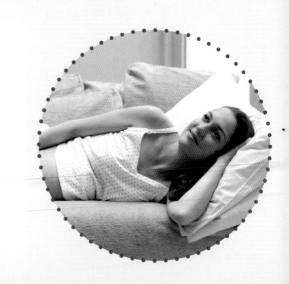

- Eat breakfast daily

- Eat frequent, small meals

- Keep hydrated (see page 108)

- Make nutritious snacks

- Eat plenty of fruit and vegetables

- Cut back on alcohol and caffeine

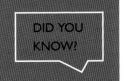
EXERCISE is one of the best stress-busters as it triggers the release of mood-enhancing endorphins – see pages 210–215 for easy, helpful pregnancy exercises.

WARM LAVENDER OIL IN A BURNER TO HELP PROMOTE RELAXATION.

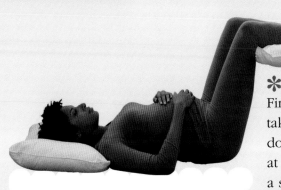

✳ Slow down

Find a window in each day to take a deep breath, relax, and do something for yourself. Look at the tips in the box, left, for a selection of ideas.

Ways to relax

- Join a pregnancy yoga or Pilates class
- Go for a walk
- Listen to music
- Lie down for a 15 minute power nap
- Take a daily lunch break when at work
- Enjoy a trip to the cinema
- Indulge in a professional pregnancy massage
- Read a book or magazine
- Have a good chat with a friend
- Take a soothing shower or bath
- Go swimming
- Try a relaxing therapy (see page 104)
- Watch a funny film or TV series

✳ Travel advice

You don't need to stop travelling just because you are pregnant, although it's a good idea to reduce the hassle if you can, and excessive travel should be avoided if possible. When travelling on a long-haul flight, help yourself by moving around the cabin, eating nutritious snacks, and drinking plenty of fluids. If commuting by train or bus, feel free to ask for a seat, and if the rush hour is particularly difficult, think about asking your boss if you can start and end your working day later to avoid it.

How do you do that?
AMAZING FACTS: PREGNANT BODY

1 ### Expanding
In just 40 weeks, the womb expands from the size of a pear to a size similar to that of a small watermelon. It increases in weight from 70g (2½oz) to around 1kg (2lb 4oz).

2 ### Creating
During pregnancy, a woman creates a whole new organ – the placenta. This is the only organ that you get rid of after use! It works hard to deliver oxygen and nutrients to the baby.

3 ### Pumping
A pregnant woman has 50 per cent more blood than usual by 20 weeks, and her cardiac output (volume pumped by each heartbeat) is 40 per cent higher. She will also manufacture 20 per cent more red blood cells to carry oxygen around her body.

4 ### Growing
The heart and liver may grow to meet the considerable demands of their extra workload; they will then return to their usual size after the birth.

5 ### Stretching
The hormone relaxin reduces cartilage and ligament density throughout the body so that the pelvis will be flexible for delivery. It also allows the rib cage to expand and accommodate an increased lung capacity.

BEING ABLE TO GROW A NEW PERSON in just 40 weeks is pretty amazing. There is a whole range of changes going on in your body to help you perform this incredible feat.

6 Glowing

The fabled pregnancy glow is real – a combination of enlarged blood vessels, increased blood volume, and more active oil glands causes a softer, rosier complexion.

7 Detecting

Expectant mothers have a heightened sense of smell, thought to have evolved to help detect the small amounts of toxins in food and drink that could be dangerous to an unborn baby. It can put you off the smell of cigarettes, coffee, and alcohol.

8 Consuming

An extra 200 calories a day is sufficient for a pregnant woman to nourish her baby, who takes whatever nutrients he needs first, leaving her with the leftovers. In order to ensure maximum absorption of nutrients, digestion slows down during this time.

9 Beautifying

An expectant mum's hair gets thicker and glossier due to the oestrogen receptors it contains, and the fact that hair loss is reduced. It will also grow quicker, as will fingernails and toenails.

10 Protecting

By 39 weeks the womb will contain around 1 litre (35fl oz) of amniotic fluid. At 37.5°C (99.5°F), this protective bubble of fluid is warmer than your body temperature, and is a little like saltwater. It is replaced gradually, every three hours during pregnancy.

MONTH 2

Weeks 5–8
DAD'S SURVIVAL
GUIDE

DID YOU
KNOW?

Raging hormones

Pregnancy hormones are kicking in, so your partner might experience "morning sickness" (a misnomer as it can occur any time), tiredness, mood changes, and nausea, or she may be lucky and sail through it all.

✳ Swings and roundabouts

A cocktail of pregnancy hormones is flooding your partner, and she may start to feel the side effects. She may be irritable one moment and elated the next, full of energy and enthusiasm at lunchtime and exhausted after work. This is due to a chemical reaction in the brain that affects the mood-regulating neurotransmitters, which in turn can destabilize her moods. Combine that with any anxiety about the coming months, and it can be a pretty tiring time for you both. Talking about your partner's concerns can help her to cope, and bear in mind that it probably isn't you she's getting angry with.

✳ Dawning sickness

The same hormones that cause mood swings can also make some women feel very sick, known as morning sickness. This affects people differently – some women may vomit, while others have an intense sensation of nausea akin to motion or seasickness. It can occur in the morning, or be stronger when tired at the end of the day, or during the night. Some expectant mums feel terrible

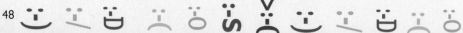

SOMETIMES dads can develop Couvade syndrome (phantom pregnancy).

MOST WOMEN suffer from nausea at some point, but the good news is that it usually subsides by the fourth month of pregnancy.

BRING YOUR PARTNER A GINGER BISCUIT IN BED TO HELP WITH NAUSEA.

IF YOUR PARTNER has lost her appetite, cook something delicious containing ginger to help alleviate nausea. A stir-fry would be great.

around the clock. If your partner feels nauseous you need to be aware of just how debilitating it can be to feel so ill – imagine a crippling hangover! Nausea can make it hard to continue with everyday life, such as travelling, cooking, and eating your usual meals. It can also bring an awareness that her body is no longer her own, and that lack of control can be pretty scary.

✳ Your growing baby

By the end of month two, your baby is now a "fetus" and has tiny arm and leg buds and facial features. His central nervous system and heart are developing. He is starting to move, but you and your partner won't be able to feel this yet as there is plenty of space in there!

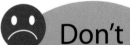

Do

Encourage your partner to rest, and help with shared jobs as much as possible. Get some early nights.

Go out and enjoy yourselves when you both feel like it.

Take a walk together for some fresh air and exercise.

Don't

Eat or cook strong-smelling foods as this may trigger her nausea.

Call the midwife every time your partner is sick. But if she can't keep food or drink down, then make an appointment with your doctor.

Smoke near your partner as this may be absorbed by your growing baby. Try to cut back.

Noticing changes

There's no pretending now – this month you'll see a difference in your body as your breasts grow, your skin starts to change, and your waist thickens. Your anomaly scan should help to make everything seem more real.

✳ Need some support?

Your breasts have probably been the first part of your body to look and feel different: full, super-sensitive, and definitely larger. You might find a sports bra more comfortable than your regular bra now. Even this early in pregnancy your body is preparing your breasts to feed your baby. Until now this has been caused by increased levels of oestrogen and progesterone, but there's a new hormone in the mix – **human placental lactogen** (HPL), produced by the placenta. This increases the amount of sugar in your blood in order to transfer nutrients to your baby. It also prepares the mammary glands for making milk. You'll probably have noticed the areola (the area around your nipples) becoming larger and darker. Can you spot any new little white bumps there? Known as **Montgomery's tubercles**, these enlarged sebaceous glands produce a protective antibacterial oil that keeps the skin clean and smooth.

✳ Feeling dizzy?

The blood vessels in your body have been relaxing and getting wider (dilating) over the last few weeks, thanks to your increased hormones, particularly progesterone. This dilation allows your veins to hold more

23%

MORE BLOOD is pumped to your uterus by week 12 than before you were pregnant.

GOOD TO EAT

Eggs for B vitamins and choline, and to boost folic acid absorption.

blood, ensuring all the new blood vessels in the placenta have a plentiful supply and that those organs that are working harder, such as your kidneys, are well supported. Your body is manufacturing more plasma and red blood cells this month, but neither are up to capacity, meaning your blood pressure is likely to be lower than usual. So if you stand up quickly you may feel dizzy. Try to bring your head up last in order to give the blood time to reach your brain. Faintness may also result from dipping blood-sugar levels; snacking on carbohydrates can help, and don't skip meals.

NEW WORDS

- HPL
- Montgomery's tubercles
- Spider naevi

✳ Is it hot in here?

Have you noticed you feel warmer, particularly your hands and feet? Are there tiny new veins on the surface of your skin, especially on your breasts and legs? The two changes are connected: more blood is flowing to your skin through the veins (called **spider naevi**) to release the excess heat generated by your increased metabolism and blood flow.

✳ Where's the bathroom?

Though you might not notice a huge difference in your figure yet, your uterus has started to enlarge and thicken. It's likely to be pressing on your bladder, which can make you want to wee at unexpected moments. You may find you're having to get up at night, too – your kidneys are working harder to filter the extra blood circulating, which means more urine. Unfortunately, this is an aspect of pregnancy that, as your baby and your uterus enlarge, will only get worse!

51

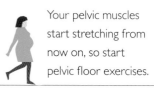

Fact or fiction?

You may be getting plenty of (un)welcome advice at the moment about the most ordinary things. Is it really dangerous to eat cheese, or paint the baby's room? Does your cat have to move out? What are the facts?

✳ Weighing up the risks

Parenthood is about assessing risk: getting acquainted with facts and opinions, working out what you and your partner think about them, and trusting your judgement enough to put those thoughts into action. Often you are just going to have to do your best.

✳ Getting drunk before the test

Did you have a few drinks too many before you knew you were pregnant? Studies in the media sometimes suggest this might be risky for your baby, so if you are really concerned chat to your doctor. However, try not to worry as most women find everything is fine. Instead, channel any anxiety into positive change, such as giving up for now.

✳ Dodgy decorating

There's convincing evidence to stop you renovating rooms that haven't been touched since the 1970s as the paint is likely to contain lead, and sanding or stripping it releases this heavy metal into the air. Exposure may harm your baby's developing brain and nervous and reproductive systems. Choose paints, thinners, varnishes, and sealants with low volatile organic compound (VOC) content, which is clearly marked on the container. And if you are concerned, it's a great excuse to put your feet up and have someone else do the work – using eco-friendly materials, of course.

* Sex in pregnancy

You might have got the idea that sex during pregnancy could be harmful for baby. Actually, sex is something you can enjoy throughout pregnancy, unless your doctor says otherwise. Thanks to your hormones you may feel like more of it than ever before!

* Household chemicals

A 2013 report by the Royal College of Obstetricians and Gynaecologists warned pregnant women to avoid chemicals in cleaning products, cosmetics, and common plastics. Conversely, toxicologists and the Royal College of Midwives state that no substantiated research backs up the findings. So how do you know what to do? Maybe avoid items bearing a big red cross and the words "danger" or "caution", such as bleach and bug sprays, because the chlorine, ammonia, solvents, and pesticides that necessitate these cautions can trigger nausea, irritate your skin, and respiratory tract, or affect the central nervous system.

* Furry creatures

There is no reason to ask your cat, dog, or chickens to move out, but you do need to be super-conscious about hygiene now you are pregnant. Avoid dealing with cat litter or poo of any kind, and wear gloves for any mucky jobs. Avoid flea treatments and get advice from your vet about natural options.

Your baby is already a boy or a girl although you wouldn't be able to tell on a scan for a few weeks yet.

All in place

A tiny person is starting to emerge from the cells. Your baby's organs are already grown and are starting to work, and she has the most enormous head!

✳ Over the first hurdle

By the end of week 12 your baby will have completed the first and most vital stage of the journey, when critical development takes place in every body system and all the basics of human physiology are put in place. Your baby now looks like a proper tiny person!

✳ Heart-to-heart

By week 10, your baby's heart will have developed into the definitive four-chambered heart. The two atria receive blood from the fetal circulation, while the ventricles pump blood out to the lungs and the rest of your baby's body. Valves develop at the exit of all four chambers to ensure that the blood is always pumped in one direction.

✳ Stretching out

By now your baby's trunk looks straighter. The arms and legs are fully formed with visible elbows, wrists, and ankles that can move, and the

Baby's progress bar: you are now 30% complete

LOADING ...

10%   20%   30%   40%   50%

BY WEEK 12 your baby weighs 15–30g (¹/₂–1oz). Moving around inside you helps her develop a strong skeleton and muscles.

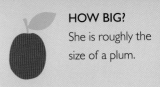

HOW BIG?
She is roughly the size of a plum.

limbs are lengthening. After week 10, tiny fingernails and toenails will appear and webbing between the fingers and toes will disappear.

✳ Muscle action

The first movements a fetus makes are small involuntary twitches, as the nervous system is not yet developed enough for the brain and body parts to talk to each other. Movement starts to increase in frequency in the third month, though you won't be able feel it for another month or so.

✳ Home sweet home

Your baby continues to float freely within amniotic fluid, which cushions her from knocks and bumps. The amniotic sac is surrounded by an inner and outer layer, which are separated by a space that contains the yolk sac.

✳ Future generations

Externally, the genitals are well developed by week 12, while inside the fetus, cells are growing that will eventually form sperm or eggs.

Mouth can open and close.

Heart rate is about 160 beats per minute.

Ears are nearly in their final position on the head.

The umbilical cord will grow to an average length of 50cm (20in).

The placenta

By the end of this month, the placenta is fully developed, ready to support your baby until birth by delivering nutrients and oxygen, taking away waste products, and providing protection.

✳ Layering and connecting

The placenta began its development in month one, just after implantation, when layers of chorion and amnion membrane were forming on the wall of your uterus around the embryo. Those layers have now thickened and extended to form a flat, oval sac filled with amniotic fluid, usually attached to the top or side of your uterus. By week 10 you have about 30ml (1fl oz) of amniotic fluid (mostly water). This increases little by little until you eventually have around 1 litre (35fl oz) towards the end of the third trimester.

✳ Life-support system

The main role of the placenta is to supply your baby with oxygen and nutrients and to take away waste. Within the chorion membrane are 200 villi, containing blood vessels, grouped like bunches of grapes. Longer villi reach deep into the wall of your uterus to bring in oxygenated blood from your arteries. These have widened and are delivering more blood to your uterus than before pregnancy, thanks to the extra blood circulating and your increased heart rate. Your blood pools in the placenta. Here the bunches of smaller villi bathe

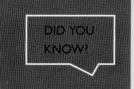

DID YOU KNOW?

SOME COMPANIES OFFER the opportunity to pay to store stem cells from your baby's umbilical cord to treat future diseases.

At 37.5°C (99.5°F), amniotic fluid is hotter than your body temperature.

in it and absorb oxygen and nutrients via their tips where the layer of cells is very thin. At the same time, waste products, including carbon dioxide, transfer to your veins and are carried away to your lungs and kidneys to be processed and expelled.

✳ Umbilical cord

Your baby is connected to the placenta by an umbilical cord, which starts at his navel and is also now fully developed. Within the cord is a main vein, transferring fresh blood filled with oxygen and nutrients into your baby's bloodstream. It also houses two arteries that carry used blood, containing carbon dioxide and other waste, away out to your body. These three vessels wind around each other to create a coil covered in sticky jelly and a layer of membrane.

✳ Protective shield

Amniotic fluid provides a cushioning, temperature-controlled environment for your baby, while the surrounding membranes create a barrier from harmful substances, from bacteria to environmental toxins. Later in pregnancy, the placenta passes on antibodies to protect your newborn. However, the placenta cannot protect against viruses, such as rubella, listeria bacteria (found in soil and some soft cheeses), or heavy metals, such as lead, that may enter the bloodstream.

✳ Hormone factory

From now on, the placenta is responsible for manufacturing the hCG, oestrogen, and progesterone required until the end of pregnancy to prepare your body for childbirth and breastfeeding.

You can now have 3D scans and video recordings of the dating scan, although this tends to be offered in private clinics only.

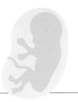

You will find out your estimated date of delivery (EDD).

The dating scan

Around 12 weeks you may be offered a "dating" scan. This is an ultrasound scan that enables you and medical staff to see your baby for the first time.

Q What's it for?

This scan helps your medical team to calculate your baby's exact age and to estimate when he might be born – his EDD (Estimated Date of Delivery). This preliminary scan also helps check other things, such as how many babies you are carrying (one or more!), and your baby's heartbeat. Although the scan is not specifically for picking up abnormalities, sometimes problems can be detected.

NUCHAL TRANSLUCENCY SCAN

This scan may be offered during 11–14 weeks of pregnancy to screen for Down's syndrome and other conditions. It measures the thickness of the pocket of fluid (the nuchal fold) behind your baby's neck and, combined with a simple blood test, can be used to calculate risk.

Q How do I prepare?

You might be asked to have a full bladder, as this helps to push your womb up to give a clear image on the scan. Be aware that occasionally scans can show unexpected things, but otherwise, just look forward to it!

Q What happens?

A sonographer will do your scan. You will be asked to lie down on a couch and pull your top up, and possibly your trousers or skirt down a little to expose your abdomen. The sonographer will smooth a gel over your tummy and

TOP TIP

LOOK FOR THE LETTERS CRL on your scan. This is your baby's "crown-to-rump length". This figure gives an accurate estimate of age.

5%

OF BABIES ARE delivered on their predicted due date.

then press down with a handheld device linked to a computer screen. He or she may move the device around to get a clearer image of your baby.

Q Will it hurt?

It shouldn't hurt, though the gel rubbed over your belly might feel cold and the probe might prod a little; at worst it may just feel a little uncomfortable. Baby won't be able to feel anything!

Q Who can I take?

Usually you are allowed to bring one adult with you. You may want to bring the baby's father, your mum, or a close friend. Children are sometimes not permitted, depending on your healthcare provider.

Q How do they do it?

The device sends high frequency sound waves, inaudible to the human ear, into your abdomen and records the echoes which bounce back with a tiny microphone. A 2D-image is built up from the echoes.

Your scan picture

You may feel that you are supposed to know just what is what in your baby's first image, but if you find the blobby white and dark patches of your scan bewildering, rest assured you would not be the first parent to feel this. Solid structures, such as bone and muscle, appear as white or grey, while soft tissues, such as the eyeballs or empty structures, including the heart's chambers, will appear dark red or black.

This baby's profile is very clear. You can see the nose, mouth, and eyes as he moves around.

The eye sockets appear as dark hollows in the clear profile of the skull. Eyes are soft tissue so appear dark.

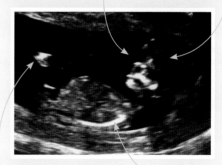

Is that a foot or a hand? Solid white areas show bone, and if the areas are moving it is likely to be a foot or hand.

The spine is clearly visible as a solid, white, curved line.

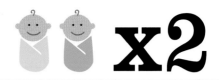

Expecting more than one?

You've just got used to the idea of being pregnant, when you discover that it's not just one. Wow! It's perfectly natural to feel overwhelmed as well as excited; there is a lot to take onboard.

✳ Tip-top care

Your pregnancy will most likely go smoothly with few, if any, complications but you will be offered extra antenatal appointments to help ensure that all is well. The chance of you developing high blood pressure, pre-eclampsia, and diabetes is raised, and so you will be monitored for these conditions. Extra scans will check that your babies are growing at a similar rate. This is especially relevant when identical twins share a placenta as more blood may circulate to one baby (twin-to-twin transfusion syndrome).

✳ How are you feeling?

High levels of the pregnancy hormone hCG can lead to you experiencing nausea, sickness, and tiredness, and it is usually worse when carrying more than one baby. The good news is that this should improve after the first trimester. Two or more babies means there is less room in your body, which can lead to heartburn and indigestion as your uterus presses against other organs. Eating small and regular meals can alleviate this. There's also a greater risk of developing anaemia than with one baby, so eat plenty of iron-rich foods. If you experience back and pelvic pain seek help from your midwife – supportive clothing and correcting your posture may help.

✻ Room for two

Your tummy will probably expand sooner, and by as early as 10 weeks it can be hard to conceal a bump! You will almost certainly gain more weight than with one baby due to the extra amniotic fluid and larger placenta/s, but the figures may not be as dramatic as you expect. Women carrying one baby gain around 11kg (24lb); an extra baby usually means a weight gain of just an extra 4.5kg (10lb) or so.

✻ Planning the delivery

Your delivery is likely to be at, or before, 37 weeks, so you need to plan to leave work earlier, get your hospital bag packed, have two car seats sorted, and have baby clothes chosen as soon as you can. 37 weeks is considered full term for a twins pregnancy; the placenta/s have worked hard and you are probably feeling ready to deliver! While a Caesarean is likely, there's no reason not to plan for a natural delivery providing your babies are in a good position, with the first twin head down (cephalic position).

IVF TWIN RATES
The rise in IVF treatments has increased twin rates dramatically. Recent figures show the rate of multiple births with IVF is 23.6 per cent – more than 10 times the rate with natural conception.

There is regular debate about the ideal age at which to have a baby. After 35 years of age the number and quality of your eggs is reduced. But then again, it takes only one to make a baby!

Older mums

Many women now have babies later in life, with almost half of babies in the UK born to mums aged over 30. Is it really something to worry about, and what is the truth about the risks and benefits?

✳ A solid start

Studies of older mums highlight many convincing arguments for delaying motherhood. Becoming a mum slightly later in life means you are more likely to be in a settled, stable relationship, be better educated, and more financially secure. You're also more likely to have achieved goals in your professional life and to have reached a satisfactory status, making it easier to put your career on hold, and easier to return to it after the baby is born. Motherhood is likely to be something you embrace wholeheartedly as you're ready to focus on family and you are less likely to feel tied down or fear you are missing out on other aspects of life. And long-term, you're more likely to achieve a fulfilling work-life balance.

✳ Confident parenting

Accruing life experience before embarking on motherhood increases self-confidence, and older mums are likely to have the necessary life skills and perspective to cope well with the ups and downs of

DID YOU KNOW?

WOMEN WHO GIVE BIRTH when over 40 years old are four times as likely to live to be 100 than younger mums.

29.7

THE AVERAGE AGE OF WOMEN IN THE UK HAVING THEIR FIRST BABY IS 29.7 YEARS.

parenting, as well as having a clear parenting style in mind. One study found that children of older mothers tend to do well academically.

✳ What about the health risks?

If you are 35 years or older and expecting your first baby, you are termed "elderly primigravida"; you will be monitored closely during your pregnancy and offered extra checks for genetic abnormalities. Women in this age bracket are more likely to develop conditions such as high blood pressure and diabetes, and run a higher risk of having a low-lying placenta. During labour, medical interventions and Caesareans are also more common. Try to see this extra level of care as a bonus; you and your baby are in safe hands. And remember, the majority of older women have healthy pregnancies and babies. Also, as older mums are likely to have a good fitness regime, eat healthily, and be less likely to smoke than younger women, this will help you to deal with any extra tiredness you may feel when baby arrives!

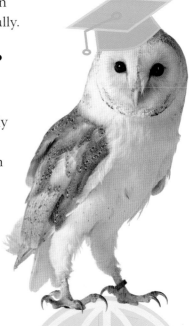

IN THE US, the birth rate has fallen in recent years, while the average age of first-time mums has risen to 23 years.

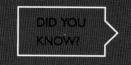

The secret's out

It's nearly time for the dating scan (see page 58). Once you have confirmation that all is well you can start shouting the news from the rooftops and it will all seem more real.

✳ Say cheese

The 12-week scan will be the first of many images of your baby. The purpose of this scan is to check that this is a viable fetus that is developing normally. The good news is that in most cases all is well and once you have heard the heartbeat for the first time the risk of miscarriage drops to just five per cent. Scans are not harmful to your partner or baby; they can be slightly uncomfortable though as she will need a really full bladder for the scan to work effectively. The sonographer will take measurements to predict the due date more accurately; he or she will also check whether there is just one baby (or maybe more!), and look for any abnormalities in the development of spine, limbs, and organs.

✳ Start spreading the news

If you've been keeping the pregnancy secret until this point, now is the time to start broadcasting your happy news. Do you tell the grandparents, siblings, or close friends first? Perhaps wait until all the key

YOUR PARTNER MAY START to get heartburn and indigestion as pregnancy hormones have relaxed the valve at the top of her stomach, allowing acid to escape.

YOUR BABY HAS JUST DEVELOPED REFLEXES AND MAY RESPOND TO GENTLE TOUCH.

Do

Move mountains to attend the scan. It's a once-in-a-lifetime experience that you should see.

───────────

Ask questions if you want to. It can be quite hard to tell what is what on the scan.

───────────

Buy the picture. People will love to see it, and it's a great souvenir!

Don't

Panic at the scan. Chances are that everything will be just fine.

───────────

Worry if people are shocked at your news. Your happiness is what matters.

───────────

Forget to tell all your key players first. You need to keep them on-side as their support will be crucial in the months and years ahead.

players in your life have heard it directly from you before you announce it on the internet. Don't worry if everyone's reaction isn't what you thought it would be; you might have friends who tell you it's hard work or you'll never sleep again, and some might even be jealous. Everyone has a different life plan, so don't take it personally.

✳ Talking it out

Now that the news is out, you may find you are on the receiving end of advice. There is so much information out there (the internet is a mixed blessing) that it can be great to allay concerns by canvassing opinion from people you trust. Experienced dads can be great sounding boards, and talking to someone who knows what you're going through can be reassuring. Later you'll meet other parents at the antenatal classes – you will obviously have at least one thing in common with them.

WHAT ARE YOUR PLANS for when baby arrives? Who's going to look after him and for how long? Maybe you'd like to?

Starting to bloom

Welcome to the second trimester of pregnancy! The most disorientating part of the journey is over, and any nausea should start to lift now. Most exciting of all, you will start to develop a visible bump.

✳ Looking pregnant at last

Depending on your body shape and the strength of your core muscles, you should start to develop a tiny bump by week 16. Your doctor or midwife can now feel the uterus in your abdomen. Though your breasts will stop feeling so tender, they too are developing – by the end of this month the milk-producing glands will be fully primed to manufacture breast milk.

✳ What's going on inside?

Your red-blood-cell count is increasing rapidly to carry the extra oxygen your body needs to feed the placenta and baby. You also have additional plasma to cope with the increased blood flow to your organs, skin, and kidneys. Your heart is working twice as hard, while your digestive system is slowing down.

✳ Health niggles

Symptoms including a stuffy nose, blocked ears, swollen, bleeding gums, and snoring are all common at this stage of pregnancy. Feel reassured, they are a sign that your body is doing just what it needs to keep you and your baby healthy. Increased circulation sends more blood through your mucous membranes, which causes slight swelling in all the tissue lining parts of your body that are in contact with the air, such as your nose, windpipe, and lungs.

❋ Help, I'm changing colour!

It's quite normal for your nipples and genitals to get darker since you now have more pigment-bearing cells. You might notice a fine line developing down your tummy from your navel to your pubic bone – this is called the linea nigra. You may also develop darker or uneven patches of skin on your cheekbones, forehead, nose, and chin, called melasma or chloasma (years ago it was called the "mask of pregnancy"). All skin pigmentation changes usually fade once the baby is born, so don't worry too much. They do, however, increase and get darker with exposure to sun, so use a high-factor sunscreen to help minimize any long-term changes. Your skin is more sensitive, too, so you need extra protection against burning and long-term damage.

STRETCH MARK ALERT

Up to 80 per cent of pregnant women notice reddish-brown streaks, called **striae gravidarum**, caused when the body grows rapidly. These spider-like lines fade to silver, but to keep skin stretchy and to reduce the amount of lines or any itching, gently massage your belly, breasts, hips, and thighs with a rich body lotion. Olive or argan oil are both used for this purpose worldwide.

Sex is extra pleasurable this month as overactive mucous membranes increase lubrication!

Spreading the news

As your energy returns this month and mood swings calm down, you're likely to feel less anxious and more able to relax into your pregnancy. You might be ready to tell friends and colleagues at work.

✱ Relax and settle in

Your hormones are starting to calm down and the risk of miscarriage is far lower than in the first trimester, so this tends to be when people start spreading the news. You're likely to feel more positive and energetic, and you can channel this into practical matters, such as researching options for birth, or booking childbirth classes.

✱ When to tell

It's tempting to shout the good news to friends, family, and colleagues right away, but once the news is out it can dominate conversation and social

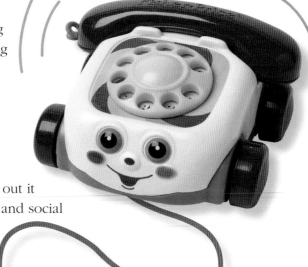

DID YOU KNOW?

YOU ARE LESS LIKELY to need to wee so frequently now as your uterus has grown and moved out of the pelvic cavity.

45%

BY THE END OF THIS MONTH YOUR BODY WILL CONTAIN 45% MORE BLOOD.

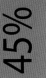

events, so make sure you are ready. If your bump is not showing yet, you may wish to keep quiet at work while you find out more about employment rights. Pregnancy can affect workplace politics as colleagues may start to reassess your capabilities or manoeuvre into position for when your maternity leave begins.

Your breasts are already making colostrum – baby's first milk.

✳ Treat yourself

Mark this new stage of your pregnancy journey by buying clothes that flaunt and flatter your changing shape. Low-cut jeans, long tops, and stretchy wrap dresses can work just as well as maternity wear, especially in the early months. You'll need maternity clothes by the third trimester and post-delivery, too, and will get heartily sick of them, so adapt your regular clothes for as long as possible.

✳ Coping with the attention

Once you tell all, you'll find you become public property. Being the focus of good wishes, gifts, and smiles can be delightful, and it can be a great way to meet new people and chat to colleagues you've never met before. But everyone has a birth horror story or tales of sleepless nights to share, and some may want to hug or pat your bump. Prepare some polite but firm responses to preserve your privacy, just in case!

A baby girl will have about 2 million minuscule eggs in her ovaries.

A tiny person

Your baby has completed perhaps the most tricky part of the pregnancy journey. By week 13, all the major organs and body systems have developed, and her muscles are growing stronger.

✷ Communication system

Nerves to and from your baby's brain are being coated in a protective layer of fat, called myelin, which will allow messages to travel between the brain and muscles in the rest of the body.

✷ Getting active

Muscles are able to contract and relax now, so your baby can move, stretching out her limbs, turning around inside you, and clasping both hands together. This can be detected on an ultrasound scan, so you can enjoy watching the movements at your 12-week scan. If you press your belly, your baby will respond by wriggling, though you can't feel it yet because of the amniotic fluid that cushions her.

Baby's progress bar: you are now 40% complete

LOADING ...

| 10% | 20% | 30% | 40% | 50% |

DID YOU KNOW?

BY 16 WEEKS your baby weighs about 90g (3¼oz) and is 10–12cm (4–5in) long. Your baby will grow 5cm (2in) this month.

HOW BIG?
She is about the size of an orange.

✳ Drinking and weeing

The kidneys start to work this month, and your baby will swallow the amniotic fluid she is floating in. She starts to make urine, and passes it out into the amniotic sac.

✳ Independent living

By the end of this month your baby will be creating red blood cells inside her body – in the bone marrow, liver, and spleen – rather than depending on an outside source. Your baby and placenta are also now producing hormones themselves (taking over from your ovary), including oestrogen and all the progesterone required until birth.

✳ Boy or girl?

Your baby is now visibly a boy or a girl, since the "differentiation" process is complete by week 14. Ovarian follicles, or a prostate gland, have started to appear and the external sex organs are evident although they are too small to see on a scan.

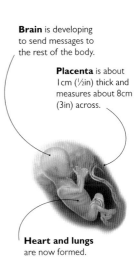

Brain is developing to send messages to the rest of the body.

Placenta is about 1cm (½in) thick and measures about 8cm (3in) across.

Heart and lungs are now formed.

60%   70%   80%   90%   100%

New sensory world

Your baby's eyes and ears develop rapidly this month and he will be able to hear and see. Taste buds and nerve endings develop, too, so he can feel things as he moves around. But it's probably too soon to taste.

"It's pretty noisy in here!"

✳ Sound

Your baby's ears are moving into position on the sides of the head and the tiny bones inside are hardening. Once this happens, your baby can hear you from the inside (your beating heart, whooshing blood, and rumbling tummy), and can also detect sounds from the outside world, including your voice. His own vocal folds, or cords, develop in week 13.

BONDING WITH YOUR BABY starts before birth. Tune into his patterns of movement – speak softly to him when he is quiet and sing lively songs when more alert.

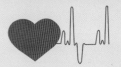

✳ Sight

Although your baby's eyelids remain closed, the eyes are fully formed – tiny eyelashes and eyebrows are even visible – and the retinas become sensitive to light. Your baby can see bright light coming in through your abdomen, which may start to help with distinguishing between night and day.

✳ Taste

Taste buds are emerging on his tongue, and 32 tooth buds are developing in the jawbones. Your baby is also practising sucking in and swallowing amniotic fluid.

✳ Touch

Your developing baby can wiggle his toes and curl up his tiny fingers. His arms are long enough to make thumb-sucking possible.

✳ Expressions

The facial bones and muscles are all in place and your baby's face moves through a series of expressions – frowning, smirking, squinting, wrinkling the forehead, and pursing the lips – even though the brain isn't fully controlling any of the movements yet.

IN THE DEMOCRATIC REPUBLIC OF CONGO, mothers sing to their unborn babies, repeating a single song until the birth. After birth the mother will sing the same tune to comfort the child. It sounds like a great idea to try.

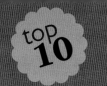

top**top 10**

I forgot. Sorry!
COMMON COMPLAINTS
IN MID-PREGNANCY

1 Forgetfulness
You have suddenly turned into an airhead and keep forgetting things.

2 Clumsiness
You keep dropping your car keys, banging into things, and are generally clumsy.

3 Wind
You are bloated, windy, and uncomfortable.

4 Heartburn
Acid reflux, a burning pain in your chest or tummy, feeling sick. Ugh!

5 Hair and nails
Your nails are brittle, your hair has gone curly, and you are growing a moustache.

WHAT TO DO

Write things down in a notepad or on your smartphone, or reduce the number of things you need to remember by delegating (though this is perhaps easier said than done!).

Proceed with care. Slow down, use extra caution in the bath or shower, keep hallways and stairs clear, and don't even think about standing on any chairs to reach things.

Reduce your intake of fizzy drinks and baked beans, and sip on warm water instead. Small, simple meals are best. Exercise helps, too, as does wearing loose clothing.

Eight out of 10 women experience heartburn during pregnancy. Avoid triggers, such as orange juice, chocolate, or spicy food. Eat little and often. Antacids are safe to take.

You can safely pluck facial hair, but don't use bleaches and hair-removal creams. Wear rubber gloves for housework to protect your nails.

YOU SHOULD BE FEELING a lot better this trimester, and less tired. The extra oestrogen you produce now may bring new symptoms.

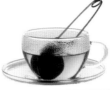

TOP TIP
Try herbal teas to keep hydrated and alleviate heartburn.

WHAT TO DO

6 **Skin changes**
You seem to be looking at a different face in the mirror. Is it really you?

Acne, spider veins, and pimply eruptions are all common in pregnancy. Use a cleanser to clear up spots, and a high-factor sunscreen to protect your skin when sunbathing.

7 **Pain in your groin**
There are sharp stabbing pains in your groin and side.

This can be a sign of symphysis pubis dysfunction (see page 233) so ask your midwife for a physio referral. Take care when getting in and out of the car or bath, and try not to do any heavy lifting.

8 **Stuffy nose**
You haven't got a cold, but you feel blocked up and snuffly.

About 30 per cent of pregnant women suffer from rhinitis during pregnancy. Try placing hot towels over the bridge of your nose or inhaling steam. Saline nose drops help, too.

9 **Nosebleeds**
If it's not a stuffy nose, it's a nosebleed!

Nosebleeds can happen much more frequently due to increased blood flow to the tissue lining your nose. To try to avoid nosebleeds, blow your nose gently, one nostril at a time.

10 **Hot and sweaty**
You wake up boiling hot, or suddenly feel hot and sweaty.

Wear layers of clothes – then you can shed them one by one if a hot flush hits you. Hot flushes will pass – at least until you hit menopause!

Top 10

TIME TO GO SHOPPING

BORROW items if you can; newborn clothes and toys rarely wear out.

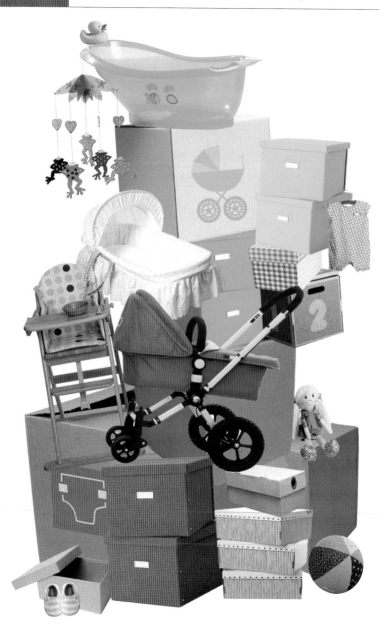

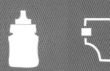

The bare essentials

You're getting ready for your great adventure into parenthood, but what will you need to get you through the first few months? In Finland, every new baby receives a cardboard box containing essential clothes and kit; the box then becomes a cot. That shows you how little you need. Here is our guide:

Basic kit (pages 92–3)
The equipment you will need in the first few weeks, from car seat and cot to baby monitors and a baby bath.

Hospital bag (pages 122–3)
You may be in hospital for a while so make it as comfortable as you can. Remember your medical notes!

Baby's wardrobe (pages 150–1)
Vests, sleepsuits, and a few hats. Newborns don't need a huge wardrobe, so save your money for the teenage years!

Getting busy

Right now you're heading into the second trimester. This part of the pregnancy should be easier for you and your partner since morning sickness should subside. She may get her energy back, and feel more like her usual self.

✳ Do a little dance

Both of you need to be in good shape for looking after a small child. There is also evidence to suggest that your partner will have an easier labour and birth if she is fit. Three or four sessions of cardiovascular activity a week will do both of you a power of good, physically and emotionally (see page 210). If neither of you are sporty, get into the habit of taking brisk walks. You need to be careful with sports where she might fall, or very intense exercise that raises her body temperature. That can all come when baby is older!

✳ Make a little love

There is one other great form of exercise you can do together – sex. Many women experience an increase in their usual sex drive during pregnancy due to hormonal changes. If your partner is one of the lucky ones, go ahead and enjoy the opportunity to bond. There are going to be plenty of changes once your baby arrives and your sex schedule may get somewhat disrupted by the ensuing sleepless nights.

EXPERIMENTS suggest women are more attracted to men who like babies.

BECAUSE YOUR PARTNER'S LIGAMENTS ARE MORE FLEXIBLE SHE IS SUSCEPTIBLE TO INJURY. IF YOU EXERCISE TOGETHER, TAKE IT EASY.

YOUR BABY is now 12cm (5in) long and his rubbery skeleton is forming into real bones.

Some women feel the opposite, however, so if this is the case find other ways to be close.

THE ANOMALY SCAN is fast approaching. Are you going to find out the sex of your baby, if your hospital allows it?

✻ Get down tonight

Many men wonder whether sex is safe in pregnancy and the simple answer is yes. Your baby is well protected in the amniotic sack as well as by the strong muscles of the uterus. You may find your libido is affected – maybe you find her swelling femininity highly erotic or maybe you have started seeing her body as more functional than fun. Both of these are entirely normal; either way you should celebrate the connection you share now you have created a new life together.

Do

Go away for the weekend together, and make a fuss of your partner.

Enjoy lie-ins together – these will be harder to come by in the years ahead.

Try out some new sex positions that are comfortable with the bump!

Don't

Worry if she doesn't feel like sex. Tell her how sexy her new curves are and she might change her mind.

Take your partner on a 10-mile jog or anything else too strenuous.

Forget that you need to be fit. There is a lot of running around to come in the future.

MONTH 5 · **Weeks 17–21**

MUM'S JOURNEY

Halfway there

Week 20 is the halfway point in your journey and a cause to celebrate! You may feel baby flutter for the first time, which can be both weird and exciting. Your energy levels are high so enjoy it and get active.

✳ Tickled from the inside

The lovely word "quickening" is used to describe the sensation of feeling your baby's first movements. It can be tricky at first to recognize these fluttery, rolling sensations: is it your baby wiggling or is it wind? Quickening generally happens during weeks 20–25, but many second-time mums sense it sooner, from as early as week 13.

✳ Get moving

Make time for gentle exercise (see pages 210–215), especially if you felt too under the weather during your first trimester. Walking, swimming, yoga, and T'ai Chi are all suitable. Pregnancy yoga classes can teach you a lot about how your body is changing, and you can learn breathing, relaxation, and movement techniques that are useful in labour.

✳ Aching sides

If your sides are aching, it might not just be down to overdoing it. Extra oestrogen softens the connective tissues around your body, while progesterone relaxes your muscles and loosens ligaments and tendons.

80

BABIES MOVE more when you are sitting quietly, lying down, or in the bath, so if you want to feel your baby these are perfect opportunities.

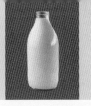

GOOD TO EAT
Milk offers a bone-friendly combination of calcium and vitamins D and K.

A stretching pain in your lower belly, on one or both sides, is probably a result of the ligaments around your uterus stretching. You might also notice a jabbing or dull ache if you stand suddenly, twist, or cough. To alleviate any pain, inhale slowly, imagine oxygen nourishing those stretched ligaments, and then consciously relax the area as you exhale. Resting forwards onto a cushion offers relief, too.

✳ Changing posture

Now your belly is really growing, your centre of gravity moves forwards to accommodate the extra weight up front, and from your breasts, too. This exaggerates the curve in your lower back, which is further exacerbated by stretched core muscles that no longer offer support. Being aware of how you sit and stand can prevent back and neck ache later (see page 214). When sitting, whether at home or at work, place both feet flat on the floor with your thighs resting on the seat and your lower back supported to get your spine in a good alignment (an extra cushion may help). Rest your shoulder blades against the chair if you can, to open your chest and relieve shoulder tension.

Making plans

This is usually the calmest time of pregnancy, which makes it a perfect time for planning. Why not book a relaxing holiday as a couple, think about where to give birth, and consider your maternity leave options?

✳ Take a trip

Holidays with a baby aren't exactly relaxing – in fact, by this time next year, your notion of a holiday will feel completely warped. So make the most of this window of opportunity to enjoy one last holiday with your partner (see pages 106–107) or a group of girlfriends. Flying is easiest before 28 weeks, after which you may need a doctor's note to fly and long journeys will be less comfortable. Relaxing by the coast might be more enjoyable than a hectic city break or action-packed adventure treks. Use the time to read, daydream, and chat about the future. Being away from the hassle of regular life often puts things into perspective and makes decision-making less daunting.

✳ Visit maternity units

You are entitled to time off work for maternity care, so use it to research the places you might choose to give birth.

DID YOU KNOW?

YOUR UTERUS has now grown so high in your abdomen that it is level with your belly button!

BY WEEK 20 your cardiac output (amount of blood) increases by 30–50%.

Do consider all the options, even if you already have a preference for a high-tech hospital or homely birthing centre. You can do a huge amount of research online, and personal recommendations are also useful, but nothing beats visiting a place in person. Talk about home birth with your midwife, too. When visiting a hospital, take your partner with you, or a friend – preferably one who has already given birth and who will know exactly the questions to ask. Join an organized tour, or you may prefer an informal visit that might reveal a less glossy picture. While you're there, look out for details of possible antenatal groups, pregnancy yoga, or relaxation classes offered on-site.

✳ Work matters

Now everyone can see your burgeoning belly, it's time to make serious plans about when to stop work and, if you're self-employed, how to hold things together while you take time off. It's advisable to keep all your options open for the moment. You might feel sure now that you'll return to work full-time or take all your allotted leave, but you may change your mind for various reasons once the baby arrives. Some parents use this opportunity to change their working arrangements, so investigate options for part-time, job-share, and freelance work. You might even contemplate ditching your current job to set up your own business or return to study. If you're not sure about your entitlements and options, the Human Resources (HR) department or the trade union in your workplace should be able to point you to good sources of information.

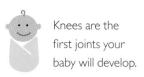

Knees are the
first joints your
baby will develop.

Splashing around

During this month's scan, enjoy the magical sight of
your baby moving around. Her muscles and joints
are developing so she can stretch, turn, and kick.

✳ Growing strong muscles

While your baby was still an embryo she developed a small number
of primary muscle fibres. These set the template for the secondary
fibres that formed in the fetal stage. Now, these secondary fibres are
increasing in mass, making the movements of the skeletal muscles
– the ones she will eventually be able to control – more powerful.
The movements are not yet purposeful, since the parts of the brain
that control movement don't develop until early in the third trimester.

✳ Bending the knees

Developing babies don't initially have joints. The skeleton forms first
as cartilage tissue, which eventually hardens into bones, but there is
a gap where two bones meet. In a developing baby, the points that
eventually become moveable joints – the elbows, knees, neck,
shoulders, hips, knuckles, thumbs, and wrists – fill with a higher
density of cells, and are known as interzones. The cells at these

Baby's progress bar: you are now 50% complete

LOADING ...

10%	20%	30%	40%	50%

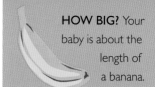

DID YOU
KNOW?

BY 20 WEEKS your baby weighs about 225g (8oz). She will grow 3–5cm (1¼–2in) this month.

HOW BIG? Your baby is about the length of a banana.

junctions then have to "commit" to becoming part of the joint and not the surrounding cartilage. The first joint to establish itself is the knee.

✳ **Working together**

The muscles become increasingly active as more neural impulses are delivered to them by motor neurons in the central nervous system. This causes the muscle fibres to contract, applying force to the bones and making them move. This has a critical influence on the developing joints; the mechanical stimulation prompts the cells in the interzones to segment, with some turning into a joint rather than following the regular pathway that turns them into cartilage. The more your baby moves, the more successfully the joints will form.

✳ **Varying movements**

The different types of joint developing will allow your baby a full range of movement, from hinging elbows and knees forwards and back to rotating sockets in the hips and shoulders.

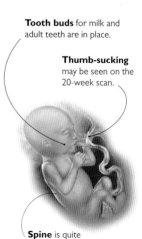

Tooth buds for milk and adult teeth are in place.

Thumb-sucking may be seen on the 20-week scan.

Spine is quite straight, with visible vertebrae.

This month, your baby doubles in weight, which is mostly due to fat.

Snug as a bug

Your baby's skin is translucent at the moment, but as he starts to develop layers of fat, the skin gradually becomes more opaque. This fat will protect and keep him warm after he is born.

❋ Staying warm

While your baby is in his bath of amniotic fluid, his temperature is regulated for him, but in the outside world he'll need a good layer of fat to help him stay warm. Deposits of fatty tissue, or "brown fat", start to develop now, especially around his torso, to act as insulation. Brown fat is also an essential source of energy should your baby need resuscitation at birth or become unwell in the first days.

❋ A protective varnish

During this month a white, waxy coating develops over your baby's skin, known as vernix caseosa, a Latin term that translates literally as "cheesy varnish". That gives you a clue to its texture! This greasy covering emerges from your baby's sebaceous glands and mixes with dead skins cells, shed by your baby in the same way that our own skin constantly renews itself. Vernix protects the baby's skin from the effects of spending nine months in a bath of amniotic fluid, which contains quite concentrated fetal urine by the end of a pregnancy. Vernix also acts as a lubricant during the birth.

HUMAN BABIES are the only primates to develop sweat glands over the entire body during their development.

THE SHAPE of a baby's hair follicles determines whether he has straight, wavy, or curly hair.

✳ Keeping cool

Two types of sweat gland develop this month. Eccrine sweat glands, which emit an odourless sweat, now develop on the palms of his hands and soles of his feet – by month seven, more of these glands will emerge all over your baby's body to help him cool himself. Apocrine sweat glands (responsible for smelly sweat) also start to form all over his body this month, but most of these will disappear by month seven, leaving only those under the arms, pubic area, lips, and nipples. These glands then lie in wait until puberty kicks off.

✳ Hairy baby

As early as week 12 your baby had eyebrows and lashes, then around week 16, hair follicles erupted on his scalp in a characteristic pattern, determining his future parting and the height of his hairline. By 20 weeks, a layer of fine fluffy hair – lanugo – has developed over your baby's body. No one really knows what purpose it serves: one opinion is that it helps maintain warmth; another is that it protects the layer of vernix. Hair growth begins on the upper body and moves downwards, so by the time it sprouts on his legs, the hair on your baby's arms can be quite long. Don't worry – it falls off by week 36. And from week 24 "real" hair starts covering your baby's scalp.

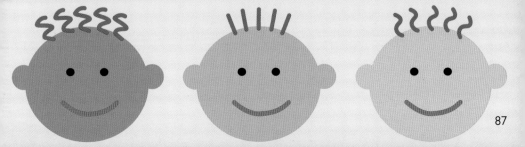

You may see your baby sucking her thumb, yawning, and stretching. She may even look a little like you!

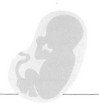

The position of the placenta is checked.

The anomaly scan

Your baby will have grown a lot since the last scan. The sonographer has several checks to make, and you might be able to find out if it's a boy or a girl.

❋ What's it for?

This detailed scan, also called the 20-week scan, is usually offered between 18–21 weeks. It is primarily to see if your baby is developing and growing properly and to detect as soon as possible any physical abnormalities, such as spina bifida or heart defects. Checking two babies will take extra time! The location of the placenta is also checked; a low-lying placenta could affect your chances of a natural delivery. If this is the case you may be offered another scan at 36 weeks to see if the placenta has moved up and out of the way.

If you didn't have a dating scan (see page 58), this scan could give an expected date of delivery, though it is less accurate at this gestation.

> **74% OF PREGNANT MOTHERS**
> opt to find out their baby's gender from their scan, according to a 2009 UK study published in the journal *Ultrasound*.

❋ What happens?

Just like the dating scan, a sonographer will put gel over your abdomen and use a handheld device linked to a computer screen to get an image of your baby.

❋ When is the due date?

A length measurement can no longer give baby's age accurately. Instead, your baby's age is estimated by taking measurements of her "bi-parietal" or

DID YOU KNOW?

GENDER-REVEAL PARTIES are becoming popular in the US and UK. One idea is to slice into a cake to reveal a pink or blue sponge to guests!

50%

THIS SCREENING SCAN picks up around 50% of major abnormalities.

head diameter, and/or the head circumference, and the length of her femur or thigh bone.

✳ Pink or blue?

At this scan, the sonographer should be able to tell the baby's gender, if there is time during the scan, though whether you are told depends on your hospital's policy and whether you want to find out. Bear in mind, they can occasionally get it wrong! If the baby is lying in an awkward position where it is difficult to see clearly, the sonographer will only be able to give you a best guess.

✳ What if the screen picks up something?

If your scan detects a problem, a trained counsellor in the area of diagnosis and screening should be available. Together with doctors and other members of the health team, they can help parents understand risks and make decisions. In most cases, everything is just fine.

A clear picture

In the 20-week scan your baby will look even more human. She has well-developed limbs, fingers, and toes, and you may even be able to make out her facial features. Her head will look disproportionately large compared with the rest of her body, just as most babies do when born. Now your baby is bigger, she may appear to be a snugger fit in your womb, with less room to move around in there. This can lead to her stretching her limbs while you watch.

Facial features can be seen clearly now; does she look like you?

Space is limited so baby needs to fold her limbs. This is a leg, folding at the knee.

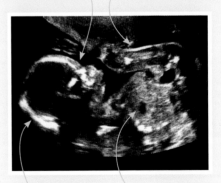

The hard bones covering the skull appear white.

The heart is checked to see if it is working well and has four chambers.

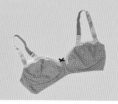

MONTH 5

After the exhaustion and possibly the nausea of the first three months, this trimester is all about looking and feeling fantastic. Time to buy a few new clothes!

Fashion and photos – work it baby!

As your pregnancy progresses, you will find you need a few new clothes. And why not celebrate your new curves by having photos taken?

tight jeans?

You can buy maternity skinny jeans, which fit under a growing bump. Later on you might also want trousers with a stretchy waistband to go over your bump so you feel warm and secure. For work, invest in well-cut trousers that you can sell later.

Three tips for perfect pictures

Photos of your pregnant figure make a fantastic record of this time in your life, and will be fascinating to your child later on. You are blooming this month, so go for it!

1

Location, location, location Choose a garden, beach, professional studio, your home... anything goes. If you feel relaxed, you will probably look your best.

2

Looking good Plan the photo shoot for after you've had a haircut. Put on a little make-up and wear simple, elegant clothing, which ensures you are looking your best!

3

Lighting Flattering lighting can make a huge difference to your appearance. Choose soft, natural light if possible. The sun setting behind you can create a lovely silhouette.

YOUR BREASTS will change shape and size during pregnancy and when breastfeeding, so you will need to get fitted for new bras. Put any underwire bras away for a while as they can cause milk ducts to block. For now, comfort and support are the most important considerations.

Your feet and back are carrying more weight now, plus your feet may get wider for a while. If your shoes feel tight, you need to go shopping!

Your centre of gravity changes when your bump is larger, making walking in high heels difficult. Make sure you can walk easily in your shoes so you won't trip over.

new shoes?

Pumps and low wedge heels are practical options. Shock-absorbing trainers are great for later in your pregnancy.

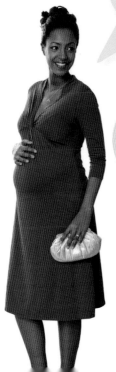

It's exciting buying maternity clothes; it feels like a rite of passage to motherhood. These days you don't have to sacrifice style for comfort.

No-one needs pregnancy clothes for long, so they rarely wear out. Borrow or buy secondhand, particularly for special parties or weddings.

fashion trends!

Cotton undies are the most comfortable.

5

Essential lists

BABY BASICS

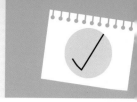

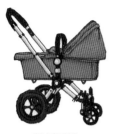

BUGGY

Can lie flat, suitable for
a sleeping newborn.

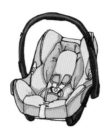

CAR SEAT

Rear-facing; removable
so you can carry baby.

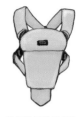

BABY SLING

To take baby anywhere,
and leave you hands free.

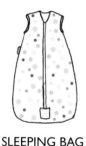

SLEEPING BAG

Cosy; prevents lost
blankets in the night.

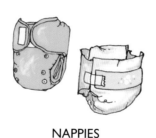

NAPPIES

Either washables (including
liners) or disposables.

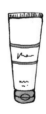

BARRIER CREAM

To protect baby from
nappy rash.

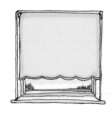

BLACK-OUT BLIND

To help with restful
sleep in your room.

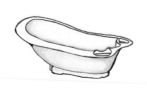

BABY BATH

Place inside your bath; saves
water and suits baby's size.

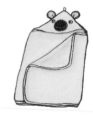

HOODED TOWEL

Soft and new, with a
hood for after bathtime.

SHOPS ARE FULL OF EQUIPMENT to buy, but you definitely don't need everything on offer: somewhere for baby to sleep, some way of carrying him easily, and ways to keep him clean are the basics. Borrow as much as you can!

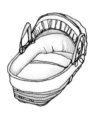

MOSES BASKET
Needs new mattress; ideal for the early weeks.

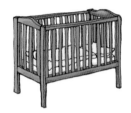

COT
Can be used from birth up to two years.

COTTON SHEETS
To cover the mattress of a Moses basket or cot.

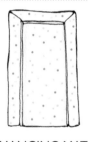

CHANGING MAT
Choose something soft and easy to clean.

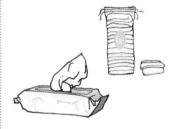

BABY WIPES
Wipes, or cotton wool, for cleaning baby's nappy area.

BABY MONITOR
So you can hear when baby wakes up.

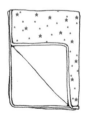

SWADDLE BLANKET
Made of cotton, for swaddling baby or to lie on.

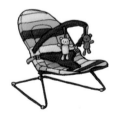

BOUNCY CHAIR
A secure place for baby to watch you.

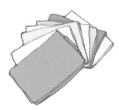

MUSLIN SQUARES
To protect you from dribble, milk, and vomit.

The halfway mark

Your partner now looks pregnant, and it all seems very real. This month is the anomaly scan where mum's and baby's progress will be checked. Your baby actually looks like a baby, and it can hit home that it's not long now.

✳ Blooming beautiful

You might think it's amazing and fascinating to see the changes to your partner's body, but some women can feel less than enthusiastic. She's probably worked hard to stay in shape over the years and now her waistline is expanding every day. If your partner is feeling fed up, be supportive; it's a great sign that baby is growing well.

✳ Hey girl, hey boy

Depending on hospital policy, this scan may bring the moment you find out whether you are having a son or a daughter. If you have decided to find out, it's best not to have any expectations. All the old wives' tales about bump size or position meaning boy or girl have no scientific basis. If you have a strong preference you have a 50 per cent chance of feeling extremely disappointed; if you stay open-

Do

Offer to smooth some stretch mark cream or oil onto her growing bump every day.

Make healthy smoothies for you and your partner to boost nutrient and vitamin intake.

Continue talking to the bump so your newborn baby recognizes your familiar voice.

YOUR BABY will start to look like a miniature newborn and can hear!

YOUR PARTNER'S CENTRE OF GRAVITY IS SHIFTING, SO SHE MIGHT FEEL A BIT OFF-BALANCE. A GREAT EXCUSE FOR HOLDING HANDS.

Whether you have a boy or girl will be determined by which of your sperm meets the egg.

WHY NOT START considering names? How will your ideas sound with your surname? Will baby even have your surname? Can the name be shortened or turned into a nickname?

Don't

Make jokes about her changing shape – she is unlikely to enjoy being compared to Humpty Dumpty or Homer Simpson.

———————————

Forget to keep an open mind about your baby's gender – girls can be good at football, too. Chances are you won't care one way or the other when baby arrives.

minded, you have a 100 per cent chance of happiness. Most parents-to-be don't care whether they get a boy or a girl as long as their baby is healthy, and that is a good place to be.

✳ Checking everything is just right

The purpose of the 20-week scan is to check the development of the baby, rather than find out the sex. The sonographer will check the position of the placenta to make sure it isn't blocking the cervix, which is the baby's exit (placenta praevia, see page 232). The baby's head, limbs, and abdominal circumference will be measured to find out if she is growing as expected for her age, and her spine will be checked to make sure it is aligned. The sonographer will also check how your baby's major organs, such as the lungs, heart, brain, stomach, and bowel, are growing. A repeat scan may be necessary if baby is in the wrong position to make all the checks. If there is any problem you will be told straight away and given support by professionals. Be reassured that most babies are born healthy so it is unlikely that the news will be anything other than positive.

The glowing time

Minor pregnancy complaints are usually outweighed by positives now – as well as that beautiful bump, your hair may be thicker and glossier, and you might be developing a fabulous pregnancy "glow".

✳ Glossy hair

Oestrogen encourages hair to linger in its growth phase, which makes it appear longer and in better condition. Since the strands aren't shed as fast as normal, it looks thicker, too. Make the most of this by getting a really good hair cut. You might want to book another appointment just before the birth to take you through the early days of babyhood when there's little enough time to wash hair, let alone style it!

✳ Healthy nails

Like hair, nails get stuck in a growth phase during pregnancy and can lengthen remarkably. If you're trying to avoid the toxic ingredients often used in nail polishes, opt for an old-fashioned

SPEND 15 MINUTES at the end of every day with your feet up. This will counteract any swelling in your legs, feet, and ankles.

GOOD TO EAT
Figs give you an energy boost, are a gentle laxative, and contain a great mix of minerals.

manicure and buff your nails to boost circulation. As your bump swells and your feet get further away, consider a pedicure. Book the luxury option and treat yourself to a foot massage, which is brilliant for your circulation.

✳ Beautiful skin

Skin tends to plump up and glow in pregnancy because of all the extra circulating blood. The increased hormones encourage your skin to retain moisture, filling out fine lines, too. You are also much less likely to get spots at this stage of your pregnancy. You might get a few tiny spider, or thread, veins on your cheeks, caused by the rapid dilation and constriction of blood vessels, but these tend to fade a few months after birth. As your belly continues to swell, your skin may begin to feel tight and stretched, so rub moisturizer or olive oil all over while your skin is damp after a bath or shower.

✳ Relaxing is essential

Retained moisture might be great for plumping cheeks, but you might find it affects your ankles and feet. You may also experience oedema, also known as dropsy, when your growing bump exerts pressure on blood vessels in your pelvis, especially on the right side, causing blood to pool in the lower body. This congestion forces the extra water downwards where it tries to escape through your feet. Gravity adds to this, making the effects most noticeable in the evening. Rest with your feet higher than your heart to help the blood circulate back to your heart. Lying on your left side, and doing ankle rotations, will help to boost circulation.

Naming and paying

Your baby is making herself obvious now as your bump gets bigger and her kicks get stronger. This prompts parents to think about baby names and also who is going to look after the baby after the birth.

✱ The name game

You might find yourselves imagining a whole little personality for your baby now, based on when and where she kicks, and how your bump is sitting. That often leads to a pet name that might be a stepping stone to a real name. If you haven't before, you might find yourself looking through baby naming sites, leaving sticky notes on books, and contemplating the expectations and associations that accompany names you are drawn to.

✱ Return to your roots

Thinking about names encourages many parents to reconnect with their own families and heritage. Names are an opportunity to make connections between families, and to celebrate the past. You may also have to confront family expectations – are you encouraged to use a first, middle, or family name that's been passed down through generations? What if you don't want to use your partner's surname? Having a baby brings together two distinct families – if you are married, you may find that naming conversations stir up as much debate as the wedding-invitation list.

DADS NOW spend far more time caring for their children. Since 1965, the average amount of time dads spend in childcare has tripled in the UK.

1/3

PARENTS in the UK spend, on average, one third of their income on childcare.

✳ Who will look after baby?

This is perhaps the most searching question parents have to ask as a child grows and circumstances change. After the initial newborn weeks, who will do the day-to-day childcare? Will one of you take most responsibility, or will you try to share tasks? Will you call in family for help, or hire a specialist? It might be a scary option, but now is a perfect time to visit prospective childminders and nurseries, even though you probably feel completely ill-prepared. The best way to find out about realistic options is to chat with parents of babies and toddlers in your area. Work out the costs, and talk to your manager at work about childcare vouchers, which can offer a tax break.

WHAT'S IN A NAME?

In Bali, every person has one of just four available names. A baby is named according to birth order and the names are the same for boys and girls. That certainly resolves a lot of discussion!

✳ Planning for the future

Despite maternity pay, your household salary will reduce once you stop working. It's easy to push this thought away, but now is a good time to plan. Work out how you might cut back, or accrue savings, to pay for baby items, and also about how you'll survive month-to-month. If you want to prioritize your thinking, plan for the living expenses – add up the cost of essential bills and food, and budget what's left over for holidays, clothes, and going out. On a positive note, despite what a flick through a pregnancy magazine might suggest, a newborn actually needs few essentials (see pages 92–93), and there's a huge amount of immaculate secondhand baby equipment for sale.

Starting to remember

Your baby's brain goes through a period of rapid growth at the start of this month. The cells that control conscious thought are developing, and with them the early stages of memory.

✳ Growth spurt

Neurons proliferate while the upper part of the brain, called the cortex, grows rapidly. This growth peaks by month six or seven. As the neurons sprout transmitters and receptors to connect with other cells and send and receive signals around the body, your baby becomes more able to move with purpose and coordination.

✳ Pruning out

Brain development is not just about cell growth – any cells that are not useful now start to self-destruct. Around 90 per cent of the cells in the cortex are discarded because they haven't formed the right connections, while those that have made the grade thrive and develop a protective coating of fatty material, called myelin, which speeds up the electrical impulses that pass through them. Your baby's motor reactions and senses now become more acute and efficient.

Baby's progress bar: you are now 65% complete

LOADING ...

| 10% | 20% | 30% | 40% | 50 |

DID YOU KNOW?

BY 26 WEEKS your baby weighs about 1kg (2lb 3oz) and is 29cm (11in) long. Your baby will grow 15cm (6in) this month.

HOW BIG? She is about the size of a cabbage.

✳ Startling stuff

Babies develop a startle, or Moro, reflex between weeks 24 and 28. This primitive reflex is an involuntary response to a sudden change in stimuli, such as a loud noise. You might notice your baby jump in reaction to a slammed door or car alarm. It is a fight-or-flight reaction, vital for your baby to deal with stress. Newborns are tested after birth, and show a response to noise by flinging their arms out to the sides and arching their backs. The reflex goes after about six months, replaced by a calmer reaction as your baby's nervous system matures and she learns to filter out unwanted stimuli.

✳ New responses

Now that your baby's senses are more acute, it's no longer just your and your partner's voices she recognizes from inside the womb. Studies suggest newborn babies recognize music they have heard in the womb.

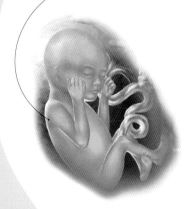

Lanugo hairs keep a layer of greasy vernix on the skin, which, in turn, is starting to develop a protective outer layer of keratinized cells.

Some women report that their unborn babies "kick" to rhythmic music.

Daytime and nightlife

Your baby has developed a cycle of sleeping and waking, and you should be able to predict when she'll be more active – although unfortunately it might not always fit in with your own sleep schedule!

✳ Rhythm of life

Your baby now starts to establish a circadian rhythm. This is the internal biological clock that governs vital body functions, such as breathing, temperature regulation, and hormonal control, over 24 hours. A master "clock" in the hypothalamus area of the brain controls other clocks in almost every body tissue to make sure that everything is working in an appropriate way for the time of day or night, and season of the year. While your baby is in the womb, your hormones help to coordinate her own developing circadian system.

✳ What's on when?

Generally, babies seem to be most active for about five hours in the morning and again in the evening. So it is likely that you'll notice your baby moving

DID YOU KNOW?

FROM WEEK 24 onwards baby might survive outside the womb, given specialist neonatal care.

0.3°C

Your baby's temperature is about 0.3°C (32°F) higher than your body temperature.

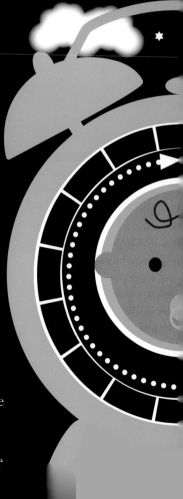

more in the evening and when you are in bed, making it seem as if she becomes more active when you are relaxing or trying to sleep.

✳ Wide awake

When your baby is in an active phase, the movements of her arms, legs, and eyes become more synchronized. Her eyes have been moving behind her sealed eyelids since about week 20, but at the end of this month, they finally open and she is able to blink.

✳ Sleeping time

Baby sleep is divided into three states: quiet, active, and indeterminate – this indicates that her brain has become more mature. Quiet sleep is similar to our Non-REM (Rapid Eye Movement) sleep, when both breathing and heart rates slow. Active sleep seems to be a precursor of REM sleep, characterized by rapid eye movements, a very active brain, dreaming, and memories. Your baby spends most of her days in indeterminate sleep, which indicates that her brain is not yet able to organize activity. During the third trimester your baby will start to spend more of her sleeping time in quiet and active sleep, getting her ready for life outside

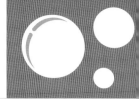

MONTH 6

SPA IDEAS AND BEAUTY TREATMENTS

Being pregnant, you may have grooming concerns – can I still use my favourite hair dye? What products should I avoid? What are the best spa treatments for pregnant women...?

Floatation tank

Unwind physically and mentally in a floatation session – you will float effortlessly in the quiet and dark, in body-temperature water. Very relaxing!

Indian head massage

If it's more comfortable to sit upright rather than lie down, try an Indian head massage, which covers your head, scalp, face, neck, upper arms, upper back, and shoulders. Research by the Institute of Indian Head Massage says it can relieve headaches, congestion, and insomnia.

Acupuncture

This can re-energize you if you are feeling tired. It can also alleviate lower back pain, and even turn a breech baby.

Facial

Pregnancy hormones can cause acne – a gentle facial may help. Facial oils can also rehydrate your skin.

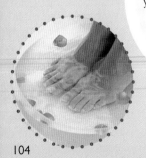

Beauty treatments

Waxing, facials, pedicures, and manicures are all safe during pregnancy, though your skin might feel more sensitive than usual.

Moisturize

Use a natural, rich cream all over your body, especially on dry areas of skin, such as elbows and heels.

Haircare

From the second trimester, people might start remarking on the thick, glossy appearance of your hair (see page 96). If you usually colour your hair, fear not, your routine doesn't need to change. The chemicals in permanent and semi-permanent hair dyes are not highly toxic. Research, although limited, shows that it's safe to colour your hair while pregnant. Henna dyes are also safe – do a patch test first as your hair may be more absorbent.

Things to avoid

- Deep tissue and sports massages are too powerful while pregnant, even on your legs.

- Steam rooms, saunas, and jacuzzis can lower blood pressure, making you feel dizzy. Raised body temperature is dangerous for baby.

- Body wraps can raise your temperature, and contain chemicals that may cross the placenta.

- Sunbeds expose your skin to ultraviolet rays, which may be linked to a breakdown of folic acid. Your skin is also more likely to burn.

- Reflexology is best avoided in the first trimester, but is okay later in pregnancy.

Alternative hair dyes

If you are concerned about using permanent hair dyes, perhaps try foil-painted highlights, or switch to wash-out colourants that contain fewer active ingredients.

Take an expensive holiday while you can before you need to pay for extra seats! Babies can travel on a parent's lap for up to two years. After that, airlines charge a full fare for children of any age.

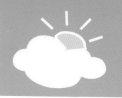

Happy babymoon

Many parents-to-be are opting to take time out to bond and relax ahead of the birth – it may be your last chance to take a trip alone for quite some time.

✳ When to go

The best time to travel is during the second trimester of pregnancy (14–27 weeks), when the waves of nausea have subsided and your bump is not yet too big. Airlines don't impose restrictions for pregnant travellers until into the third trimester, although some may request a letter from your doctor after 28 weeks.

✳ Where to go

Everyone's idea of a romantic, restful destination is different. For some, sunny beach resorts provide the perfect backdrop; for others mountain retreats or city breaks are preferred. Opt for somewhere with decent medical care should the need arise. Long-haul flights add unnecessary stress, as well as increasing the risk of DVT (deep vein thrombosis); drives shouldn't be too long either and take regular breaks.

✳ What to do

Nap in a hammock, lose yourself in a good book, soothe away muscle stress in the pool, or spoil yourself with a massage. Savour long, leisurely dinners together or spend the evening stargazing; take the time to bond and enjoy this special period of transition.

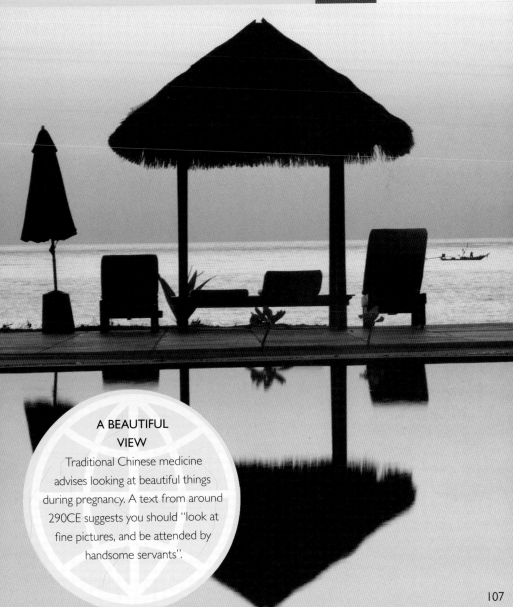

DID YOU KNOW?

MOVING AROUND on a long car, train, or plane journey will reduce your risk of deep vein thrombosis.

34

AFTER 34 WEEKS MOST AIRLINES WILL NOT PERMIT YOU TO TRAVEL.

A BEAUTIFUL VIEW

Traditional Chinese medicine advises looking at beautiful things during pregnancy. A text from around 290CE suggests you should "look at fine pictures, and be attended by handsome servants".

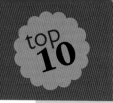

How do you do that?
GETTING A GOOD NIGHT'S SLEEP

1 Comfort is key

Lying on your left side can be more comfortable and aids blood flow to the placenta (so good for baby, too). Place a pillow under your bump and between your legs for added comfort.

2 Eating habits

Try not to eat less than two hours before you go to bed, and avoid spicy and fried food. Position a bottle of liquid antacids next to your bed to sip if indigestion keeps you awake.

3 Drink in the day

Don't drink too much, or get thirsty! The recommended amount of liquid per day is eight 227ml (8fl oz) glasses, plus one extra glass for each hour of light activity. That includes all your intake of water, herbal tea, and soft drinks.

4 Enjoy some gentle exercise

If you have done some exercise your body will be more tired and you'll feel more relaxed. Avoid exercising in the evening, though, as it can increase adrenaline, which prevents sleep.

5 Alarm trick

If you can't sleep, it can make you clock-watch. Try resetting your alarm for an hour later than usual as this can make you feel more relaxed if getting back to sleep takes a while. It's better to be a bit late for work than half asleep all day.

IS YOUR BUMP KEEPING YOU AWAKE, making sleep a luxury you can only dream about? Then follow these handy tips and you will soon be sleeping like a baby.

6 ### Dealing with worries
Having a baby gives you plenty to think about, and in the middle of the night your thoughts can spiral unchecked. If that happens and you find yourself panicking, write down what you are worrying about, then put it out of your head until morning.

7 ### Banish bad dreams
Pregnant women, especially with their first baby, may suffer from strange dreams and even nightmares. This is a natural result of a fear of the unknown and is normal. Relieving anxiety will help, so book yourself into a relaxing therapy.

8 ### A soothing bedtime routine
You can practice on yourself for when the baby appears. Try hot milk, music, reading, or lavender oil on your pillow – whatever works for you and helps you wind down.

9 ### Nighttime baby gym
As soon as you lie down to rest it may feel like the baby inside you wakes up and starts exercising! Some people say turning on the radio can help soothe baby off to sleep again; it may also distract you from the little gymnast inside.

10 ### Visit your doctor
Your lack of sleep won't directly affect your baby – so don't worry. However, if it is affecting your ability to function make an appointment to speak to your doctor for advice.

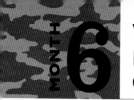

MONTH

6

Weeks 22–26
DAD'S SURVIVAL
GUIDE

DID YOU
KNOW?

Money on your mind

It's getting very real now and it's time to start thinking about practicalities, equipment, and finances. On the plus side, you can feel baby move, too!

✳ Money, money, money

Now that you are starting to shop for your new addition, you might realize how much he is going to cost you. If you haven't already, you and your partner should figure out a budget. With one or both of you taking leave from work you will have less money, and you will also be spending more on nappies, clothes etc. Make time to go through your incomings and outgoings to help avoid stress. Borrow as much baby kit as you can, and welcome offers of gifts for big-ticket items, such as a car seat or buggy. You will probably make short-term savings by having fewer expensive nights out in the months to come.

✳ Work it baby

In the UK men are entitled to up to two weeks paternity leave, plus additional time off if your partner returns to work before the end of her

In the US there is no legal right to paid paternity or maternity leave.

ALL OF HIS SENSES are developing rapidly – he can hear low-frequency sounds, responds to light, and even has taste buds!

THE AVERAGE COST OF RAISING YOUR BABY TO 21 YEARS IS £222,000. OUCH.

maternity leave. You can share the year between you and are entitled to some pay for at least part of it. If you can take extended leave to be primary carer it can be a wonderful experience. It will also give you some insight into the tough job your partner does when you are at work. Scandinavian countries also have good paternity benefits, but perhaps surprisingly, the US is very behind in offering any paternity leave, unpaid or not.

✳ Move it

Your baby's movements will start to be noticeable and the nerve pathways in his ears have formed, meaning he can hear. To get a wriggle from baby, try talking and singing to him, and you could try shining a flashlight on your partner's belly, or rest a cold drink against her if she'll let you. In the next few weeks you may be able to see baby moving as he changes position, which is really exciting and nothing for you to be fearful about.

Do

Think about taking paternity leave and your entitlements.

Write down all the things you will need to source ready for the baby.

Work out a budget based on your reduced income and decide together if you will need to make any changes to your outgoings.

Don't

Prod or poke the bump trying to get a reaction from your baby – you're likely to stress him out!

Put off thinking about a will or life insurance – get it sorted and put your mind at ease.

Moan or go for a coffee when shopping for baby items. Your input is important.

On the move

As you now enter into the final stage of your pregnancy journey, you might wonder how your body is able to accommodate your expanding baby, and where all your organs have ended up as a result.

✳ Growing bump

By week 28, the top of your uterus will be about 6–8cm (2½–3in) above your belly button, and from now on your bump will get noticeably higher and wider. As the baby puts on weight, your internal organs shift to accommodate this.

✳ Tummy troubles

Your stomach and intestines are squeezed upwards as the baby grows, butting into your diaphragm, which increases the likelihood of indigestion and heartburn. Your intestines get squashed against your back which, along with the slowing effect of hormones, makes constipation increasingly likely, too. Both kidneys increase in length as the smooth muscle relaxes and dilates.

✳ Squashed bladder

In the first trimester, weeing was more frequent, partly due to your enlarging uterus. This problem returns now as your bladder gets squashed by your uterus, especially if your baby is head-down. Your bladder muscle has also relaxed now.

IS YOUR BABY feeling long as she stretches inside you? At seven months, she is almost the length she'll be at birth.

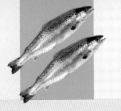

GOOD TO EAT
Oily fish with omega-3 fatty acids for development of your baby's brain, eyes, and nervous system.

✳ Opening ribs

Your ribs react to a widening uterus and higher digestive organs by expanding sideways. This can feel uncomfortably stretchy, which is exacerbated if your baby is lying head-up in the breech position.

WEIGHT GAIN slows down slightly in month seven. As your womb presses on your belly, you feel full more quickly after meals.

✳ Breathing in

A widening rib cage affects your diaphragm. This dome-shaped muscle at the base of the lungs contracts when you inhale, moving downwards to create space in the chest cavity for the lungs to expand, drawing in air. The movement is hampered by a higher uterus and stomach, so your in-breaths will feel more restricted now the diaphragm can't move to make space.

✳ Adapting spine

The column of vertebrae in your spine adapts to accommodate the increasing weight and bulk of your uterus by exaggerating its natural curves. This can cause back pain. Postural exercises can be helpful.

✳ Cramping legs

Cramps in the legs are common from week 29, especially at night; some doctors put this down to increasing pressure from the extra weight straining your leg muscles, or the effect of your growing uterus on nerves in the pelvis. Shooting pains, or tingling down the backs of your legs, can be a sign that your baby's head is pressing into the sciatic nerve in the lower part of your spine.

By the end of month seven you will have gained around 7kg (15lb).

Showers and sunshine

It's the start of a new trimester and your fast-approaching due date can feel daunting, so this is a good time to reconnect with supportive friends and family – and is an ideal time for a "baby shower".

✳ Coping with fatigue

The energy of the second trimester starts to run out now, and it's normal to feel a little disconsolate, as if pregnancy will last forever. When your increased metabolism and squeezed organs make breathing, moving, and sleeping less easy, it's no surprise that life seems more of a chore. If you've not done so already, work out what tasks you can jettison or delegate at work and at home. Then try to enjoy the latter stages of being pregnant.

✳ Stress and hormones

The third trimester brings an increase in a stress hormone called corticotropin-releasing hormone (CRH), which is released from the placenta. Although CRH brings benefits to your developing baby, as a stress hormone it can have a negative impact on you. Studies show that strong family support at this time – both material and emotional – correlates to lower levels of this hormone, and fewer symptoms of depression later. This is a good time to test out some of the support systems that you hope to rely on after the birth – there's still time to change plans if need be.

BABY SHOWER CELEBRATIONS are traditionally intended to soothe, nurture, and shower the mother-to-be with good things.

RISING LEVELS of the stress hormone CRH (see below) help your baby's brain to develop and his lungs to mature.

✳ Pack a birth bag

Getting together everything you need for the birth can also lift a weight from your shoulders, and bring a welcome feeling of control. You might want to show your shopping list to friends planning your baby shower, and make sure you go shopping yourself before walking becomes a little difficult. In particular, consider what you might want to wear during labour, and choose some nursing tops if you plan on breastfeeding.

✳ Choice friends

You might find that some single friends aren't into the baby scene, or notice that child-free colleagues are increasingly anxious in your presence in case you go into labour. This is not the time to have additional concerns playing on your mind. Try not to take their comments personally, and spend time with more nurturing people.

✳ Start classes

This is a great time to get serious about antenatal classes – knowledge of pain-relief options, relaxation techniques, and what actually happens during labour equips you to write a birth plan (see pages 138–9), and can ease common third-trimester anxieties about delivery. These classes can be bonding experiences, too – there's nothing like practising breath-control exercises and birthing positions to break the ice in a room of strangers! You may also meet a new set of parents-to-be who you'd like to spend time with through the remainder of your pregnancy and beyond – learning to pant and moan together has sparked many special post-pregnancy friendships.

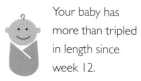

Your baby has more than tripled in length since week 12.

Are we nearly there?

Your baby is nearer to her destination – at the start of the third trimester she is lengthening and putting on weight, but there's still room to turn somersaults.

✳ Tight fit

By the end of this month, your baby's movements will feel significantly stronger; her activity is building towards its peak at 32 weeks, after which space for in-utero aerobics becomes more limited. You will feel these movements as sharp kicks to the bladder or headbutts into the ribs, all of which are perfectly normal. In the past, mothers were encouraged to monitor their baby's movements, counting the number of kicks in 12-hour periods, but there's no need to record anything nowadays; just be aware of patterns and contact your doctor or midwife if the movements reduce significantly.

✳ Visible limbs

You're likely to see your belly move dramatically now, which can be rather unnerving. This is because your baby is getting bigger and her bones are harder (they are fully developed by week 29). It is also because your production of amniotic fluid has almost ended, resulting in reduced cushioning of limb movements.

Baby's progress bar: you are now 75% complete

LOADING ...

| 10% | 20% | 30% | 40% | 50% |

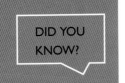

DID YOU
KNOW?

BY WEEK 30 your baby weighs about 1.5kg (3lb) and will grow up to 5cm (2in) throughout this month.

HOW BIG?
She is about the size of a pineapple.

✳ **Where are you, baby?**

The position of kicks and visible body parts gives clues as to how your baby is positioned. At the start of this month she may be lying horizontally (known as a transverse position). By 30 weeks most babies are vertical (longitudinal), often upright with a bony skull uncomfortably wedged up into your ribs. This is also known as breech position and it is quite normal this month. Between 35–40 weeks, the presentation of your baby is very important, whether she is head-down or bottom-down in preparation for birth. The ideal position she needs to get to at the end of this trimester is head-down and facing your hip. You can help gravity along from month seven by regularly getting into a hands-and-knees position or relaxing forward onto cushions so that the heaviest parts of your baby (her head and spine) drop into a good position for birth.

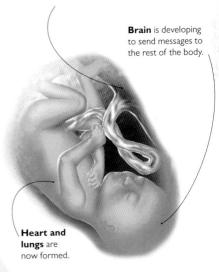

Placenta passes antibodies from you to your baby.

Brain is developing to send messages to the rest of the body.

Heart and lungs are now formed.

Getting ready to breathe

While most of your baby's body systems are relatively mature now, the lungs have some way to go before they can function after birth, so every day that goes by makes a huge difference to their development.

✳ Bigger and better

The lungs don't have to work independently until the moment your baby is born – and they spend the final trimester gearing up for this. Until last month they were completing the phase of development in which the airways branch to form bronchioles. Right now they are growing an increasing number of clusters of tiny air sacs on those bronchioles, called alveoli, which form the final subdivision of the passages inside the lungs. A network of blood vessels is forming around each of the sacs, preparing to carry oxygen from the lungs and bring back carbon dioxide to be expelled. In fact, most of a baby's alveoli form after birth, vastly increasing the surface area available for oxygen and carbon dioxide to be exchanged. This final growth phase continues up to the age of about two and a half.

✳ Super elasticity

From this month on, the smooth walls of the alveoli are receiving a very thin coating of "surfactant", an elasticating fluid that will help them to expand when they first fill with air after birth, and ensure

THE MARROW in each of your baby's bones is producing red blood cells. In adulthood, this changes and is produced in just a few bones.

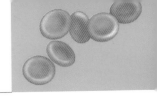

that they do not collapse when breath is exhaled. The surfactant can be detected now in your amniotic fluid. Doctors test it to find out how mature a baby's lungs are if premature birth looks likely. Rest assured, even if your baby is born prematurely, there are effective treatments that doctors can administer to help make baby's lungs more elastic.

Your baby's lungs are already practising to inhale with amniotic fluid, rather than air.

✳ Boost that blood

Deep within your baby's bones, bone marrow is now producing most of your baby's supply of red blood cells. These cells pick up the oxygen from alveoli, via the tiny blood vessels, and carry it around the body, offloading oxygen where required and picking up carbon dioxide waste to be exhaled. The process of making red blood cells first began in the egg sac, moved to the liver, and is now in the place it will stay for life. Your baby is manufacturing fetal blood cells now, which contain the oxygen-carrying pigment haemoglobin F (HbF) – it is especially good at extracting oxygen across the placenta and combines well with oxygen from your bloodstream – it will be replaced in the last few weeks in the womb by the adult form, called haemoglobin A (HbA). When newborn, a baby's red blood cells are up to 95 per cent HbF; the remainder being HbA.

Aches, pains, and veins
COMMON COMPLAINTS IN LATE PREGNANCY

WHAT TO DO

1

Insomnia
Heartburn, needing the loo, your big tummy… It's difficult to get comfortable at night.

Be careful about what you eat and drink before you go to bed, and establish a soothing sleep routine. Sleep aids, such as pregnancy cushions, can help.

2

Numb fingers
Your fingers are numb, tingling, and you have wrist pain.

You may have carpal tunnel syndrome (see page 228). See your doctor, who may refer you to a physiotherapist. Shaking your hands can help ease discomfort. Avoid activities that aggravate it.

3

Piles
You have uncomfortable pea- or grape-sized lumps inside or sticking out of your bottom.

Piles (or haemorrhoids) are often a result of constipation. Eat a high-fibre diet, drink plenty of water and fruit juice, and get regular exercise. Try not to strain when you go to the loo.

4

Back pain
Your lower back aches like mad and you are starting to walk like John Wayne.

Exercise! You may not feel like it but swimming, gentle walks, and yoga can help. Avoid standing or sitting for long periods, and if you experience severe pain or numbness contact a doctor or midwife.

5

Varicose veins
Swollen, knotty, bluish veins on your lower legs.

Avoid standing for long periods or crossing your legs. Rest with your feet and legs up, and you could try wearing support tights.

IT CAN FEEL like a struggle to reach the finishing post, but every day that passes brings you closer to meeting your baby.

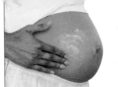

ALMOST 90 PER CENT of women develop stretch marks.

WHAT TO DO

6 Stretch marks

Narrow red lines or streaks are weaving their way across your tummy or breasts.

The big question is: will they go away? The answer is that they will fade to a silvery white and be far less visible. Moisturizing with oil or cream can help improve their appearance.

7 Swelling

Swollen ankles and feet, and fingers like sausages, especially at the end of the day.

Water retention in pregnancy causes this swelling. Put your feet up, wear comfortable shoes with no tight straps, and avoid standing for long periods. Remove rings if you need to.

8 Incontinence

If you laugh, sneeze, or cough you wet yourself a bit.

Increased pressure from your growing baby has an effect on your bladder control. Do pelvic floor exercises morning, afternoon, and night and you WILL notice results.

9 Breathlessness

You are in the middle of talking when you have to stop and pant for breath.

Sit up straight and push your shoulders back to give your lungs more room to expand. Take things easy and don't push yourself too hard when you exercise. Don't panic – it's normal.

10 Exhaustion

It's back – you feel extremely tired, all the time, again.

It's not surprising! Avoid standing for long periods or walking far (though gentle exercise can be energizing). Eat well, and rest when you need to.

Essential lists

HOSPITAL BAG

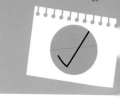

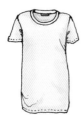

LOOSE T-SHIRT
An old, cotton T-shirt to wear during labour.

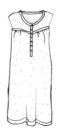

NIGHTIE
For during labour, and with buttons for breastfeeding.

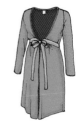

DRESSING GOWN
For on the ward; don't forget your towel, too.

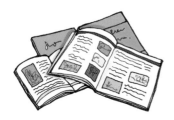

MAGAZINES
Something easy to read during labour and after.

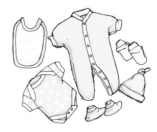

BABY CLOTHES
A few vests, sleepsuits, and a newborn hat.

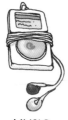

MUSIC
MP3 or CD player for distraction during labour.

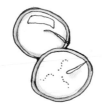

PADS
Plenty of nursing and breast pads.

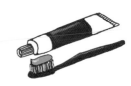

TOILETRIES
Shower gel, shampoo, comb, and toothbrush.

YOU WILL NEED a bag for the labour ward, including your hospital notes, any pain relief, such as a TENS machine or birthing ball, and a pack of newborn nappies. Plan for a one to two day stay, though you may be home sooner. Your partner can pick up anything you forget, so don't worry!

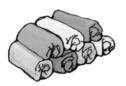

UNDERWEAR

Plenty of old, comfy or disposable knickers.

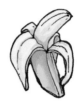

FOOD AND DRINK

Tasty and easy snacks for during labour.

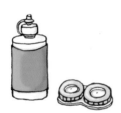

DAILY ITEMS

Any regular items you need, such as contact lens solution.

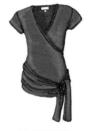

CLOTHES

For when you go home; make sure they're comfy.

EARPLUGS

For a noisy ward; check you can hear your baby!

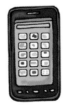

MOBILE PHONE

Fully charged, with all the numbers you need.

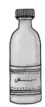

MASSAGE OIL

For your partner to give you a footrub, if you like.

PREMATURE BABIES

The early bird

Premature labour (before 37 weeks) can be a shock, leaving you little or no time to prepare for your baby's arrival. But although they may feel extra fragile, many early babies do not need special care.

✳ Is this it?

Your first reaction might be to panic, but try to stay calm until a midwife or doctor has assessed you – often, what are thought to be symptoms of early labour are something else. If labour is confirmed, your carers may try to slow things down and give you steroids to mature your baby's lungs. Medical care is fantastic nowadays and babies can survive from as early as 26 weeks.

✳ Speed is of the essence

A decision may be made to induce labour or elect for a Caesarean if your baby needs to come out quickly. Being induced means your labour may be faster than usual and you will be more closely monitored, so you may have to surrender some of your birth plan.

✳ A loving touch

Ideally you will enjoy a first cuddle straightaway, but if there are immediate concerns the doctors may have to intervene, for example, if your baby needs help breathing, or if she weighs less than 2kg (4lb 7oz). If she is taken to a special care baby unit (SCBU), touch is especially important (see Getting involved, right). You should be able to stay with your baby day and night, but if not, ask a midwife to take a photo for your bedside.

✳ In safe hands

If your baby is born before 34 weeks, or has health concerns, she will spend time in a neonatal unit, or an intensive care baby unit (ICBU). Although it is frightening, this is the best place for her, with highly trained staff and specialist equipment helping her to thrive. Be patient, she will soon be coming home.

✳ Getting involved

While you can't attend to your baby's medical needs, you will play a fundamental role in caring for her during her early days. Here are a few ways to make your time in ICBU positive for both of you.

1. Touch and stroke her – she seems so delicate, but gently stroking her can be immensely soothing and she will enjoy your familiar smell.

2. Talk to her – she already knows your voice from months inside you, so hearing you talking, singing, or just humming is reassuring.

3. Look into her eyes – holding her gaze is one of the first steps to bonding.

4. Hold her – once you are allowed to pick her up, carrying her skin-to-skin, known as kangaroo care, helps with bonding and has real benefits, actually shortening hospital stays.

5. Express your milk – this can be fed to her, providing her with immunity and super nutrition.

Entering the home stretch

Welcome to the third trimester – the home stretch. Your partner might be getting fed up with being pregnant, and there is a lot to organize.

✳ Mixed blessings

Baby will be growing rapidly, as will your partner's bump. Both of you need plenty of nutritious food, so help out by providing nourishing meals. Your partner may find it hard to sleep due to the size of the bump, and she may experience heartburn and leg cramps at night. Get used to extra pillows in the bed, and make sure she has plenty of space to move. You might need a bigger bed!

✳ Father fears

How do you feel about your partner having to go through labour? You may hate the thought of seeing her in pain, but bear in mind that labour pain is a sign that her uterine muscles are working; it doesn't mean there are problems. Perhaps you're worried that something will go wrong. This is a common fear among fathers approaching the critical point, but the

> **YOUR PARTNER** is getting achy all over. You could learn a few basic massage techniques for her head, hands, and shoulders.

MANY MEN report changes in their own sleep pattern at this point.

SOME WOMEN DEVELOP RESTLESS LEG SYNDROME NOW – REDUCING CAFFEINE CAN HELP, ALONG WITH EATING A BANANA TO AVOID CRAMP.

IF YOUR BABY is a boy his testicles will be moving down to his groin.

chance is very low. Let's be serious for a moment: in the UK these days there are only about eight maternal deaths in every 100,000, and four infant deaths per 1,000 births. These figures are the lowest ever recorded, and continue to fall, so it's a good time to have a baby.

✱ Big-ticket buys

This is the time you need to bite the bullet and buy or borrow the expensive items such as a cot, buggy, and car seat. Do online research, visit shops, read product reviews, check message boards on parenting websites, and talk to parents you know. If your partner is the one who will be using the buggy most she should be a big part of the decision-making process, even if the gadget man in you is dying to take control. It's worth buying a buggy in a shop rather than online so you can see if you can both use the thing.

Do

Make sure she gets plenty of milk or another source of calcium to help your baby form his skeleton.

Feed her lots of iron-rich food to boost her production of red blood cells, and vitamin C to help iron absorption.

Undertake any outstanding DIY tasks.

Don't

Panic if she experiences Braxton Hicks contractions (see page 129) – these are just practise for the real thing.

Worry about the birth. Research as much as you can so you can offer reassurance.

Forget to make your home safe, such as fitting smoke alarms if you don't have them.

127

On the home straight

Your body is the hottest it's ever been (literally), and ramping up for birth by whooshing extra blood around your system, while practising contractions that may take your breath away.

✳ Hot stuff!

The amount of blood in your body continues to surge through your third trimester, and it hits maximum volume at 35 weeks, at around 5 litres (9 pints). You have 25 per cent more blood than before pregnancy; it now contains up to 50 per cent more plasma (the liquid component). To cope with the extra volume, your **cardiac output** – the amount of blood your heart pumps around the body with each heartbeat – goes into overdrive. Because your blood vessels are now fully dilated, and can't relax or expand any further, they set up a resistance that causes your blood pressure to rise slightly.

✳ Can you stand the heat?

Your core body temperature has risen by almost 1°C (1.8°F) as your metabolism has speeded up, so you're more likely to sweat. Your dilated blood vessels are also working hard to cool your system and maintain a safe temperature for your baby.

NEW WORDS

- Cardiac output
- Braxton Hicks
- Oxytocin

HORMONE LEVELS are high, so you may feel elated one minute and anxious the next. Don't worry – it's your body getting ready for labour.

GOOD TO EAT
Beef for iron, B vitamins, and protein, plus chromium to support your baby's tissues.

❋ Taking the strain

All the extra fluid circulating in your body can be visible in bloated fingers and legs, as well as ankles and feet. Swollen veins may be a problem, too – blood can pool in smaller dilated veins in the lower body, such as the anus and vulva, especially as the weight of your uterus presses on the main supply veins in the pelvis. Ouch! Up to 40 per cent of women notice varicose veins in pregnancy, and this tends to be hereditary. Gentle exercise and resting with your feet higher than your heart can help, as well as eating plenty of roughage, such as prunes.

❋ Let's pretend

Have you noticed your abdomen tightening and hardening from the top down? The sensation can take your breath away and tends to last about half a minute before relaxing again. This is a **Braxton Hicks** contraction, a weak, irregular version of the contractions you'll experience in labour, and a sign that your body is gearing up for the big day. The squeezing action directs blood to your placenta and starts to prepare the cervix for action. These contractions are not generally painful, but can get quite strong through the final weeks. A warm bath or back massage can help. Not all women experience Braxton Hicks contractions, however, so don't worry if you don't feel any. Your body will perform fine on the day regardless!

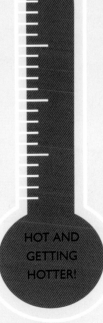

HOT AND GETTING HOTTER!

Building a nest

As your journey takes you closer to the main event, your body prepares you psychologically for parenthood in surprising ways. Even the least homely mothers-to-be can feel a compulsion to hang curtains.

✳ The nurturing instinct

The urge to nest reminds us of what we are in essence: mammals. Nesting is an instinct shared among mammals who give birth to offspring who can't look after themselves. For humans, it's an intuitive urge to establish a safe, sheltered place that best equips us to meet the demands of a helpless infant, and to exert a little control and calmness at a slightly uncertain time. Best not to fight nature: give into the urge and use it to tie up loose ends, clear the clutter, and make final decisions about how to turn your pre-baby apartment or house into a family home.

✳ Nearly time

The onset of nesting behaviour seems to be triggered by **oxytocin**, the same hormone that triggers the uterus to start contracting in the first stage of labour. In fact, your midwife will be interested to hear about any extreme urge to nest in the final weeks of pregnancy, since it is often regarded as a sign that labour is imminent.

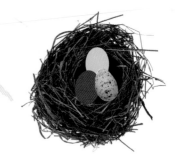

DID YOU KNOW?

MORE THAN half of dads-to-be say they experience the nesting instinct even though they don't produce the "nesting" hormone.

200

YOUR BODY will require 200 extra calories per day during the third trimester.

However, although it can be tempting to balance on ladders or wield power tools as the insatiable urge to nest takes over, the more physical tasks are best left to someone else at this stage of your pregnancy. Also avoid hardcore cleaning and decorating that involves ammonia, bleach, and oil-based paints or thinners, as they give off potentially toxic fumes.

FROM THAILAND TO WEST AFRICA the birthing room is traditionally adorned with beautiful objects – beads, mirrors, painted fabric – to please the newborn baby, and deter evil spirits.

✳ Winding down

It might be sensible to work out what aspects of your life need to start winding down. If you are working, then you'll have already set your leaving date, but you may want to start delegating any new projects and handing over existing ones to colleagues. It's also a good idea to shelve any major outstanding plans, such as a house move or serious renovation work – added stress at this stage is best avoided. Instead, make time to reconnect with family and friends – they will be your primary support network in the months to come.

✳ Final plans can wait

Are you in a dilemma about whether to prepare a nursery for your baby and wondering how you'll ever have time to get it ready? Don't worry, it will be much easier to make that decision once she's here, when you'll have clearer instincts about whether she should sleep in a crib beside your bed for a few months, or have her own space.

A tiny teenager

The adrenal glands are getting larger and more active this month, and as a result sex hormones are triggering your baby into a phase she won't hit again until puberty.

✳ Hormone factory

The adrenal glands, positioned just above the kidneys, have doubled in size since month five, and are about to double in size again. The hormones they produce are essential for maturing the lungs, and they are working overtime right now to manufacture the hormone cortisol. Your baby needs this to trigger the production of enough surfactant to coat thousands of developing air sacs (see pages 118–119).

✳ Going into overdrive

The adrenal glands in both boys and girls also secrete huge amounts of the male sex hormone dehydroepiandrosterone. The liver processes this before it is converted into oestrogen by the placenta. In addition, boy babies' testes pump out male hormones, including testosterone, which help develop the genitals. These high levels of hormones reduce after birth and are not reactivated until puberty.

✳ Birds and bees

A baby boy's testicles will probably be descending this month, dropping down from his abdomen into his scrotum. A girl's ovaries don't move into position until after birth.

YOUR BABY CAN now differentiate between sweet and sour tastes.

Women pregnant with boys eat 10% more calories than those carrying girls. Their appetite may be stimulated by hormones secreted by their babies' developing testes.

✳ Dozy baby

Also like a teenager, your baby is sleeping more this month; in fact she's out for the count for more than half the day. There's a noticeable decrease in "indeterminate" sleep and more quiet sleep now, as well as greater harmonization of her circadian rhythm (waking and sleeping times) with your own periods of rest and activity. Her sleep patterns and rhythms of day and night, activity and rest will continue to evolve during the first three to six months after birth.

✳ Beating the bugs

In preparation for life after birth, your immune system is now passing on IgG antibodies (the primary protector against invading germs and the only one of five antibodies able to cross the placenta) to your baby. You are passing on immunity against every germ you have been exposed to during your own lifetime. Sealed safely inside the womb, your baby has been protected from germs, so her own immune system won't start making IgG antibodies until after birth; her spleen and bone marrow, however, have been producing increasing levels of IgM antibodies since the end of the first trimester.

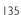

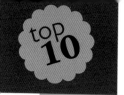

Saving a fortune
HOW TO HAVE A BABY ON A BUDGET

1 **Do your research**

Find out what you really need – talk to other parents before buying masses of kit you'll never use. Check product reviews and message boards before investing in big-ticket purchases.

2 **Mini fashionista**

Resist the temptation to buy designer baby clothes; babies grow out of them at an alarming rate, and are often sick down them, too! Buy a capsule wardrobe of cost-effective basics, and splash out on just one or two indulgent items. You're sure to be given clothes as gifts, too.

3 **Bargain hunter**

Using internet auction sites to buy expensive items, such as buggies, secondhand can save a fortune. Save your money for things you have to buy new, such as a car seat and cot mattress.

4 **Money wise**

Check your entitlements and claim any benefits or tax breaks you can. Look into savings accounts for your baby and put aside a little money each month, if possible.

5 **Help from friends**

Borrowing or inheriting from friends and family with older children can yield rich harvests of high chairs, slings, clothes, and toys. If anyone offers to buy a gift, great – you could ask for larger-size clothes, or something specific such as a monitor.

Top 10

136

THERE'S NO GETTING AWAY FROM IT, children are
expensive. With careful budgeting and a bit of know-how you
can keep the costs under control, especially in the first year.

6

Breast case scenario

Breastfeeding is a brilliant way to save money as it is free
apart from a few breast pads, so if you can make it work for
you and your baby, that's great. When your baby moves onto
solid foods you can cut costs by cooking your own baby food.

7

Nappy happy

Nappies are a significant expenditure – to make savings
consider either buying them in bulk, or using cloth ones.
The cloth route will cost you a little more in effort and washing
powder, but your wallet and local landfill will thank you.

8

Shop smart

Buy own-brand wipes and nappies. Cotton wool is cheaper
than wipes, and kinder to baby's skin, too.

9

Resale value

Unless you plan on having more children, sell anything you
no longer use. Keep boxes and instructions to increase resale
value and help with postage and packing costs. Don't take labels
off clothes until they get worn, so you can sell them easily.

10

Let me entertain you

Swimming and music groups are fun, but can be pricey.
Check out what your local library or children's centre has
to offer, or organize your own informal get-togethers.

Women who remember their birth experience in a positive light are likely to have a subsequent child more quickly.

Birth plan

It's impossible, of course, to plan the exact course of your labour and delivery, but compiling a birth plan can be a helpful process as it makes you think about your options and formulate your preferences.

❋ How does a birth plan help?

This useful tool enables you to communicate with the people looking after you throughout labour, and during possible moments when you're unable to communicate verbally. Focusing on your options and preferences for labour and birth is empowering, too, as you become informed about the process and will know what to expect. Feeling prepared makes it easier to adapt to changes on the day if events don't turn out quite as expected.

❋ What's the best approach?

You may have a vision of your perfect labour, featuring candles, a birthing pool, and some well-timed massage or, conversely, ensuring that the anaesthetist is on duty so an epidural can be administered at the earliest opportunity. The reality, though, may be quite different: events may mean a water birth proves tricky, or you may progress so fast that an epidural is not possible. Setting down your wishes is a starting point for discussion with your midwife, but

DID YOU KNOW?

BIRTH PLANS were first introduced in the 1970s, and have been shown to enhance a woman's confidence during labour.

LABOUR IS UNPREDICTABLE, SO A PLAN SHOULD BE FLEXIBLE.

be aware that a birth plan is not about achieving the perfect birth or ensuring a specific outcome; it's a document stating how you intend to cope and, ideally, how you would like events to be handled.

✳ What should it include?

Think about how you want to manage the different stages of labour. Do you want to be active in the first stage, and are there positions you would like to adopt for giving birth? Would you like to labour, and maybe give birth, in water? What type of medical pain relief would you like to try, and is there anything you would like to avoid, for example, an epidural if you want to feel in control of pushing? Also, think about who you want with you during the birth. At the delivery, would your partner like to cut the cord? And do you want skin-to-skin contact with your baby straight after birth, or to breastfeed immediately? You can always change your mind about any of these things on the day.

IN RURAL TANZANIA, women who are encouraged to make a birth plan are more likely to access health facilities with skilled professionals during pregnancy and in the postnatal period, giving their babies the best start in life.

MONTH 8

Weeks 31–35
DAD'S SURVIVAL
GUIDE

DID YOU
KNOW?

The university of life

Roll up your sleeves and put on your "swottiest" glasses; you need to do some serious preparation for the birth. Not long now, so be sure you're ready.

✳ The homework

Your partner is going to need your help in some very practical ways this month. Fancy yourself as an amateur pedicurist? No? Well, you're going to need to give it your best shot all the same as she might need your help to cut her toenails. She will also be feeling tired and uncomfortable so take over her share of the household jobs.

✳ Distance learning

Practise driving the route to hospital in bad traffic so you can time it accordingly, and know a few alternatives. If the hospital offers a guided tour, make sure you go, so you can check out what facilities are available, and so you know your way around on the big day. Find out if you are allowed to stay over night after the birth.

✳ Life lessons

It will be around now that you head to your antenatal classes, and you should go along ready to listen, make notes, ask questions, and take in as much as possible. Other dads will be there, so there is no

YOUR BABY gains up to half of his birth weight in the last eight weeks of pregnancy.

LOOK OUT FOR "MANTENATAL" CLASSES, DELIVERED EXCLUSIVELY TO DADS-TO-BE.

DRINKING MORE WATER will ease water retention, so remind your partner to drink regularly.

need to feel awkward. If you plan to be the birth partner (and most dads do these days) you should participate with your partner in practising positions and breathing. It won't be embarrassing as everyone will be doing the same, and every piece of knowledge you gain will prepare you to be a well-informed and confident birth partner. You will be your partner's advocate on the day so you need to know what happens, what's available, and what she feels about every option, particularly pain relief.

> **MAKE SURE YOU** get to the antenatal classes whether you plan to be the birth partner or not. Be prepared for anything!

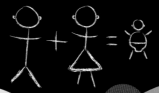

Do

Socialize with the other parents in the classes – you may make lasting friendships.

———

Add important numbers to your phone – doctor, midwife, labour ward, and grandparents.

———

Drive to the hospital at different times of the day as preparation.

Don't

Make silly jokes in the classes – this won't make a good impression on anyone.

———

Forget everything you've learned at the classes. Practise useful positions and exercises when you get home.

———

Bottle up your emotions – you're not alone if you feel tense at this point.

Keep on moving

You've made it to the final month of your pregnancy journey. Hooray! Your baby can be born safely after 37 weeks so rest easy – you're almost there.

✳ Getting comfy

Your baby is said to be "engaged" once she has dropped into a position in your pelvis where two-fifths of her head is above your pelvic bone. Once this happens you may find it easier to breathe as your ribs and diaphragm won't feel so constricted. You'll also notice a change in the shape of your bump, which may look lower. Don't worry, however, if the head has not engaged – sometimes this doesn't happen until labour starts. You may find it less comfortable to move now; having a head wedged in your pelvis affects your posture, gait, and sleeping position. Changes also occur in your pelvis as ligaments loosen further and joints become less stable in preparation for shifting apart during birth. Many women find a pregnancy belt helpful at this stage. An all-fours position can ease lower backache: tuck your pelvis under and arch your upper-back like a cat, rock backwards and forwards, and rotate your hips in both directions.

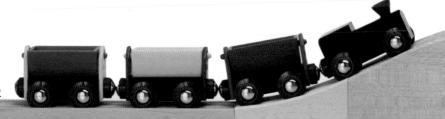

YOUR BABY DROPS deeper into your pelvic cavity this month, known in the US as "lightening".

GOOD TO EAT
Spinach for iron and vitamin C, plus vitamin K to aid blood clotting.

✳ Feeling buxom

You may notice your breasts swelling in size again as they ready themselves to produce colostrum. This thick liquid is a precursor to milk and will provide your baby with sugar, protein, and antibodies after birth in the few days before you start making breast milk. It's normal for breasts to leak a little colostrum at this stage. Now is a good time to get fitted for a new bra to take you into the postnatal days.

✳ Practice makes perfect

In the last few weeks Braxton Hicks contractions (see page 129) can increase in frequency, making labour seem all the more imminent. Obviously, you'll wonder if this is the start of labour, but if you can wonder about contractions they are probably not fierce enough to be the real thing! However, do contact your doctor or midwife if you would like reassurance.

✳ Show time

Don't be alarmed if you notice increased vaginal discharge at this time, maybe tinted pink or brown, rather like at the start of your period. This is a natural sign that your cervix is preparing for birth by softening and receiving an increased supply of blood. However, report any pain or bright red blood to your doctor immediately.

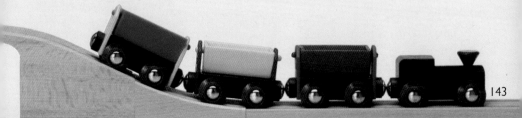

The final stretch

There's plenty to do during this final month, but it's important to set aside regular time each day to rest. Try to give up work with a few weeks to spare – this will help you to rest and mentally adjust.

✳ Take it easy

Last-minute shopping for baby items, cleaning the house, and planning for your new arrival are moments filled with excitement, but this natural "nesting" instinct, combined with the fact that you are at your maximum size now, can cause stress, raising your heart rate, blood pressure, blood-sugar levels, and increasing your breathing. In addition, the stress hormone cortisol will be coursing through your body at the end of the third trimester making it extra important to take it easy during this stage of your pregnancy. It's helpful to know that cortisol helps to mature your baby's brain and lungs, and can influence the time of birth; it also sharpens your senses, making you mega-attentive to your baby after birth. The downside, however, of having these stress hormones in such large volume is that you may suffer mood swings, insomnia, and reduced appetite. Antenatal relaxation (see Relaxation technique, right) and yoga classes can help, as they teach pregnant women how to control their breathing and how to achieve muscle relaxation (both will be useful during labour, too). Birthing hypnotherapy DVDs can also result in incredibly deep relaxation.

TAKE CARE when going up and downstairs – your centre of gravity has now altered significantly and you can no longer see your feet.

3-4cm

ACTIVE LABOUR is measured from when your cervix is 3–4cm (1¼–1½in) dilated.

✳ Relaxation technique

Progressive muscle relaxation is a simple technique that teaches your body the difference between tension and relaxation. It enables you to tap into your body's natural responses to labour, which should help you to feel better equipped to communicate your wishes. Lie on your left side, relaxing your top leg forwards onto cushions. Inhale and tense your right foot, lifting your leg. Hold the tension, then release on an exhalation – let your foot flop down, and notice the relaxation. Tense and release your calf, thighs, and buttocks; repeat on the left leg. Then tense and release your upper body. Finish by tensing your face, then exhale, allowing your jaw, forehead, and tongue to become soft and heavy. With practice you'll be able to imagine the tension and release your whole body on an exhalation. Also try scanning your body from the toes up. Wherever you spot tension, picture that body part softening.

✳ Inner peace

In order for labour to start, your pituitary gland needs to make the hormone oxytocin, which stimulates the contractions that trigger birth. It does this most effectively when you feel relaxed, safe, and at ease. When tense, you produce the stress hormone adrenalin, which inhibits labour. This is why many women find contractions halt temporarily when they reach hospital.

145

Get ready to celebrate!

By the end of your pregnancy, your large belly can be a source of sheer amazement, but you're probably ready to say goodbye to it. Buckle up, these last weeks bring you to the biggest change yet – your baby!

✳ End of an era

Labour represents an enormous emotional and physical challenge, and many women experience scary dreams and vivid nightmares during the last few weeks of their pregnancy journey. However, try not to feel too unnerved – this is a completely normal reaction to the irreversible changes your life is about to undergo – your ability to spontaneously change plans, to jump on a plane, to stay out late, or to work after hours will be curtailed when you have a baby. She will affect your relationship, too; you are a couple for a few weeks longer, then you become a family. Don't be daunted. Producing a child is the start of the best journey ever!

✳ Well-wishers

As you creep ever nearer your due date (or past it!), you are likely to be inundated with calls and texts from well-wishers. They obviously mean well, but it can be irritating to be constantly reminded that your long-awaited baby has still not arrived. If the unwanted attention is getting to you, leave a message on your mobile phone explaining you'll be in touch when you have news, then switch it off.

DID YOU KNOW?

ONLY 5 PER CENT of babies arrive on their estimated date of delivery (EDD).

700

YOUR WOMB increases 700 times in size from conception to birth.

✳ Support for the big day

You might want only your partner to be with you during the birth, but some women find that a third party, perhaps a sister or close friend, can be helpful, especially if labour is drawn out or if your partner can't get to you straightaway. Discuss it with your partner and if you would like an extra birthing partner, consider who would be best suited to the task – someone you totally trust, can confide your fears, and rely upon. Having someone who has had a good birth experience themselves is likely to increase your chances of having one, too. It's a big commitment, so show her your birth plan and perhaps take her along to a class to help her work out her role.

✳ What did you say?

In the final weeks of pregnancy it's common to become extremely forgetful. You'll find yourself standing in front of the fridge wondering why you're there, missing appointments, and zoning out mid-conversation. Some studies point at a reduction in brain-cell volume that affects short-term memory – it's not permanent, thank goodness. Your memory should return to normal once you're over the sleepless nights, but if the fogginess makes you feel scared or sad, tell your partner and chat to your doctor or midwife.

IN BENGAL, women in the last month of pregnancy have their every wish granted and are given new clothes, jewellery, and fine food to prepare them for birth.

147

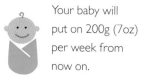

Ready to go

Month nine marks the beginning of the end of your pregnancy – your baby is almost ready to make her way into the world! She's putting on those final ounces and getting herself in position for her big trip.

✳ Head first

Most babies drop head-down into the pelvis after 36 weeks, tightly curled in readiness for birth. Space is limited, but you should still feel hefty kicks and jabs. If all movement stops, contact your midwife immediately. Baby's head has been growing in circumference as the brain folds to form wrinkled troughs and peaks. The three bones of the skull are still not joined, with gaps called fontanelles in between. During labour, these spaces allow the bones to slide over each other to compress the skull and enable it to travel through the birth canal.

✳ Bring on the air

The lungs mature in the final month until your baby is finally ready to breathe air. The number of alveoli air sacs will continue to multiply and increase in diameter in the first six months after birth.

Baby's progress bar: you are now 99% complete

LOADING ...

| 10% | 20% | 30% | 40% | 50% |

DID YOU KNOW?

YOUR BABY'S head is growing 2–3cm (¾–1¼in) per week at this stage.

HOW BIG?
She is about the size of a small watermelon.

Your baby exercises her breathing muscles by expanding and contracting the chest, and hiccupping to strengthen the diaphragm.

✳ Suck and swallow

Your baby is now equipped to process milk, and her ability to suck is well developed. Right now she's swallowing a massive 750ml (26fl oz) of amniotic fluid each day. As lanugo hair falls off into the amniotic fluid, she swallows that, too, along with skin cells. These lodge in the large intestine, compacting to form meconium (see page 186).

✳ Dinner on a plate

At its full size – both diameter and capacity – your placenta now weighs about one-sixth of your baby's weight, and is working hard to serve up oxygen and nutrients to the baby, and to carry waste back for you to deal with.

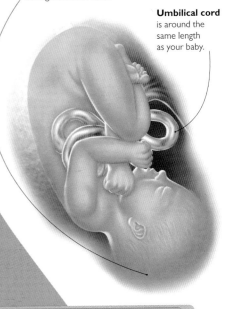

Skull bones are still separated for easy passage through the birth canal.

Umbilical cord is around the same length as your baby.

Essential lists

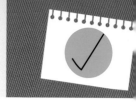

BABY'S WARDROBE

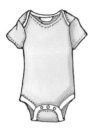

VESTS
Short-sleeved cotton,
worn as a base layer.

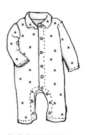

BODYSUIT
Long-sleeved
for going outside.

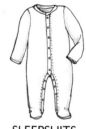

SLEEPSUITS
In-built feet keep baby cosy
at night or in the day.

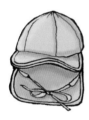

SUN HAT
With a wide brim and a flap that
covers the back of the neck.

WARM HAT
Close-fitting in natural fibres
for winter months.

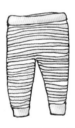

TROUSERS
Easy to put on leggings or
trousers for daywear.

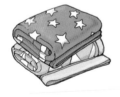

BLANKET
For an extra layer, or a
discreet feeding cover.

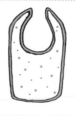

DRIBBLE BIBS
To protect baby's clothes
during bottle-feeding.

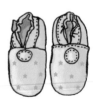

SOFT SHOES
For cold weather; choose
soft leather only.

"COMFORTABLE" AND "EASY TO PUT ON" are your mantras when choosing clothes for your baby. Opt for cotton and natural fibres. Choose vests and bodysuits with poppers, and wide, envelope necks to fit easily over the head.

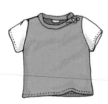

T-SHIRTS
To wear in the day over a vest with trousers.

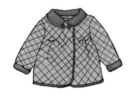

CARDIGANS
Easier than sweaters to put on and fasten.

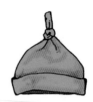

COTTON HAT
Close-fitting for wearing outside in summer.

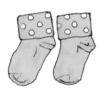

SOCKS
To keep feet warm when out and about.

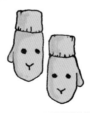

JACKET
Quilted for warmth; cotton makes it washable and practical.

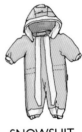

SNOWSUIT
For cold weather; always check for overheating.

SCRATCH MITTENS
To protect baby's face from sharp fingernails.

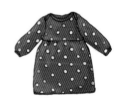

WARM MITTENS
To keep hands cosy for the winter months.

SPECIAL OUTFIT
For looking great when out and about!

Going overdue

You've reached your due date. After nine months, you're ready for labour to start, but the date comes and goes with no sign of movement. So what now?

✳ How long can you go?

If all is well with both you and your baby, your care team will usually be happy to wait up to two weeks before suggesting medical intervention to kick-start labour.

✳ What happens next?

After 40 weeks and 10 days there's an increased risk of the placenta losing efficiency, which could affect your baby. At around 41 weeks, your midwife may offer you a membrane "sweep" – an internal examination designed to stimulate the cervix and trigger the release of hormones to kick-start labour. This increases your chance of going into natural labour in the next 48 hours by

30 35 40

DID YOU KNOW?

IN DEVELOPED COUNTRIES, as many as 25% of births are induced.

25%

Contractions brought on by the synthetic hormone syntocinon are usually stronger, longer, and more painful than natural contractions.

around 30 per cent, avoiding a medical induction. If this doesn't work, an induction will be arranged, during which drugs will trigger contractions.

The late arrival

Babies who are born late look slightly different – they tend to have long fingernails and plenty of hair, they are more alert than on-time babies, and are generally quite large.

✳ Bring it on!

If you're fed up waiting and keen to avoid an induction, you may want to try some of the following:

1. Have sex – it's thought that prostaglandins in sperm affect the cervix, encouraging it to soften and dilate. And oxytocin, the hormone that triggers labour, is released during orgasm and may stimulate contractions. It's unproven, but worth a try…

2. Nipple tweaking – if the thought of sex wears you out, stimulating your nipples is a more straightforward way to release oxytocin to trigger contractions.

3. Stay active – movement works with gravity to encourage your baby down the pelvis and put pressure on the cervix.

4. Eat a spicy curry – the idea is that the spices stimulate bowel muscles, in turn stimulating uterine muscles.

MONTH 9

Weeks 36–40

FIRST SIGNS OF LABOUR

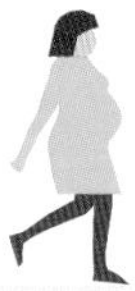

Any time now!

It's time for your baby to make an appearance, but how will you know when he's on his way? As your body gets ready to give birth, several changes happen.

✻ It's all good

Gradually, over many hours, pressure will build in your pelvis and rectum as the baby drops further down in the pelvis, and you may develop a dull, niggling backache. Although uncomfortable, these are encouraging signs that your baby is on the move.

✻ A positive sign

A bloody mucus discharge, or "show", means the mucus plug that protected the womb from infection in pregnancy has dislodged from the cervix. This can mean labour is fairly imminent, although it may be days, or more, before labour starts. Either way, it's a clear sign that your cervix is changing, getting ready for labour.

✻ The floodgates

The media portrayal of a pregnant woman's waters breaking seconds before labour starts is very misleading – in only 15 per cent of pregnancies do the waters break before contractions have started. If it does happen before contractions start, labour is imminent and you should inform your midwife, who will want to assess you now that your baby has lost his protective seal.

THE START OF LABOUR can be surprisingly hard to pinpoint and is different for each woman. No single event signals its start; instead, a build up of changes in your body work together to set it in motion.

✳ This is it...

The surest sign that labour has started is when you're having three to four strong contractions in 10 minute increments that steadily increase in intensity and duration, while the gap between each one gets shorter. This is nature's way of gently managing your body's pain tolerance level. Changing position doesn't reduce the intensity, and it's pretty hard to hold a conversation during one. These true contractions start to shorten, soften, and dilate the cervix.

✳ All systems are go

Tempting though it may be, resist the desire to rush to hospital at the first twinge. Being in a comfortable, familiar environment for as long as possible will help your labour progress naturally. Rest, move around, and eat when you feel peckish.

GO TO HOSPITAL...

- When your contractions are regular, strong, and about five minutes apart
- When your contractions last for about 45–60 seconds each time
- When your waters have broken
- If you start bleeding
- If you are concerned about your baby's movement

Phone in advance before setting off so the birthing unit can prepare for your arrival. Don't forget your hospital bag as you dash out of the door.

IN INDIA doors in the home are left wide open during birth to mirror the "opening" of the uterus.

IN MEXICO doors are shut to keep out unwanted spirits.

MONTH 9

Weeks 36–40
DAD'S SURVIVAL
GUIDE

DID YOU
KNOW?

The time has come...

At last, the final month – this is the one that ends with you meeting your baby, and the start of family life. Time to brush up on your birth knowledge.

✳ On your marks...

Maybe you think pregnancy has flown by, or you may think it has taken ages. Most likely you feel both, but one thing is for sure: your baby is coming any time now whether you're ready or not! If you are the birth partner, make sure you know as much as you can about the process and the options. Does your partner want pain relief, and what does she think about, say, a water birth or ventouse delivery? Discuss the birth plan and have a copy to hand, but remember to keep an open mind and encourage her to do the same.

✳ Get set...

Earn yourself brownie points by cleaning the house and cooking a week's worth of meals to freeze. Put the car seat in now and check it is fitted safely – you need this to bring your baby home. Your partner should have her own hospital bag prepared but be sure you also pack key items for you: camera, jumper, snack, drink, something to read/music for waiting around, and of course your phone (fully charged) so you can give everyone the happy news. As the day approaches, check in with home on a regular basis so your partner doesn't get anxious that she can't get hold of you.

YOUR BABY will be considered full term if born any time this month.

STUDIES SHOW that women who are well supported by their birth partner have a smoother path through labour and are less likely to need intervention.

WHY NOT get a haircut now before it all gets a bit too busy.

✳ **Go!**

When your partner tells you she's feeling those first contractions, don't get in such a panic that you rush out of the door before you need to! For first births, it's a fairly gradual process so you probably don't need to hurry; early contractions can take days! If the contractions are spaced well apart and infrequent, you could run a bath for your partner, or make something to eat for you both. Help your partner to stay active if she can – why not go for a short walk and make the most of the excitement of early labour. When contractions become frequent, or if you have any concerns, call the midwife. If you are having a home birth, the midwife will need some notice to get there. If you are going to hospital, wait until they give you the go-ahead, and then drive there calmly.

DISCUSS WHETHER you want to cut the umbilical cord or want a professional to do it. It's not the kind of thing you should decide on the spur of the moment.

Do

Brush up together on any positions, massage techniques, or breathing exercises you learned in antenatal classes.

Keep the car topped up with enough petrol to get you to hospital, or get taxi numbers.

Load up with plenty of coins for parking or vending machines.

Don't

Spend all month waiting – make sure you both get plenty of rest, eat well, and do some enjoyable activities together.

Plan to go out drinking with friends on the eve of the due date.

Forget to buy your partner a birthing gift, and something for the baby, too.

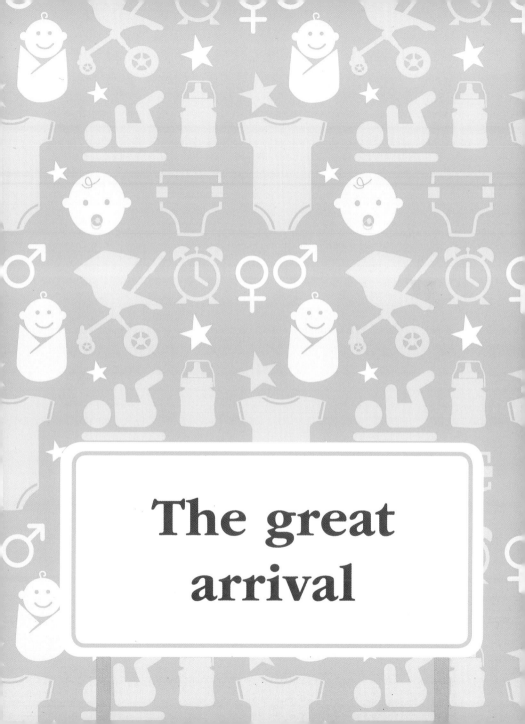

The great arrival

Amazing journey

Labour is one of life's greatest challenges, as well as one of its miracles. Your baby is almost with you – this is the final push!

✳ First few steps

At the beginning of labour, known as the "latent" stage, contractions are not frequent or long – maybe every 20 minutes and lasting 30–60 seconds; they are mild enough to doze or read through. As you progress into "active" labour, contractions become more frequent (every 10 minutes, then five, then two) and intense, spreading from the top of the uterus down. Each contraction lengthens to 60–90 seconds while the gaps between shorten. This gets your body used to the processes of labour and increases your levels of endorphines – nature's painkiller! Leaning forwards, moving around, or circling your hips can allow gravity to move the baby downwards and may help. As the contractions press your baby's head into the neck of your uterus, the cervix pulls up and thins out, opening around 1cm (½in) per hour. Finally, the cervix will draw back and your baby will pass through.

✳ On the road

The end of the first stage is called "transition"; contractions are at their most intense and frequent, with barely a gap between them. This is a sign that labour is progressing well and you are about to enter second stage – when your baby is born. The first stage transition

REMEMBER: there is no pain between contractions, so try to focus on these breathers.

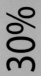

30%

DURING BIRTH you will gain 30 per cent extra space in your pubic joint by squatting, kneeling, or being on all fours.

can last for seconds or hours, as you wait for the urge to push. If you need to make noise, feel free – medical staff, and your partner, won't be fazed. If you need to have quiet around you, tell everyone to be quiet – this is your moment.

Hormones act on the cervix, so it is ready to stretch to 10cm (4in).

✳ **The final few miles**

At this stage, your baby is out of the uterus and in the birth canal. There may be a short gap, then contractions restart, and many women have an urge to bear down, breathing deeply and working with the force of the contractions to push the baby out. For first-time mums this stage can last for up to three hours. If you don't feel the urge, your midwife will show you how to breathe to make the most of your contractions. Squatting during contractions aids delivery by widening the pelvis. Rest on a chair or lean forward onto the back of the bed between contractions. Finally, the head "crowns", stretching the vagina. The sensation of tingling, or burning, is intense and your midwife may encourage you to stop pushing to lessen the risk of a slight tear to the skin. First one shoulder emerges, then another, until your baby comes out and is handed to you. Well done!

✳ **Almost there**

The final stage is like a mini birth, only this time you deliver a soft mass of placenta, one third the size of your baby; the umbilical cord is also cut. Breastfeeding can encourage this process to happen more quickly, or you can have an injection of syntometrine (a drug that mimics the hormone oxytocin).

Your baby's head is said to "crown" when the widest part of his head is visible.

The final frontier

Your baby starts labour deep in the uterus with his head engaged in your pelvic brim. The minor contractions that have been gently massaging him will now push him out into the world.

✳ Ebb and flow

Each muscular squeeze of the uterine muscles contracts the uterus in size, forcing your baby down towards the neck of the womb – the top of your baby's head has to push open the exit. This motion might break the sac of amniotic fluid, if it hasn't done before now, causing a rush of liquid – this is your waters breaking. Your baby's head presses further into your cervix, which dilates until he can pass through, moving out of the uterus into the birth canal.

✳ Do the twist

As your baby descends into the pelvic cavity, he hits the pelvic floor and a slope that forces him to twist, rotating by 90 degrees. This takes advantage of the extra room between your pubic bone and the coccyx, a small triangular bone at the base of the spine, which moves out of the way. Your baby then has to rotate again to pass underneath, bending his head back so the tip of his chin leads the movement. Once this has been negotiated the head returns to the front and his face sweeps past your pelvic floor until the crown of his head is exposed and he emerges head first followed by shoulders.

YOUR BABY'S SKULL is, on average, 1cm (½in) larger in circumference than your fully open cervix. Thankfully, the bones of the skull overlap at the edges to allow the head to fit through.

CONTRACTIONS are measured from beginning to end.

✳ A safe arrival

Your baby may experience this squeezing as intensely as you – babies sometimes kick in reaction to contractions. The skull is pressured (the sliding edges of the bones protect the brain) and the placenta and umbilical cord are compressed by each contraction, reducing the amount of blood and oxygen delivered to your baby. As a result, his stress hormones are probably higher than yours. Don't worry, this serves a purpose – in a mirror image to you, your baby's stress hormones slow his heart rate and direct blood and oxygen away from his muscles towards his brain. This is a protective reaction. The hormones, called catecholamines, also trigger the lungs to step up production of surfactant, preparing the alveoli to breathe air. Your baby is monitored during birth for signs of distress, including low or high heart rates or an irregular beat. The frequency and strength of your contractions might also be recorded to see how your baby's heart responds to them.

✳ Nudging along

If your baby isn't progressing on his journey along the birth canal as expected, your midwife might break your membranes, which can speed things up, or give you a synthetic version of oxytocin by drip to make your contractions more regular. The final stage of delivery may be assisted (see pages 224–225), and your baby will be monitored continuously as he nears his destination.

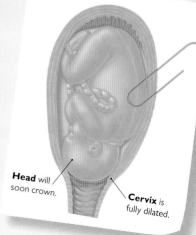

Head will soon crown.

Cervix is fully dilated.

What should I expect?

LABOUR IS UNPREDICTABLE

WHAT TO EXPECT

1 **It's not time yet!**

Not quite 37 weeks but contracting every 5–10 minutes for at least an hour? Had a show, bleeding, or abdominal pain? Call the midwife – it's important to be assessed quickly. If your waters break, phone the hospital.

2 **Waters have broken**

If labour doesn't begin within 24 hours of your waters breaking and you are more than 35 weeks pregnant, put on a pad and check the volume and colour of the discharge. You may have to be induced because of the risk of infection.

3 **Labour just won't start**

If you are very overdue, you may be offered a "sweep" (the midwife sweeps her fingers around the membranes through your cervix), amniotomy (artificial breaking of the membranes), or an induction via a stimulating pessary or induction drip.

4 **Bottom or feet first**

If your baby's head doesn't press into the neck of your uterus, contractions may be ineffective at stretching the cervix wide enough. For babies in breech position your doctor may try to turn the baby, or recommend a Caesarean section.

5 **Wrong way round**

If your baby's back is against your spine (posterior position), contractions may be less efficient. Moving and leaning forwards may help. Baby can turn once in the birth canal, or your doctor may use forceps or ventouse vacuum extraction.

LABOUR CAN START late or early, and can stop once started. It's probably best to expect the unexpected and be flexible with your birth plan at this stage...

WHAT TO EXPECT

6 **Labour is slow**

Doctors and midwives often prefer you to dilate within a set time frame and may speed things up in the first stage by breaking your membranes or giving a synthetic hormone, syntocinon. In second stage labour, you may be offered an assisted delivery.

7 **Flexible birth plan**

Planned a water birth or no medication, but it's tougher than you thought? Birth plans are great because they make you research the options and articulate what you want, but not if they make you feel stressed or guilty. Be open to all options.

8 **I need a poo!**

It's normal for you to wee or poo at the end of the second stage – and while this may sound like the ultimate humiliation, you will neither care nor notice! In any case, the midwives will have seen it all before.

9 **I need to push!**

At the end of the first stage, you may be 1–2cm (½–¾in) away from full dilation but already feel the pushing urge. Pushing too early can make the cervix swell, so your midwife may suggest panting and getting onto your hands and knees.

10 **Checks on baby**

Some babies may need a vigorous rub to get their breathing started. Midwives will keep you informed if your baby needs any extra help in resuscitation.

MOST LABOUR PAIN is caused by cramping as the uterine muscle contracts.

A positive delivery

Think about giving birth and you're likely to imagine pushing out your baby's head: ouch! Each woman copes differently – you may find natural methods see you through, or you may need something stronger.

✱ What's a good approach?

Experiencing pain is stressful, causes tension, and impedes oxygen flow to the muscles, which then makes the pain harder to bear. It's therefore universally agreed that letting go of the fear of pain is the most positive approach to labour. The more prepared you are, knowing what to expect and how you might deal with discomfort, the more likely you are to relax and have confidence in your ability to cope.

✱ As mother nature intended

Lots of women opt for natural pain relief, either just in the early stages of labour or all the way through. There are many natural therapies (see page 226) that are effective at easing pain, have no nasty side effects, and enable you to experience every moment of your labour.

✱ Medical assistance

When natural pain relief isn't cutting in, there are various medical pain relief options that can be administered to help you cope. These range from drugs that take the edge off (gas and air), to those that block out all pain (an epidural).

During the first stage of labour, contractions grow in intensity. Breathing techniques and other natural methods may carry you through most of this stage, or you may like to try gas and air, a TENS machine, or hypnobirthing.

If you're really struggling, you can request opioid drugs, such as pethidine, or an epidural can be put in place.

Remember to empty your bladder regularly. A full bladder can slow labour down.

Once your cervix is fully dilated and you enter the second stage of labour, you can continue to use gas and air, but pethidine won't be given this close to the delivery as it can affect your baby's breathing. If an epidural is in place, this can be topped up.

One of the most pivotal supports during labour is that of a reliable birth partner who can help you physically and emotionally. Whether it's your partner, a close friend, or a combination, being supported helps you deal with stress.

It is increasingly common for women to pay for a doula, a woman with training in childbirth who stays with you, supporting and guiding you throughout.

Change your position every 30 minutes, swaying in rhythm with your breathing.

Use a birthing ball, which you can lean on for support, or bounce on to encourage contractions.

If planning a water birth at home, establish whether the floor of the room will sustain the weight of the filled pool. Make sure you have a tap and hose nearby to fill it, and an easy way to empty it.

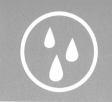

Water birth

Soothing, relaxing, relieving: all words we associate with warm water, so it's little surprise that many women choose to labour, and sometimes give birth in a pool.

✳ How water helps

Immersing yourself in warm water during labour can be incredibly therapeutic. The warmth soothes muscles, releasing held-in tension, and increasing your ability to relax, which in turn helps you cope with the pain of contractions. The natural buoyancy of the water supports your weight, lifting pressure off your back and making it easier to move around and change position. It can be easier, too, to position yourself upright, such as when squatting, which enables you to work with gravity to help your baby move down the birth canal. In combination, the elements of warmth and buoyancy make for a more efficient, less tiring labour. Statistically, women who labour and give birth in water have fewer episiotomies and a shorter second stage of labour – all pretty compelling stuff!

✳ Making it happen

You can harness the soothing effects of water simply by spending part of early labour in a warm bath at home. However, if you wish to use water as your main form of pain relief, and intend to give birth in a pool, check what arrangements are needed before your due date. If you're booked in for a hospital birth, enquire about the birthing pool

MILLIONS OF YEARS AGO the ocean's seawater shared the same salinity, 0.9%, as amniotic fluid.

5cm In hospital you will need to wait until your cervix is 5cm (2in) dilated before getting into the pool.

facilities and whether midwives are trained in water births; if facilities are limited, see if there are birthing centres close by with pools. If you're planning a home water birth, you will need to hire a pool in advance: your midwife can give you details of companies who hire out pools. You'll need a suitable space to set up the pool, where you can fill it easily and where the midwife will have space to move around the edge. Check, too, if your midwife is experienced in water deliveries.

✳ Water slide

At hospital, you may not be allowed to get into the pool until you're in established labour (see pages 160–161) or until your cervix is 5cm (2in) dilated. The water is kept at, or just below, 37.5°C (99.5°F), which ensures you don't overheat and potentially cause distress to the baby. The midwife will monitor your baby with a waterproof, hand-held sonicaid, and may check how far you are dilated. If you give birth in the pool, your midwife will wait until the baby is completely delivered before lifting him to the surface for your first cuddle.

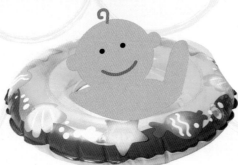

THE GROWING POPULARITY of water births today has roots in 1960s France, where the obstetrician Michel Odent promoted labouring in warm water as a "gentle" birthing experience.

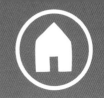

Home births

A home birth can offer the opportunity to give birth in familiar, comfortable surroundings and to have a greater degree of control over your birthing experience.

✳ The heart of the family

If your pregnancy is straightforward, and you have no medical complications, giving birth at home is a safe option. You may have known early on that you would like a home birth, or perhaps it is a decision you came to only recently – either way, you can change your mind at any point. Being in your own home, supported by your partner and midwife, offers a safe environment for a challenging event, and this can reduce tension, making it easier to cope with pain. You're more likely to be active, making labour more efficient: studies suggest that home births are quicker than those in hospital. Staying in one location can also prevent a "stop-start" labour, which can happen when women move to hospital, possibly because this interrupts the flow of hormones. At home, you'll enjoy care from one midwife, and ideally be joined by a second midwife for the birth. Statistically you are less likely to have medical interventions or a postnatal infection.

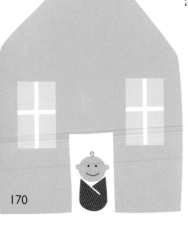

✳ Getting clued up

Before your due date, your midwife will visit you at home to drop off a home-birth pack with everything she'll need for the birth, including gas and air, pain relief, a blood-pressure monitor, and a sonicaid or stethoscope to monitor your baby. She will also discuss any last-minute arrangements. When you go into labour, your midwife will stay with you, monitoring your progress and your baby's heartbeat. As well as the medical pain relief she provides, you can use any natural pain-relief methods including a water birth (see pages 168–169).

✳ Shared care

If your midwife has any concerns, for example, if your baby becomes distressed and she feels ill-equipped to deal with the problem, you will be transferred to hospital.

Getting ready

Designate a "home birth" area in your home and assemble these items for the day:

- Plastic sheeting and old towels
- Bright lamp or desk light for the midwife
- Clean, warm towels and a blanket for your baby
- Any props you want, such as candles or a birthing ball

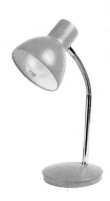

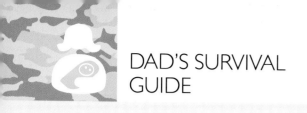

Exit via the gift shop

During your partner's labour, it may be hard to imagine that you'll look back on this as the best day of your life! But if it gets tough, remember it will all be worth it in the end.

✳ Stage One: Bring it on

As soon as your partner's contractions start, you should time both how long they last and the gaps between them. This stage can last a while so you may as well put on some music or a film and try to relax. Make some food, even at 3am, and stay hydrated. She may want you to run her a bath, which will help with the pain. During strong contractions, your best tactic is to stay calm and be quietly encouraging. She may want you to rub her back or try out some of the positions you learned in antenatal classes; or she may not want you to touch her at all! If seeing her in this much pain is upsetting you, just remember that every contraction brings you both closer to meeting your baby.

✳ Stage Two: Baby coming through

After some time she will feel the urge to push or be encouraged to do so by the midwife. Once the cervix is fully dilated it might take as long as an hour for pushing to commence. Position yourself close to your partner's head and hold her hand, telling her you know she can do it (she will be feeling pretty exhausted at this point). Remember to stay out of the way of the professionals. Don't be horrified by the

EVERYONE WILL WANT news of the birth as soon as possible, and this job will probably fall to you. Charge your phone, and only send photos of your partner to all and sundry if she wants you to!

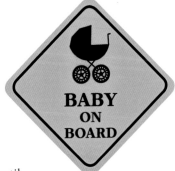

BABY ON BOARD

sight of your squashed, slimy baby the first time you see him – this is all perfectly normal and he'll soon be looking cute. Your partner will probably want him on her chest first, but you can stay close and share his first moments.

✳ Stage Three: You're a dad

Your partner will continue having contractions until she delivers the placenta. If she has a tear or cut, she will need stitches. Your role is no longer as simple as it was earlier – you now have two people to care for. She may want you to continue holding her hand, or she may want you to follow baby's progress as he is assessed and weighed. Once everything is done the three of you will be left alone together to recover – as a family. Enjoy this precious moment before you start sharing it with the world.

Do

Take plenty of photos (nothing too graphic please).

Accept the necessary changes to the birth plan – as long as the baby is safe that is all that matters.

Give your baby a first cuddle! You can strip off and be skin-to-skin, or hold him in a towel.

Don't

Take it personally if your partner shouts at you – she is in pain and doesn't mean it!

Get so distracted by keeping others up to date that you miss the birth.

Over-react if your baby is born with a birthmark. It will probably soon fade.

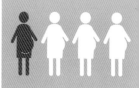

In the UK, 25% of women deliver by C-section, whether out of necessity or choice. The most important thing is that mum and baby arrive safely at their journey's destination.

Destination baby

The rates of Caesarean (C-section) births are rising in many countries. You may want a natural birth, but remember C-sections are usually carried out when they are the safest delivery option for you and your baby.

✳ Planning ahead

A C-section is referred to as "elective" if it is planned ahead of your EDD. Usually this is because your doctor or midwife think it is unsafe for you or your baby to go ahead with a natural birth, for example if the baby is in a breech position, your placenta is covering the opening of your cervix, or you are expecting more than one baby. In the UK, C-sections will not be performed on maternal request in the absence of non-medical causes. If you are extremely anxious about giving birth, you may be counselled by a specialist midwife who will highlight the risks and benefits of both modes of delivery.

✳ A change of plan

An emergency C-section is carried out when things do not go to plan during a normal labour and there are risks posed to either you or your baby by continuing with a natural birth. This may feel like a shock, especially if you had expected to give birth naturally, but rest assured, once you have your baby safely in your arms, you will not care by what method she got there.

Reasons for a C-section

• Baby is upside-down

If your baby has forgotten to turn head-down in the weeks before birth ("breech" position) your midwife or consultant may try to manoeuvre her by applying pressure to your abdomen. If your baby remains breech, you might be offered a C-section, although some babies turn during labour contractions.

• You have twins or more

Multiple babies can make natural birth more difficult if, for example, your babies share a placenta, or one is much bigger than the other.

• Big baby, small pelvis

Very rarely, a baby's head may be too large to fit through the birth canal, so helping her out with a C-section may be the safest option.

• Placenta is playing up

A planned C-section may be safest if your placenta is lying too low, or covering your cervix ("placenta praevia"), which would make birth difficult. In around one in 150 deliveries, the placenta will begin to peel away prematurely from the uterus ("placental abruption"); you may be monitored, or opt for a C-section.

• Get me out of here!

If your baby is in trouble, for example, if her heartbeat becomes irregular during labour, it may be a sign that she is not coping well with labour and a C-section may be necessary to get her delivered as quickly as possible.

• You need looking after

You may be advised to have a C-section if you have an existing medical condition, such as a heart problem or high blood pressure.

• Labour is taking ages

Despite you trying your hardest, your baby is still not coming out, and you are both really tired and fed up, known as "in distress". A C-section may be advised if you are not fully dilated and have become too exhausted to carry on labouring.

• Personal choice

We live in the 21st century and many women argue they should be able to choose how they give birth – be it in a birthing pool, at home, or by having a C-section. Some US doctors suggest C-sections for fear of malpractice suits with a natural birth. In the UK, most hospital trusts won't fund a C-section for non-medical reasons.

If you have a C-section, you may still have a natural birth next time. Every delivery is different, and you have a 60% chance of having a natural birth with your second child.

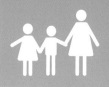

Having a C-section

Whether planned or not, going into hospital for a Caesarean section can be a little daunting – it is an operation, which carries an element of risk. Just remember that C-sections are performed every day.

❋ The nitty gritty

A C-section is an operation where a surgeon cuts through the abdomen and uterus to deliver the baby. The cut, which falls lower than the bikini line, is made horizontally (a "transverse" incision). Vertical incisions are now rarely used as they take longer to heal.

❋ You won't feel a thing

You will be offered a regional or "local" anaesthetic, such as an epidural, to numb the lower half of your body. If there is time before an emergency operation, this will also be the first option. A local anaesthetic works fast, and leaves you awake to experience your baby's delivery. It also helps you to recover more quickly. Occasionally, doctors may use a general anaesthetic, which will make you unconscious, if they think it is the quickest and safest option.

❋ Getting prepped

Surgery sounds scary, but remember your partner should be with you throughout and at the end of it all you get to meet your baby. You will need to wear a hospital gown, and remove any jewellery or nail varnish. Your pubic area will be shaved (you may be asked to do this in advance for an elective C-section), and a catheter inserted into your bladder so you don't need to worry about going to the loo. You will also have an intravenous drip attached to your hand or arm to provide medication and fluid during and after the operation.

✳ Gently does it

You will sit on an operating table, and the table may be tilted sideways a little to take pressure off your womb and abdomen. This is to reduce the risk of your blood pressure dropping. A screen will be placed across the lower half of your body so you can't see the operation, but you will be able to see when your baby is lifted out. A midwife will stay near your head, and tell you what is going on, and check that you are ok. You may feel a slight tugging (like someone rummaging around in your tummy) as the surgeon lifts your baby out of the small incision, but it won't be painful.

✳ That was quick!

Your baby may be delivered as quickly as five to 10 minutes into the operation! While you hold and get to know your baby the surgeon will take another 30–40 minutes to remove the placenta, sew up the incision, and apply a dressing. Any scar from the operation will eventually fade to a thin, white line that is almost invisible.

✳ Baby bonding

A midwife will ensure your baby is dried and kept warm since babies get cold quickly and theatres tend to be cold. Skin-to-skin contact with baby is encouraged as soon as possible after any birth and this is possible after C-section, too. You should be able to breastfeed your baby in the recovery room soon after the operation.

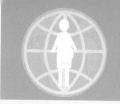

Caesareans have saved the lives of countless mothers and babies worldwide. A rise in C-sections is due to an increase in the number of older mums, more multiple births, and obesity.

The road to recovery

You may be feeling delighted with your new baby and eager to get back to your pre-pregnancy life, but you've just had an operation, so allow yourself plenty of time to recover at your own pace.

✱ A short stay in hospital

You will stay in hospital for a few days to check you have recovered fully. Your dressing will be changed after about 24 hours, and you will be given painkillers to make you comfortable as your body heals – place a pillow over your belly if you need to laugh or cough as this will ease any pain. As you'll need to rest in bed for much of the first few days, you may need to wear support stockings (just like flight stockings) to reduce the risk of deep vein thrombosis (DVT). You are, however, encouraged to be mobile as soon as you can, and gentle activities, such as taking a shower or walking to the loo, will help to reduce the risk of blood clots.

✱ Rest and recuperation

When you get home, don't rush around trying to do everything you did before. Allow yourself time to rest, yet also try to go out and enjoy some gentle walks. Your midwife will give you advice on how to take care of your wound, keeping it clean and dry to prevent infection. You may have dissolvable stitches, or your midwife may visit you to remove them, which takes just a few painless seconds.

YOUR PELVIC FLOOR won't have had as tough a time as during a natural birth. However, you still need to do your pelvic floor exercises!

Getting on with things

Your midwife and health visitor will check your scar when they visit you at home. Once you are signed off from the midwife team, you will have a postnatal check with your doctor at six weeks. She will look at how your scar has healed – most women feel much better by this time. After the all-clear, many women feel well enough to get back to normal activities. Your body will get stronger month by month, but everyone is different, so take your time to recover.

 # Do

- Rest as much as you can, especially in the first two weeks.
- Spend time cuddling your baby. Being less mobile than usual has its advantages – you can lie on the bed or sofa with your baby and enjoy the special first days together.
- Wear large, cotton knickers and comfortable clothes to let your scar "breathe" and heal.
- Ask other people to help you with moving the buggy, making dinner, carrying washing, or putting out the rubbish.
- Accept a lift, or take a taxi or public transport when getting out and about.
- Take gentle exercise, such as yoga or swimming, when approved by your doctor.

Don't

- Lift anything heavier than your baby for at least six weeks, since your muscles and wound are still getting back to normal.
- Forget to keep mobile – although you need to protect your scar you also need to slowly strengthen your muscles. Keeping mobile is also important to avoid blood clots or medical complications.
- Feel guilty that you aren't able to do everything you hoped with your new baby; time spent cuddling is ideal for bonding.
- Drive in the early weeks. There used to be a six-week ban, but now you can decide if you feel you can brake the car quickly without hurting yourself. Check with your insurance company and your health visitor as to when she thinks you are safe to drive.

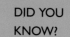

The road less travelled

In the UK, one in four births is via Caesarean section, whether planned or emergency. Surgeons perform C-sections every day; they know what they're doing.

✳ Use an alternative route

You both may be feeling worried in the run-up to the operation, but remember you would probably be feeling pretty nervous even if your partner was having a natural birth. If your partner is having problems giving birth and the doctors have decided this is the best course of action, they will ask for her consent to proceed and she should definitely be supported in her decision. While it may not be on the birth plan for either of you, the chips are down, and the priority is getting your partner and baby safely through the day.

✳ Action stations

Wherever possible an epidural or regional anaesthetic will be used, so your partner will be awake but pain-free for the operation. There will be a surprising number of people present but they are all there to help the process go smoothly – this also applies to all the beeping machinery and equipment. A screen will be erected between your partner's head and bump, and you will stay near her head, holding her hand. A cut will be made just above her pubic bone and your baby will be handed to the midwife to dry and wrap. This will happen a few feet away and should take only a short time. Your partner will

C-SECTION incisions heal quickly, but your partner will have stitches for at least a week.

40% OF C-SECTIONS are planned before labour starts for medical reasons. The remaining 60% are decided during labour, for example, if the baby is getting distressed.

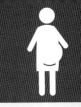

be able to hold baby if she feels able, and you can help her to do this. It can take up to 40 minutes to complete the operation now, but this is the perfect time for you both to meet your baby. Your partner can try skin-to-skin contact which is great for encouraging breastfeeding.

✳ Recovery and moving on

After the operation, the three of you will be moved to a recovery room. Your partner's body temperature may have dropped during the operation, but it is nothing to worry about – the nurses will provide blankets (sometimes a hot drink) and any shivering won't last more than half an hour. Depending on the circumstances your partner may be disappointed by the way things went – you will need to reassure her that it is not the journey but the destination that counts. Because of her scar and stitches she may be less mobile and could find it difficult to get comfortable enough to feed, and your help will be invaluable.

 Do

Reassure your partner that having to depart from her birth plan doesn't matter; focus on meeting the baby.

Remember to take photos of your partner and baby. Not necessarily in the theatre, but in the recovery room and ward.

Request feedback if you feel you need it.

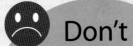 Don't

Be afraid to ask for music in the theatre if it is calming, or have it switched off if it's not to your taste.

Watch the operation if you know you might faint – concentrate on your partner!

Forget that your partner has had a major operation and will need time to recover.

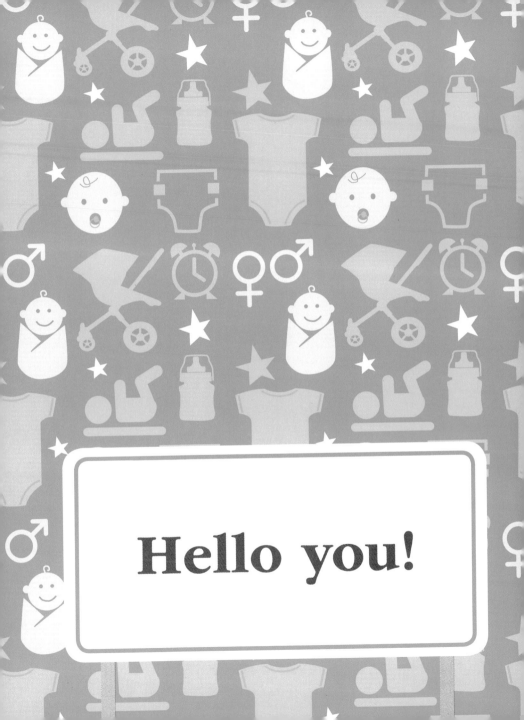

Hello you!

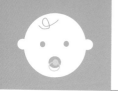

After the birth

Finally, the moment you've thought about so often has arrived – you're meeting your amazing baby! After an initial cuddle, she'll need a quick medical check – don't worry, she'll be back before you know it.

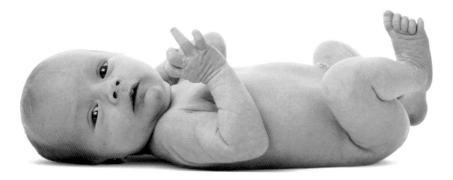

❋ Safe and sound

Within minutes of the birth, the midwife or doctor will assess your baby to make sure she doesn't need any immediate medical attention. Her pulse and breathing are checked, reflexes and skin colour noted, and her movement assessed. She will also be weighed, something newborns really don't like! These tests take just a few moments and you may not even notice them happening as you recover and take everything in. You're a mum!

DID YOU KNOW?

SKIN-TO-SKIN CONTACT after birth has impressive benefits, including regulating your baby's temperature, and even reducing sensations of pain for you.

70

YOUR BABY IS BORN WITH AROUND 70 REFLEXES.

✳ Baby MOT

Within 72 hours of the birth, your baby will have a complete top-to-toe check (see below) to ensure all her parts are in good working order. It's most likely that she will be the picture of health, but if anything is spotted, picking it up at an early stage will ensure that help can be given quickly, and any problem rectified.

 Head The circumference will be measured and the soft spots, called fontanelles, will be checked.

 Ears It may sound odd, but the ears will be looked at to check they're in the right position. Your baby may also be given a hearing test now, or this will be done in the first weeks.

 Eyes A light is shone in your baby's eyes to check the "red" reflex, which rules out cataracts.

Top of the mouth The palate is checked to make sure that it is complete and the tongue moves easily.

 Heart A stethoscope is used to check the heart rate: a newborn baby's heart should beat more than 100 times per minute.

 Hands and feet Digits are counted, reflexes checked, and the position of the feet looked at to check there's no twisting, a condition known as club foot.

 Lungs These will be listened to with a stethoscope. Breathing is checked for slow, irregular, or laboured breathing, and to make sure baby doesn't need to make an effort.

 Hips These are gently rotated (don't worry, this won't hurt) and bent to check they aren't "clicky", a sign of dislocation or dysplasia.

 Spine Your baby will be held face-down so the doctor or midwife can have a good look at her spine to check that it is straight and there are no irregularities.

10

Don't panic, it's normal
THINGS NOT TO WORRY ABOUT WITH YOUR NEWBORN

Top 10

1 ### Black poo
Newborn babies produce a very dark, olive-green poo called meconium. The colour and texture of your baby's poo will progress to yellow and brown as he takes in more milk.

2 ### Possetting or vomiting
Babies often sick up a small amount, or even a large amount, of their feed. It's likely to be due to wind, but if it's shocking and projectile, take baby to the doctor. As long as your baby keeps down most of his feed and is gaining weight, don't worry.

3 ### Milk spots
Around 40 per cent of newborns develop tiny whitish pimples on their face, neck, and scalp. These milk spots, called milia, are caused by the sweat and oil-secreting glands springing into action. Don't be tempted to squeeze them; they will disappear.

4 ### Mysterious blotches
Raised, red blotches can appear almost anywhere on your newborn baby's body and are another harmless result of sweat and oil glands starting to work. The condition will almost always disappear within the first four or five days.

5 ### Is that dandruff?
Cradle cap looks like crusty scales on the scalp. Don't pick or poke at it as baby's skin is sensitive; it will disappear on its own. Gently rub olive oil into his scalp then shampoo it off.

186

SPOTS, BLOTCHES, AND BLACK POO can all be slightly alarming if you're not forewarned. Here are 10 things your newborn baby won't be worrying about, and neither should you.

6 Scaly skin

Dry, flaky skin is common, especially in overdue babies. Keep bathing to a minimum – one bath a week should be enough and rub olive oil or baby moisturizer into his skin afterwards.

7 Mongolian blue spot

Large blue marks on a baby's bottom or lower back are very common in babies of native American, African, Asian, or Hispanic descent. They are totally harmless and disappear within a year or so.

8 Pulsing fontanelle

Your baby's skull bones are not yet knitted together, allowing his head to fit down the birth canal more easily. The soft part at the front is called the fontanelle and may pulsate in time with his heartbeat – this is normal (if a little unsettling!).

9 Stork marks

Around half of all babies are born with small areas of redness on the nape of the neck, forehead, or eyelids. These are known as stork marks and will eventually fade away to nothing, though it can take up to a couple of years.

10 Blood in a girl's nappy

During pregnancy, high hormone levels can stimulate a baby girl's uterus to shed a tiny amount of blood within the first week of life. A smear of blood in her nappy is nothing to worry about.

Newborns in a nutshell

Over the following days and weeks, you and your partner can spend time getting to know your new baby – prepare for an emotional rollercoaster!

✳ Love at first sight?

Bonding with your baby follows its own timetable, so enjoy the journey. You may experience an overwhelming sense of love and emotion at the birth, or you may feel exhausted. Sometimes the joy, or shock, of having a baby only hits you when you get home from the hospital. Remember, there is no "right" way to feel, as everyone responds differently.

✳ Babies can look funny

Your baby may have a cone-shaped head, be red and wrinkly, or dry and scaly – don't worry, this is all perfectly normal. It's amazing how quickly a baby's skin and head shape change after the birth. Take guidance on caring for your newborn from midwives and doctors. Ask plenty of questions; the more you know, the more confident you will feel. Soon you will be at home without their help and getting on with being a wonderful parent!

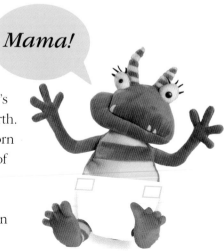

Mama!

DID YOU KNOW?

NEWBORNS BREATHE around 40 times per minute. An adult breathes in and out between 12–20 times per minute.

UNDER SIX WEEKS, A BABY CAN FOCUS ONLY 20–30CM (8–12IN) AWAY.

✳ The first six weeks

Leaving hospital can be nerve-wracking, so accept all offers of help. Then, once at home you can focus on your baby. For the first six to eight weeks some newborns sleep for most of the day (see pages 196–7). You may find it hard to cope if your baby is more wakeful at night than in the day, but he is born with a set of skills to help him get your attention, and to encourage you to care for him. The easy days will become more frequent as your baby grows bigger. And then, at about six weeks, you will be blown away when he first smiles.

IN ARMENIA,
it's customary for women to remain in the house for 40 days after the birth. Only those in the household can see the baby.

NEPALESE FAMILIES take their newborn to a priest to choose the name.

SURVIVAL **TACTICS**

1. Being born is thirsty work and your baby will want feeding with milk soon after.

2. Within one hour of being born, your baby needs to feed every two to three hours. Don't worry about setting your alarm for every feed – he will let you know by crying.

3. A newborn loses five to eight per cent of his birth weight within the first week, but should gain it back quickly.

4. Newborns can be noisy sleepers. Don't worry if he snuffles, snores, and hiccups.

5. If you are breastfeeding, get as much help and advice from experts as you can.

6. If bottle-feeding, have some packaged ready-made milk available as a back up, but don't make feed too far in advance.

7. Your baby will poo several times a day and wee every one to three hours, though less often if breastfed. Change his nappy to avoid a rash.

8. It's amazing how time-consuming a newborn baby can be, so any help with cooking or cleaning should be accepted gratefully.

9. Refer to pages 150–1 for your baby's wardrobe list. Having a supply of clean clothes and nappies on tap is a life saver.

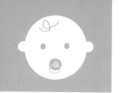

Breast milk is the right food for your baby; nothing can replicate it exactly. However, breastfeeding doesn't work for every new mum, which is when formula makes sense.

Breastfeeding or bottlefeeding?

Breast milk is the ideal first food for your little one. But why is this, and does it mean that your baby misses out if breastfeeding isn't for you?

✳ Why breastfeed?

• Your milk adapts constantly as your baby's needs change. From the nutrient-packed "pre-milk", known as colostrum, which is produced at birth, to the higher-fat, calorie-dense milk that comes through several days later, its composition evolves to ensure your baby grows and thrives.

• Breast milk boosts immunity, too, providing antibodies and white blood cells that protect your baby in the first vulnerable weeks and months. This can't be replicated in formula.

• Breastfed babies have fewer ear infections, respiratory problems, and eczema than bottle-fed babies.

• Breastfeeding is a clever system of supply-and-demand – as your baby sucks, nerve endings in your breasts are stimulated, triggering the release of the hormone prolactin, which signals your body to make more milk. You should always produce exactly the right amount of milk for your baby.

• Breast milk is thirst-quenching, as well as filling. At the start of a feed, your baby enjoys more watery "foremilk", and as your breasts empty, richer, fattier "hindmilk" is released.

• Mums benefit, too. Breastfeeding triggers the release of the hormone oxytocin, which causes your womb to contract back after birth. Together with the calories used, many women report rapid weight loss. Longer term, breastfeeding may lower your risk of various cancers and osteoporosis in later life, too.

• Breast milk is easier to digest than formula, and babies are less likely to be constipated.

• It's convenient; you can feed your baby anywhere, producing milk at the right temperature.

• Breast milk can help to stimulate your baby in the day and relax her at night.

190

THE FIRST FORMULA was developed in 1867 and has evolved over the years, with many companies investing in research.

1867

✳ Why bottle-feed?

• If you decide to bottle-feed, you can be confident that formula, derived from cow's milk, provides a high-quality alternative to breast milk. Designed to replicate breast milk as closely as possible, formula meets all your baby's nutritional needs. Choose a formula with more whey protein as it is easier for baby to digest.

• It can be reassuring to know exactly how much milk your baby is drinking.

• Bottle-fed babies have steadier, more predictable weight gain than breastfed babies. There is a variety of bottle sizes, so you can match the bottle to your baby's appetite, but make sure you don't overfeed her.

• You can share the experience with your partner, taking it in turns to do night feeds and having a little more sleep.

• There are no sore nipples, embarrassing leaks, or worries about whether what you eat and drink will affect your baby.

5 BEST WINDING TACTICS

1. Hold your baby upright, her head over your shoulder, and rub her back in a circular motion.

2. Sit her on your lap, supporting her in an upright position, and lean her forwards slightly while rubbing her back.

3. Lie her face-down across your lap, supporting her securely under the arms with one hand while you rub her back.

4. Lie her down on her back and rotate her legs back and forth in a cycling motion.

5. Cradle her face-downwards along your forearm, supporting her head with your hand, and rub her back while gently swinging her.

IN 2010,
83 per cent of new mums in the UK breastfed their babies after birth.

THE US, FRANCE,
Italy, and Spain have the highest rates worldwide of bottle-fed babies.

Feeding your baby
GREAT TIPS FOR BREASTFEEDING

Your midwife will show you how to help baby latch on.

1 Are you sitting comfortably?

Feeds can last from 10 minutes to an hour, so sit comfortably with your back well-supported. Place baby on a U-shaped feeding cushion, or pillow, so you don't get tired arms.

2 Gather everything you need

Have a glass of water (to replenish fluids), a book, your phone, or the TV control to hand as feeding may take a while. Then when your baby is latched on, sit back and try to relax.

3 Is baby ready?

Gently stroke your baby's cheek with the back of your fingers to trigger her rooting reflex, which makes her open her mouth and turn, or "root", for your nipple.

4 Latch on

Getting your baby to latch on is the key to easy feeding. Place her nose opposite your nipple; when she opens her mouth, bring her towards you. She should take the areola (dark area around your nipple) as well as the nipple into her mouth and start drinking.

5 Take your time

Leave her on your breast until she has finished, so she gets both the watery hydrating "foremilk" at the start of a feed through to the thicker, nutrient-dense "hindmilk". Then change breasts.

BREASTFEEDING is simple once you've mastered it, but it can be tricky when you first get started.

MOST MUMS produce more milk through their right breast, but you must use both!

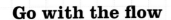

6
Go with the flow
Young babies need to feed at least every two to three hours as their tiny tummies hold only a little milk. Feeding on demand is best for your baby and your milk supply.

7
Wear a fitted maternity bra
Your breasts will feel uncomfortably full at times, so a supportive bra is essential. A clip or zip opens the cups for quick access!

8
Sore nipples?
Air your breasts between feeds if you can, and apply lanolin-based nipple cream to soothe.

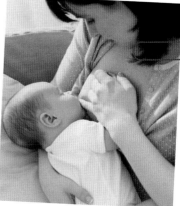

9
Sore breasts?
If your breasts become engorged, feeding can relieve fullness. It shouldn't last long.

10
Keep going!
The first few days, or weeks, can be challenging, but once you've got the hang of it breastfeeding provides instant food for your baby anywhere.

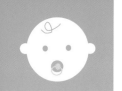

Ways to soothe baby

WHY IS HE CRYING?

CRYING IS OFTEN MORE FREQUENT in the late afternoon and early evening.

Hush little baby

Hearing your newborn baby cry can be distressing, especially if you aren't sure what is wrong. As you get to know your baby you will soon find out why he is crying and learn how to soothe him.

✳ Rock-a-bye baby

Even if you're unsure what's wrong, a nice cuddle will always be welcomed. Pop him in a sling and gently bounce or walk about – this usually helps. Alternatively, try driving him round the block or taking him out for a walk in a buggy; the motion is soothing.

✳ Keep calm and carry on

Babies can pick up on stressed vibes, so keeping calm is important. If incessant crying is getting to you, take him out of the house: a change of scene will do you both good. If you are really starting to lose it, put your baby down in a safe place and let him cry for five minutes while you leave the room, take deep breaths, and remind yourself "this will pass". Look at the checklist, right, for signs of why your baby might be crying.

The length of time a baby spends crying increases until about six weeks after birth, followed by a gradual decrease in crying until three to four months. After that, crying remains relatively stable.

Soothing solutions

VOICES
Sing or talk to your baby in a low, calm voice.

WHITE NOISE
Turn on a ceiling fan, hair dryer, or static radio.

BATHING
Some babies love baths, even in the middle of the day.

BARE UP
Snuggle your baby against your bare skin and heart beat.

SUCKING
Offer a dummy, or a clean finger or knuckle.

PHONE A FRIEND
Go on a visit or invite a friend over.

FRESH AIR
Go outside.

CRYING CHECKLIST

Hungry?   Smacking lips, rooting, eating hands – Feed

Tired?   Yawning, avoids eye contact – Sleep

Dirty nappy?   Check and change

Wants to be held?   Calms when picked up – Cuddle

Tummy trouble?   Crying after a meal, knees pulled up – Wind

Too cold?   Cold torso – Change clothes or wrap in a blanket

Too hot?   Red and sweating – Strip off a layer of clothing

Wants less stimulation?   Passed around a lot, loud noise – Sleep

Wants more stimulation?   Been doing the same thing for a while – Play

Teething?   Red cheeks, hard nub of a tooth breaking through – Rub on teething gel

Not feeling well?   Nappy rash, temperature, a cold or cough – Take temperature

RUN THROUGH this list to see if you can work out what's upsetting your crying baby – then act accordingly.

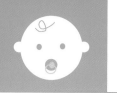

Newborns sleep for an average of 16½ hours per day, evenly divided between day and night. By three months he should sleep for about 10 hours at night, breaking for feeds, and five in the day.

Blissful sleep

You may also be astonished by how much a newborn sleeps, and it can be weeks before he works out day and night. For the first few weeks let your baby dictate proceedings, and then move towards a routine.

✱ Soothing space

A baby's brain slowly learns to distinguish day from night. Keep night feeds as restful as you can in order not to wake your baby too much. If you need a light on, make it dim and keep him wrapped up – you're both more likely to get back to sleep if warm and relaxed. Don't bother changing him, unless his nappy is dirty, and no talking.

✱ Where to sleep

For the first six months it's safest for baby to share your room in a Moses basket or cot – babies learn to roll over very young, making a bed or sofa risky. Place your baby on his back to sleep, with feet touching the end of the cot. Tuck in a sheet or blanket securely, no higher than his shoulders. There's no need for a pillow or hat, and layered sheets and blankets or a baby sleeping bag are safer than a duvet. Don't overheat the room – 18°C (64.4°F) is

DID YOU KNOW?

THE IDEAL POSITION to lie your baby during daytime naps is flat, rather than in a car seat or buggy, but don't worry about keeping too quiet or darkening the room.

A MOSES BASKET OR CARRYCOT IS IDEAL FOR YOUR NEWBORN.

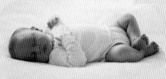

ideal. Current advice is to avoid co-sleeping (sharing a bed) but if you do, you need to know that babies who live in a home with a smoker, or who share a bed with someone who drinks alcohol, takes drugs, or is on medication (these all interfere with normal sleep patterns) are at most risk. Never sleep with a baby who was born prematurely or had a low birth weight. If you choose to co-sleep, keep pillows and covers to a minimum.

✳ What to wear

Baby sleeping bags are popular across northern Europe, preventing infants from pulling covers over their heads or sliding beneath blankets. In the summer, or in hot climates, dress your baby lightly and check for overheating by feeling his tummy.

✳ Bedtime routine

Putting a baby to bed in the same place, around the same time of day, builds associations between bedtime and rest. Bedtime routines work from around three months: maybe try a bath followed by massage, then a feed with soothing music. Place your baby in his cot while sleepy, but not exhausted, so he can drift off on his own. Try to avoid rocking your baby to sleep and then laying him down: babies who fall asleep in mum's arms can find waking alone in a different place disorientating and they may need settling again.

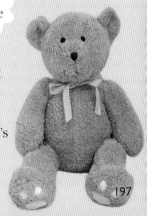

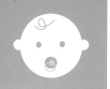

A bath cushion is a great piece of kit to have if you are nervous about holding your baby and washing her at the same time. There are several styles and designs available on the market.

Bathtime!

Babies don't need a daily bath – a quick "top-and-tail" wash will do. But some love bathtime so much that it turns into playtime, and on days when you both feel tired there's nothing more soothing than a shared dip.

✳ How to bath a new baby

You will need a baby bath or plastic bowl, a soft, clean flannel, cotton wool, and a soft, hooded towel. You don't need shampoo or baby bath products for tiny babies, though you can use them if you like, and olive oil is useful as a "soap" for wiping away any dirt. Make sure the room is warm and your baby is alert and happy.

1. Half-fill the baby bath with tepid water (around 38°C /100.4°F). Undress your baby to her vest and nappy. It's easiest to do this on a soft towel placed over a changing mat on the floor.

2. Moisten a piece of cotton wool and carefully wipe one eye from the centre outwards (babies often have gunky eyes). Wipe the other eye using a new piece of cotton wool. Repeat around the ears and nostrils, if necessary. Be firm but don't press too hard on your baby's delicate skin.

3. Soak a flannel, squeeze out most of the excess water and wipe her face gently, avoiding her eyes. Then wipe around her neck creases where milk and sweat can build up and cause dirt and irritation. Pat dry with a warmed towel.

4. To freshen her hair, hold your baby with her head supported by your hand or the crook of your arm, above the bathwater. Scoop water over the hair until any cradle cap is washed away. You don't need baby shampoo every time. Pat dry.

DID YOU KNOW?

IN TURKEY, MOTHER AND BABY are traditionally taken to the hammam baths on the 40th day after birth for a celebration of ritual cleansing, song, and feasting.

A GOOD TIME TO BATH YOUR BABY IS BEFORE HER LAST FEED OF THE DAY.

✳ Sharing a bath

Some babies hate being naked. If this is the case for your baby, try bathing together. Step into the bath and check the temperature is tepid (body temperature). Have your partner pass you the baby, cupping the back of her head and bottom. Rest her back against your chest, her bottom in your lap to support her. When ready to get out, pass the baby to your partner before getting out yourself.

5. Take off her vest and nappy (wiping away any mess). Lower your baby into the water, supporting her neck and shoulders with one hand. Swish water over her with your other hand. Sing and chat while you wash.

6. Uncurl her fingers to clean her hands. Wash beneath her arms and clean around her bottom. Lift her out, supporting her head and bottom, and wrap her in a warm towel. Pat dry, rub lotion into dry skin, and put on a clean nappy and clothes.

CAUTION: Never leave a baby in the bath alone, even for a few seconds.

199

New mum's survival guide

PLAN YOUR DAY

1 ### Sling it!

Babies love being held by both their parents, and enjoy the closeness and safety. Carrying your baby in a sling when out and about can be enjoyable and avoids having to take a buggy everywhere you go.

2 ### Day tripper

When feeling cooped up at home, make plans to go out for the day, perhaps to meet up with a friend or relative who lives further afield. If you're nervous about going on a bus or train, travel by car or take someone with you on the first trip.

3 ### Cultural stimulation

Your newborn baby may sleep for hours in the daytime, so take advantage of this down time and go out and do some of the things you never normally have time for – visiting museums, galleries, or a local attraction.

4 ### Me time

Being a new mum is wonderful, but you also need time to yourself in order to stay sane. Plan for your partner to look after the baby one night while you spend some time with your friends. You can still enjoy a glass of wine even if you are breastfeeding.

5 ### Meet and greet

Most first-time mums will be experiencing the same emotions so it is a great time to connect with new people. Invite postnatal friends over for a coffee or out to a baby event, such as daytime "baby" screenings at your local cinema.

IT'S GREAT FUN BEING a new mum, but it can also be daunting. Here are a few hints and tips on getting to grips with parenting, and enjoying life with your new baby.

6 **Regain your shape**

The nine-month wait is over and your baby has been born – but you still look pregnant! Now could be the time to start exercising and eating healthily in order to regain your figure. Don't diet if breastfeeding, however, as this may affect your milk production.

7 **Feeling blue**

Most new mums will feel very emotional during this hormonally turbulent time and for some this can turn into baby blues, or even postnatal depression. Talk to your partner about your feelings, or seek help from a professional.

8 **Baby classes**

Sign up for mother-and-baby classes as they are a great way to meet first-time mums like yourself. Try baby yoga or massage, fitness and swimming classes, or baby music time. Both you and your baby will love it!

9 **Bonding**

You may feel that you are running around all the time and need a rest. Take time out just to stay at home and hold your baby; let him touch your skin and gaze into your eyes as this bonding has a very positive effect for both him and you.

10 **Work-life balance**

Although you may not be using them at the moment, don't forget that your work skills and interests are still there – you are just taking a break. Don't feel guilty about not working; being a new mum is wonderful but it is still a tough job!

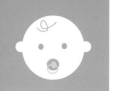
PROMPT MEDICAL SUPPORT makes all the difference if suffering from postnatal depression.

Looking after you

Babies are brilliant, but they take plenty of looking after – and so do new mums. Your hormones are still all over the place, and tiredness can make you wonder where "the old you" has gone.

✳ Those pesky hormones

Remember what your body has achieved: you have successfully created a new person, and now you are trying to get back to a sense of normality. However, your hormones are running amok, so it's really common for new mums to get "baby blues" a few days after the birth. It is thought to be caused by a huge drop in oestrogen and can make you feel overwhelmed with emotions. Baby blues can peak

 Do

Read cheerful magazines and books to keep you entertained when baby is sleeping.

Stock up on healthy snacks that are quick and easy to eat, such as fruit, muesli, and nuts.

Give yourself a mood-boost, such as visiting a beautiful place.

 Don't

Feel you have to invite every member of the family round – you are still recovering.

Watch the news: take a break from depressing stories for a while.

Soldier on in silence. If you are feeling exhausted, anxious, or just not yourself, tell your doctor.

DID YOU KNOW?

A GLASS OF FIZZ to celebrate the arrival of your baby is just what the doctor ordered, but if you are feeling depressed, then any more won't help.

ONE IN SIX new mums has an episode of the "baby blues".

three to 10 days after birth (see below if you feel fed up for longer than this). Sleep can really help so if you can, get someone to look after baby so you can catch up on rest – you will feel much better.

✳ Sharing the load

Perhaps more than at any other time of your life, right now you need TLC, nutritious food, and sleep – but with a newborn to care for that is a tall order! Welcome all the help you can from your partner, friends, or family. Perhaps your partner can be in charge of settling baby at night at the weekend, or organizing dinner. Maybe a friend can sit with baby while you have a bath. Get shopping delivered; employ a cleaner; ask someone to walk the dog. If you are used to being with work colleagues then suddenly the day can seem quiet, even with a new baby in the room. Invite people round and don't worry about suggesting a time limit if you need to rest. Even if you don't feel hugely sociable, at least try to get out every day and talk to people. There are plenty of clinics or parent-and-baby groups to go to; try as many as you can to find which you enjoy the most.

✳ Something more serious?

If life feels overwhelming, or if you experience any of the following symptoms, then talk to your doctor for support:
• Finding it hard to see the funny side of things
• Feeling lonely and bored
• Crying and feeling fed-up
• Getting scatty; turning up late and forgetting things
• Finding it hard to sleep even when you are really tired

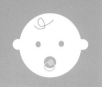

The six-week check-up

FOR YOU AND YOUR BABY

Your postnatal check-up

Your doctor will check that your body has recovered from the delivery, and that you are coping with sleep deprivation and the new-mum hormonal rollercoaster. After a number of routine checks (see below), you will be signed off from postnatal care to a local health visitor team.

Urine test

Prepare to wee in a pot. A urine test ensures you haven't got an infection (it's okay to admit to leaks, and feeling scared to poo). You may also be reminded to do your pelvic-floor exercises.

Weight and blood pressure

If you are unsure about the best diet for breastfeeding or losing baby weight, do ask. You might have questions about starting to exercise (if you can find time).

Abdomen and pelvis

The doctor will check that your uterus has contracted and any Caesarean scar, tear, or episiotomy has healed. An internal examination shows whether your cervix has closed. You'll be asked about your discharge (mention anything heavy, smelly, or painful), and be advised when to have a smear test.

Breast check

Ask the doctor to check your breasts if you are worried about anything, whether breastfeeding or not. Milk ducts can easily get blocked.

The sex question

Try not to laugh too much when asked about contraception. Lack of sleep, squirty boobs, and a baby in the room may mean sex is the last thing on your mind, but some women are pregnant at their six-week check. You can be fertile again before your periods start!

IN MANY CULTURES women stay at home for a while after the birth, but by six weeks – if you haven't already – it's time to venture out into the world and show off your new baby.

Your mental health

How are you coping generally? It's not shameful to admit to bouts of crying or rage against your new lifestyle (see pages 202–3). Sleep deprivation makes everyone feel terrible.

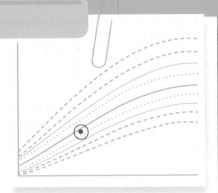

Your baby's check-up

This takes places separately, often at a baby clinic, six to eight weeks after birth. It's a good time to ask about feeding, vaccinations, and anything that's concerning you. You'll be asked to undress your baby for weighing.

Weighing and measuring

Your baby's length, weight, and head circumference are plotted on a graph in a baby book. Remember to take this book to every check-up to keep a record. Don't worry if your baby isn't on a specific percentile (growth measurement) – not everyone is average. The key is that he's growing.

Reflexes and muscle tone

The doctor checks that your baby can hold his head in line with his body and balance his head when pulled to a sitting position. Reflexes in the eyes are also checked.

Body systems

Your baby's heart, lungs, head, spine, ears, eyes, palate, hips, legs, and genitals are all checked in turn for development. The doctor will check for signs of inherited problems, such as congenital heart disease, dysplasia of the hip, glaucoma, or cataracts. Boy babies are checked to ensure that their testes have descended into the scrotum.

A whole new world

You've made it home with your brand new baby.
Welcome to this uncharted territory, full of unfamiliar
sights, sounds, and smells. Have no fear – you will
soon learn the customs and feel completely at ease.

✳ Trying to sleep

As comfortable as your bed may be, you will inevitably find getting
a good night's sleep a challenge at first, so grab any opportunity
for 40 winks. If Granny arrives and offers to do some housework or
take your baby for a stroll, say yes, and snuggle into bed with your
partner for a power nap. Don't drink endless cups of coffee to help
you stay awake or it will be harder to snatch that bit of sleep when
you can. Remember though, your partner is more tired than you, so
fill a bottle with formula or expressed milk and give her the precious
gift of a few hours of undisturbed sleep.

✳ What to do all day

Your partner will be busy caring for the baby, as well as recovering
from the delivery, so you need to care for her. If she is breastfeeding,
take her cushions, and fetch a drink and the remote control. Once
your baby is fed she can hand her to you, the new resident burping
expert. Burping is a good technique to learn and it means that your
baby will get to know your sounds and smells and become bonded
to you. You could also take charge of baths for the time being –

YOUR BABY will make a swimming motion with her arms and legs if she is placed in water. This is a survival reflex and doesn't mean she's an Olympic hopeful. Don't try this without holding her firmly!

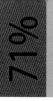

71%

OF PARENTS and babies across the world co-sleep (see pages 196–197).

Do

Take responsibility for a couple of aspects of the babycare.

———————————

Leave work on time and cut back on commitments temporarily to give you and your family time to acclimatize.

———————————

Arrange for food to be delivered each week from an online supermarket.

Don't

Be too hard on yourself – it'll take time to learn the skills and demands of fatherhood.

———————————

Feel down about your loss of sleep and leisure time – this doesn't last forever!

———————————

Assume your partner knows all the answers; you are on this strange journey together!

having a regular routine will help your baby settle and feel happier, and it's a good way to get quality time together. Cut back on your exercise regime or leisure commitments temporarily, but do take the time to relax by going out for a walk or gentle jog. If possible, rearrange your work schedule or book some leave – spending time at home now will mean you can help establish routines. Offer to take baby out in her sling and your partner can have a break while you're gone. It's a great opportunity to get out and show off your baby.

✳ **What's on the menu?**

Keeping yourself and your partner well fed is likely to be your responsibility, so make time for nutritious meals and plenty of water. You don't need to be a Michelin-starred chef, but producing something edible will earn you major hero points. Once back at work, eat healthily at lunch to look after yourself, too.

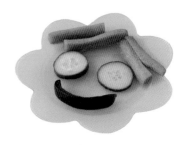

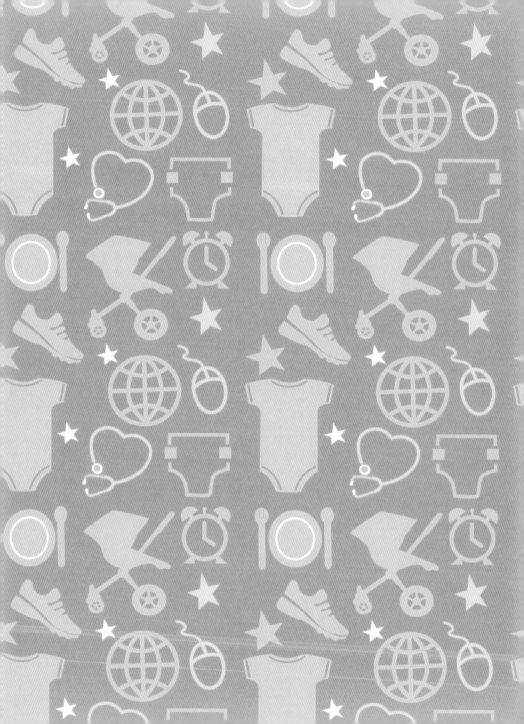

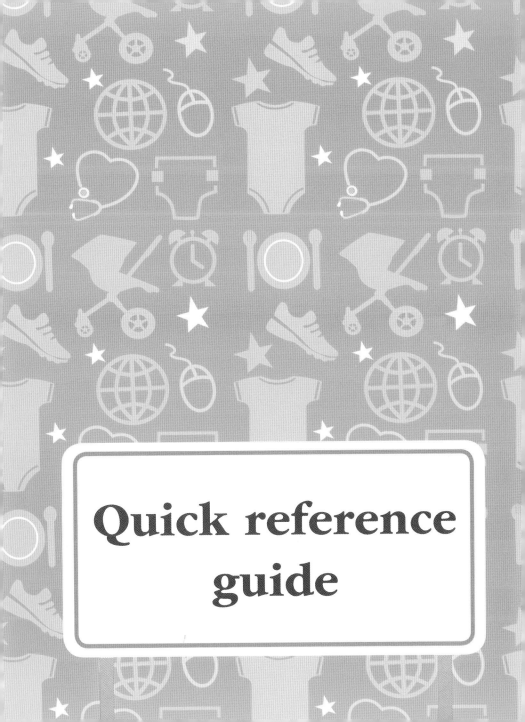

Quick reference guide

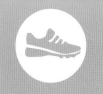 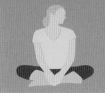

EXERCISE

Working out your workout

Many people think of pregnancy as a time for taking it easy, but while rest is important, you need to make sure you are fit and well for the journey ahead.

Rest is best?

The changes in your body during pregnancy can put it under enormous strain, and giving birth is one of the most physically demanding things you will ever do. Your path through labour and delivery is likely to be smoother if you feel fit and strong. You do also need to rest, and if you take part in a lot of exercise, you might need to listen to your body and rest more.

Body benefits

Regular cardiovascular exercise will help prevent your weight gain from going too far above the average (10–12kg/22–26lb). It also boosts the function of body systems such as your circulation and digestion, which are under pressure at this time. Gentle

exercise, such as swimming and yoga, can help prevent problems with joints and tendons. What's more, maintaining a good level of fitness during your pregnancy will make it easier to get back into shape once baby is born.

Making adaptations

It is possible to exercise throughout your pregnancy and in most cases there is no real need to change your usual regime. You can run, dance, and cycle, though common sense would suggest you minimize your risk of falls by choosing even paths and switch to a stationary bike or running machine. If you feel like your body is telling you to stop or slow down, then listen to it. If you are a gym regular, get a new gym programme that suits your body,

TOP TIP

CAN YOU STILL TALK? You should be able to hold a conversation when exercising. If you become too breathless to talk then your activity is too strenuous.

20% **INCREASE IN HEART RATE** during pregnancy equals that of low-level aerobic exercise.

and switch to lighter weights. Contact sports, such as basketball and judo, or any sport where you could fall (such as horse riding or skiing), should be put on hold. If you don't have a regular exercise plan you can put one into action while pregnant, but discuss it with a doctor or midwife first.

Walk, swim, and stretch

Cardiovascular activity, such as brisk walking or swimming three or four times a week, reaps real benefits. You may find your energy levels improve and you sleep better at night. Just 30 minutes of brisk walking or swimming will be effective. Swimming is usually safe throughout pregnancy, and the sense of weightlessness can be a real tonic when gravity is no longer a friend. Yoga and Pilates are ideally suited to pregnancy as they combine relaxation and stretching with core-strengthening movements that target the muscles that are most under strain in pregnancy. Seek out classes specifically for pregnant women.

 # Do

- Stay active every day, even if just walking. Aim for at least 30 minutes most days.

- Tell the instructors of any classes you attend that you are pregnant. There may be safe variations you can try.

- Learn exercises to strengthen your pelvic floor (see page 215).

- Find a yoga, Pilates, or aquafit class designed for pregnancy. You will be able to exercise safely and meet other expectant mothers.

 # Don't

- Stop exercising. Find exercise that feels good, safe, and keeps you active.

- Forget to listen to your body; if you start to feel nauseous or dizzy take a break.

- Exhaust yourself – you may have to tone down the intensity of your usual exercise routine; your body will give you clues!

- Do anything too strenuous in hot weather or allow yourself to become dehydrated.

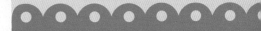

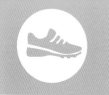

Gentle strengthening

STRONG CORE MUSCLES are vital during pregnancy as they support your spine and help you maintain the correct posture.

Exercises First trimester

These toning and stretching exercises are designed to develop the muscles you use most in everyday life and need to be strong during pregnancy: your core abdominals, thighs, and glutes (buttocks).

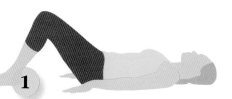

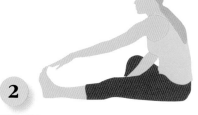

1 **CORE STRENGTH** Inhale, and as you slowly exhale push your lower back down until it is flat on the floor. Hold the position for five seconds, then repeat eight times.

2 **FLEXIBILITY STRETCH** Take hold of your toes. Inhale, and exhale as you lean forward for a gentle stretch down the back of your leg.

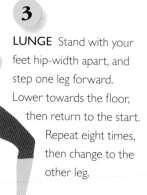

3 **LUNGE** Stand with your feet hip-width apart, and step one leg forward. Lower towards the floor, then return to the start. Repeat eight times, then change to the other leg.

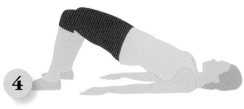

4 **BRIDGE** Raise your hips, bring your knees together, while tensing your buttocks. Open and close your knees 10 times before slowly lowering your hips.

Move to improve

IF INITIAL NAUSEA has settled down, use this time to stay active with three gentle cardiovascular activities each week, such as swimming or walking.

Exercises Second trimester

Energy levels are higher in the second trimester, so these exercises are more dynamic. You are advised not to exercise on your back after the first trimester.

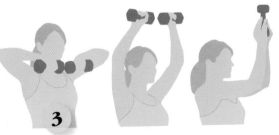

1

THE SLING Inhale, and as you exhale draw your muscles up and in towards your back, as if lifting your belly. Gently return to the starting position, and repeat 20 times.

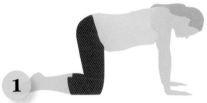

2

SUPERMUM Lift your left arm and right leg and hold for a count of five while still breathing. Lower slowly and repeat on the other side. Repeat on both sides eight times.

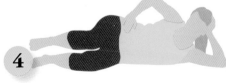

3

UPRIGHT ROW Inhale, and exhale as you raise your weights (1¾kg (4lb) each) slowly above your head. Bring your elbows together, then apart again. Inhale as you lower slowly. Repeat 16 times.

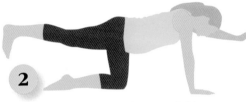

4

LEG IT Lift and lower your top leg slowly, without raising it above hip level. Repeat 30 times. Turn over to repeat on the other leg. Add a pillow under your belly as support if you feel like you need it.

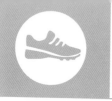

Looking after your back

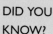

Exercises Third trimester

Your changed body shape and an increase in tiredness can affect your mobility and balance. Check your posture and keep your back strong and supple.

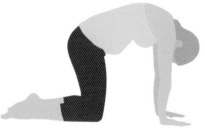

ENJOY A CAT STRETCH Your hard-working back will benefit from a gentle daily stretch. This exercise will also activate your abdominal muscles. Inhale as you pull in your abdomen and round out your back. Let your head and neck relax gently downwards. Hold this position for five seconds, while breathing and without locking your elbows. Exhale as you flatten your back. Repeat eight times.

THE IMPORTANCE OF GOOD POSTURE

Good posture will help take the strain away from your back.

SHOULDERS Relax your shoulders, and try not to let them hunch forwards.

BACK Keep your back straight and don't be tempted to exaggerate its curve.

HIPS When standing, keep hips square and bottom tucked in.

KNEES These should be soft when standing and you should avoid crossing them when sitting.

FEET Keep your feet hip-width apart and flat on the floor when standing or sitting.

STRONG LEGS will prepare you for beneficial labour positions, such as squatting and staying mobile when you are tired.

ONE IN THREE WOMEN experience some pelvic floor weakness during or after pregnancy, such as stress incontinence. Simple exercises can help avoid this. You can do them any time, any place!

Don't ignore your pelvic floor

Your pelvic floor is a muscle that stretches like a sling from your pubic bone to the base of your spine, holding your bladder in place and controlling urine flow. Pregnancy can weaken your pelvic floor, leading to stress incontinence and reduced sensitivity during sex. Building up your pelvic floor strength during pregnancy can help prevent the development of these issues.

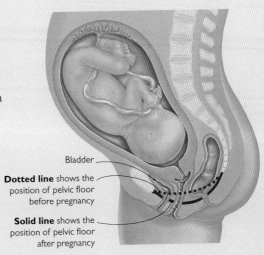

Bladder

Dotted line shows the position of pelvic floor before pregnancy

Solid line shows the position of pelvic floor after pregnancy

PELVIC FLOOR TONING Sit comfortably, stand, or get on your hands and knees. Focus on the muscles you would use to prevent yourself from passing wind or urinating. Squeeze and lift the muscles, then relax. Take care not to hold your breath or to tense your buttocks, thighs, or stomach as you lift. Once you get used to the feeling, try holding for a few seconds at a time. Repeat 15 times. Add more squeezes each week. Continue this during and after pregnancy to maintain your strength.

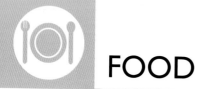

FOOD

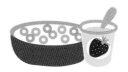

Breakfast

We all know that breakfast is "the most important meal of the day", and this really is true during pregnancy. By morning you haven't eaten for eight or so hours, and you need to break this fast.

If you are feeling sick in the mornings, or you are in the habit of skipping breakfast, then you need to find some simple, appealing ideas that you can introduce into your daily routine. Aim for as much variety as possible – perhaps one morning you will have time to make a simple cooked breakfast, such as poached eggs or grilled bacon. Other days, a bowl of cereal or toast will be all you have time or appetite for. To make this important meal as nutritious as possible, choose wholegrain breads and cereals. Many cereals are packed with sugar, so if you can make your own muesli or granola at the weekends to eat during the week, you can save on unwanted sugars.

• Porridge can be very soothing to a turbulent tummy. Measure out the oats the night before, and pour over water or your choice of milk (cow's, soya, or almond are all good options), so the oats are well soaked by morning. Simply heat through in a pan and stir for three minutes or until the porridge is ready. Top with dried or fresh, chopped fruit.

FIBRE AIDS NUTRIENT ABSORPTION and will help keep your blood-sugar levels steady. Roughage is easily available at breakfast time with wholemeal toast and cereal. Aim for 25–30g (1–1½oz) of fibre per day.

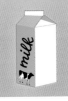

TWO SERVINGS of dairy produce every day give you the calcium you need.

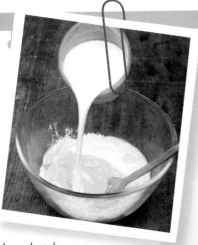

Pancakes

MAKES ABOUT 6 PANCAKES

If you are not feeling great, pancakes are easy to digest. Mix together to form a batter:

125g (4½oz) flour
pinch of salt
1 egg
300ml (10fl oz) milk

Fry for 2–4 minutes, turning once.

• Bake a batch of muffins using wholemeal flour. Add any combination of flavours, such as sunflower seeds, dried fruit, nuts, and fresh berries.

• Eggs make a quick and nutritious breakfast. Buy free-range eggs that are omega-3 enriched. Serve with toasted seeded bread for extra vitamin C and fibre. Stir in frozen, chopped spinach while cooking.

• Keep a selection of rye, seeded, and wholemeal breads and bagels in the freezer. Top with avocado, nut butter, or smoked salmon instead of jam.

• Make a smoothie. Whizz together a handful of frozen berries, a chopped ripe banana, and 100ml (4fl oz) yogurt or milk.

• To make your own muesli, mix together oats and wheat flakes, dried apricots, sunflower seeds, and almonds.

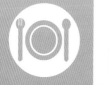

FOOD

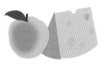

Main meals

If your appetite is affected by your pregnancy, or you prefer smaller meals at the moment, aim for variety and pack in plenty of nutritious ingredients.

When planning your meals, aim for a variety of ingredients so you and your baby get everything you could possibly need – carbohydrates, proteins, and fats – this is not the time to cut anything out (see pages 30–1 for more information). Think about ways you can add plenty of vegetables to every meal: frozen, tinned, and fresh all count!

Aim for at least three different types of vegetable each day, and two or more fruits. If you are feeling tired, don't feel you have to cook a hot meal every day; a substantial salad or soup packed with pulses and vegetables would give you everything your body needs. On days when you, or your partner, have energy, cook extra so you have meals in the freezer for days when you're tired or for after baby is born. Pasta sauce, lasagne, fish pie, roasted vegetables, tagines, and stews all freeze well. Include brightly coloured fruit and vegetables as they contain vitamin C and carotene, which may increase the production of infection-fighting white blood cells to prevent viruses.

DID YOU KNOW?

YOUR BABY can taste what you eat as early as 13 weeks – strongly flavoured foods can be tasted in amniotic fluid.

50% OF YOUR FOOD SHOULD COME FROM CARBOHYDRATES.

Asparagus, broccoli, and ginger stir-fry

A quick and easy meal to boost iron, and to help alleviate nausea. Add a portion of protein, such as cashews, tofu, chicken, turkey, or beef, to vary the recipe. White rice is a quick and easy accompaniment, but ideally serve with brown rice for extra nutrients and fibre.

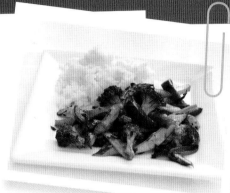

SERVES 2

- **1 tsp vegetable oil**
- **1 fresh red chilli, deseeded and finely chopped**
- **2.5cm (1in) piece of fresh root ginger, sliced into fine strips**
- **½ bunch spring onions, cut into 5cm (2in) lengths**
- **1 garlic clove, finely chopped**
- **½ red pepper, deseeded and sliced**
- **150g (5oz) broccoli, cut into small florets**
- **½ bunch asparagus spears, halved**
- **1 tsp sugar**
- **salt and ground black pepper**
- **½ handful of fresh mint leaves**

1. Heat the oil in a wok or large pan. Add the chilli and ginger and toss for a few seconds.

2. Add the spring onions and garlic. Stir-fry for 5 minutes or until softened. Add the red pepper and stir-fry for a few minutes.

3. Add the broccoli, and stir-fry for a few minutes more, before adding the asparagus. Continue stir-frying for 1–2 minutes. Sprinkle over the sugar, season well, and stir-fry for a few seconds to dissolve the sugar. Stir in the mint.

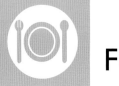
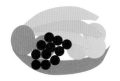
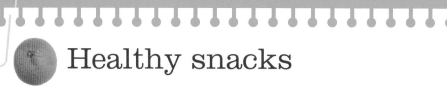

Healthy snacks

Eating little and often can help to reduce the symptoms of nausea, alleviate hunger, and give you an energy boost. Ideally, aim to eat something containing protein to regulate your blood sugar.

• Chop up fresh vegetables, such as carrots, peppers, and cucumber for crunchy crudités. Sugarsnap peas are delicious, too.

• Make hummus, guacamole, and salsa. Eat with strips of pitta bread, crudités, or rice cakes. An easy way to get a little extra protein.

• Bake a batch of flapjacks, and add some seeds or dried fruit. The oats, seeds, and fruit will give you useful energy.

• Buy a variety of fruit, such as melon, mango, raspberries, and kiwi. Make up a fruit salad, and help yourself when you need to. Add yogurt for protein.

• Choose wholegrain bread wraps and rolls.

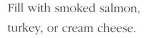

Fill with smoked salmon, turkey, or cream cheese.

• A handful of nuts and seeds is packed with protein and fibre.

• A small square of 70 per cent dark chocolate contains nutrients and can help boost energy.

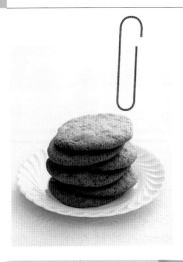

Ginger biscuits

MAKES ABOUT 35 BISCUITS
225g (8oz) butter, at room temperature
175g (6oz) light soft brown sugar
I tbsp syrup from a jar of stem ginger
I large egg
350g (12oz) self-raising flour
I heaped tbsp ground ginger
3 balls of stem ginger in syrup,
drained and finely chopped

1. Preheat the oven to 190°C/375°F/Gas 5. Line two baking trays with baking parchment. In a bowl, mix together the butter, sugar, and syrup until creamy.

2. Mix in the egg, flour, ground ginger, and stem ginger to form a soft dough.

3. Roll the dough into 35 walnut-sized balls. Place on the baking trays and flatten with your fingers. Bake for 12–15 minutes, or until golden brown. Transfer to a wire rack to cool.

Snack attack

Take nuts, fruit, and chopped vegetables to work each day so you get a variety of snacks – don't rely solely on biscuits! If you have a long commute, take a small packet of nuts, such as almonds, and a bottle of water with you to keep you going.

Restaurant guide

SAFE EATING

Enjoying a night out

Eating at restaurants can become a bit of challenge when you're pregnant, so here are some hints and tips on which foods you can still enjoy and which you should avoid for a short while.

Main course

✔ Smoked salmon is safe to eat.

✔ Shellfish is safe to eat as long as it is cooked. Tuna is fine, but only in moderation as it contains mercury: no more than two tuna steaks or four small cans per week.

✘ Game meat, such as venison, rabbit, and pheasant, is best avoided as it may contain lead shot.

✘ Shark, swordfish, and marlin due to high levels of mercury.

✘ Liver and pâtés.

✘ Avoid rare and undercooked meat – check burgers are cooked.

✘ "Homemade" mayonnaise, hollandaise, and béarnaise sauces contain raw egg, so avoid them.

Cheeseboard

✔ Hard cheeses, such as Cheddar Edam, Emmental, Gouda, Gruyère, Jarlsberg, and Parmesan are fine.

✔ Stilton contains blue mould but is safe because it is pasteurized. If concerned, only eat it when cooked.

✔ Cottage cheese, mozzarella, feta, cream cheese, paneer, ricotta, and halloumi are fine, so long as they are pasteurized.

✘ Mould-ripened cheeses, such as Brie, Camembert, and soft, blue-veined cheese (such as Danish blue, Gorgonzola, and Roquefort).

✘ Goat's cheese is best avoided if uncooked, such as in salad, but fine when cooked, such as a baked quiche.

CAFFEINE?

It's fine to keep enjoying tea and coffee if you are pregnant, but you are advised to limit your intake of caffeine to 200mg per day. Some large-sized coffees sold in cafés contain more than 300mg in one cup, so be vigilant. Remember, too, that caffeine may lurk in other drinks (see right).

Measuring caffeine

8fl oz filter coffee = 180mg

"energy" drink = 80mg

12fl oz cappuccino = 75mg

mug of tea = 75mg

hot chocolate = 70mg

can of cola = 40mg

Desserts

✔ Cooked puddings or desserts containing pasteurized cream.

✔ Fresh fruit, if washed or peeled.

✔ Processed soft ice-cream.

✔ Manuka honey, along with other types of honey.

✘ Homemade ice-cream, mousse, tiramisu, and soft meringue should be avoided because they contain raw eggs. Hard meringue is fine as the egg white is cooked.

✘ Uncooked cheesecakes should be avoided as they are made with raw eggs, but cooked ones are fine.

✘ Pastry dough contains raw eggs so make sure it's thoroughly cooked.

Alcohol

Even if you're accustomed to a glass of wine with dinner, it is advisable to avoid alcohol during your pregnancy, and with good reason: alcohol has been linked to preventable birth defects and mental retardation, and it increases the risk of miscarriage and low birthweight.

SUSHI

Food safety regulations in the UK require shops and restaurants to freeze raw fish used to make sushi at -20°C (-4°F) for at least 24 hours, but it's worth double checking. Vegetarian sushi options are safe.

ASSISTED DELIVERIES

When help is needed

It may not feature in your ideal birth plan, but roughly one in every eight women has an assisted birth, and the midwife will only suggest it when it is completely necessary. If your baby is in an awkward position, if there are concerns about his heart rate, or if you are simply too exhausted this may be the best course of action.

What's available?

Assisted deliveries are performed either with forceps or ventouse (see below) – these instruments connect with your baby's head and help to ease him out of the birth canal. You will be offered local pain relief.

Forceps

One of the most common methods for assisted birth, forceps are like a pair of tongs, or two large spoons, that are eased onto either side of your baby's head to allow the doctor to lift him out gently or rotate him slightly while you are pushing. They have a high degree of success but may cause some tearing, or you may be offered an episiotomy (a small surgical cut to gain access). Don't worry, everything will be repaired and will heal. Forceps will often leave marks on your baby's head but these will fade.

Ventouse

This method works by attaching a plastic "cup", which acts as a suction device, to the top of the baby's head. The cup is connected to a tube that the doctor will pull on during a contraction to deliver the baby. A baby born via ventouse may

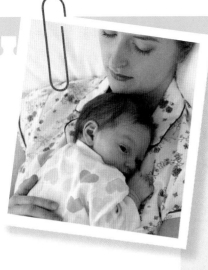

"The moment you hold your baby in your arms you realize that nothing matters except that he has had a safe delivery."

have a raised bump on his head (called a chignon), but it will disappear within 24–48 hours. The advantage of having a ventouse delivery is that the baby can still rotate automatically as he descends through the pelvis because the head has yet to "crown" (emerge).

Can I avoid an assisted delivery?

Unfortunately the short answer is no, not if your midwife or doctor has advised one. Assisted deliveries are only called into play when there is little chance of your baby being born safely without one. There are, however, ways you can reduce the

likelihood of needing one – stay active as long as possible to keep labour progressing; eat snacks so your energy does not flag; and make use of gravity by trying upright positions.

Moving on

Ask to speak to a midwife or doctor if you have questions after delivery or had a bad experience. Your health care provider won't want you to be anxious, and can advise about delivery interventions that were needed. You will recover quickly and there is an 80 per cent chance you won't need intervention the next time around.

Pain relief in labour

WHAT ARE THE OPTIONS?

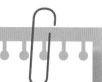

Natural remedies and medical choices

During labour, the body's naturally occurring painkiller, endorphins, reach the same level as those recorded in male endurance athletes at the peak of their treadmill workout. However, you might need a little top up on the day. Getting clued up now on your pain relief options for labour will help you feel prepared.

Nice and natural

There is an array of natural pain relief options that provide considerable benefits with no side effects.

Being immersed in warm water is soothing and supportive. The buoyancy frees movement and lifts pressure from the back and pelvis, while the warmth relaxes muscles and relieves tension (see pages 168–169).

A firm, sweeping back massage will release your natural, painkilling endorphins. However, on the day you may find touch unbearable.

A natural reaction to contractions can be shallow breathing, impeding the oxygen flow to the uterus and the release of oxytocin, the hormone that progresses labour. Controlled rhythmic breathing helps you focus, conserve energy for pushing, and releases tension, allowing your birthing muscles to work as intended.

Hypnobirthing combines breathing with positive thinking and visualization techniques to help you embrace the "surge" of each contraction that sweeps your baby along. Studies show that this technique can result in a shorter labour, fewer medical interventions, and a more positive birth experience.

You might like to try a TENS (transcutaneous electrical nerve stimulation) machine. This simple device uses electrical impulses to block pain messages, and can be effective during early labour. Pads are attached to your back so you can freely move around.

Drugs now please!

Labour is not an endurance test, so if it all gets too much there are effective medical pain relief options that can help make your birthing experience easier to cope with.

Easy to administer and suitable throughout labour, gas and air – Entonox – is a mixture of oxygen and nitrous oxide. Simply inhale at the start of a contraction and let it take effect, reducing pain as the contraction peaks. It doesn't affect the baby, although you may feel queasy; the effects are short-lived.

"Heat relaxes muscles in labour – microwaveable 'hotties' mould to your body's contours, providing localized warmth."

Longer-lasting, effective pain relief is provided by opioid drugs, such as pethidine. Usually injected, these work quickly and last several hours.

For a total pain block, an epidural injection delivers regional anaesthesia into the space between the spinal cord and column, numbing the lower half of your body. It can slow progress, though, so you might be encouraged to forgo an epidural if delivery isn't far off.

A spinal block is a one-off shot of anaesthetic in the spine. However, it can cause a drop in blood pressure and slow the baby's heart rate.

Pregnancy complications

Most pregnancy aches and pains are just a passing inconvenience and should clear up following delivery. However, some problems, where medical intervention may be required, are summarized here with possible symptoms and treatments. A high-risk pregnancy will always be closely monitored, so you will always be in safe hands.

Anaemia (iron deficiency)

Having more plasma (the fluid element) in your blood means diluted red blood cells and less effective oxygen delivery. Symptoms include exhaustion and paleness and affect a third of women in the third trimester. Iron supplements may be prescribed.

Carpal tunnel syndrome

Fluid retention in the wrists can result in pins and needles and weakness in the thumb and fingers for 50 per cent of pregnant women. Wrist splints or steroid injections may be prescribed.

Chickenpox (varicella zoster)

Up to 28 weeks, exposure to the varicella zoster virus in the womb can affect a baby's developing eyes, brain, limbs, bladder, or bowel; up to 36 weeks, a baby may get shingles as a toddler; after this, babies can be born with a severe form of the virus. The infection is transmitted to the mother by droplets spread during face-to-face contact. Ninety per cent of women are immune to the virus; if you are not, an immune-strengthening inoculation will be offered.

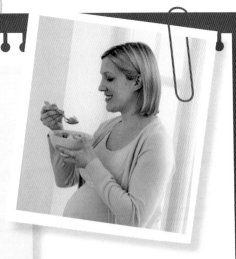

> *"If you eat healthily you are less likely to suffer from illness during pregnancy."*

Deep vein thrombosis (DVT)

Blood clots are more likely in pregnancy (when blood easily clots to prevent bleeding). Symptoms include pain and swelling in one leg, heel pain, and tender, warm skin. Treatment is required before a clot blocks a major blood vessel, and includes compression stockings, exercise, and anticoagulation drugs.

Ectopic pregnancy

In 1 per cent of pregnancies, the fertilized egg implants in the fallopian tube, outside the uterine cavity, where it cannot grow. Symptoms from week six onwards include severe lower abdominal and shoulder pain, and bleeding. If a doctor suspects an ectopic pregnancy, he will suggest an ultrasound. A ruptured tube is life-threatening, requiring immediate surgery or a laparoscopy.

Essential hypertension

Raised blood pressure is a common problem in pregnancy, mostly after 20 weeks. It's a symptom of pre-eclampsia (see page 232) and linked to growth problems and premature birth. Low-dose aspirin and calcium supplements may be prescribed and a 34-week scan will check the baby's growth and amniotic fluid.

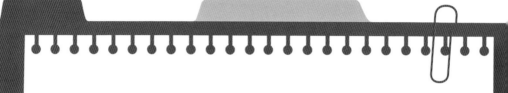

PREGNANCY-RELATED PROBLEMS

Fibroids

These are benign growths in the uterine muscle wall and can vary in size from a small pea to a large melon. They are more common in Afro-Caribbean women. They can cause late miscarriage or premature labour. They usually shrink in size post-delivery and will be monitored by a doctor throughout pregnancy.

Gestational diabetes mellitus

If insufficient insulin is produced to meet the extra needs of pregnancy, blood-glucose levels rise, usually after 24 weeks, risking early induction, diabetes, and metabolic syndrome for the mother, and birth injuries due to the size of the baby. Treatment includes healthy diet, exercise, and sometimes insulin injections.

Hyperemesis gravidarum

This most severe form of morning sickness affects less than 1 per cent of pregnant women. Regular vomiting lasts for weeks, not days, leading to dehydration and sometimes liver problems. It usually resolves by 16–20 weeks. Rest and small, frequent meals help; in severe cases, anti-vomiting medication or steroid therapy is given.

Listeria

This is a food-borne bacteria that lurks in some soft cheeses, pâtés, and undercooked food; it can cause late miscarriage. Avoid the risk by cooking meat and fish thoroughly and avoiding soft cheeses (see pages 29 and 222), deli meats, and alfalfa sprouts.

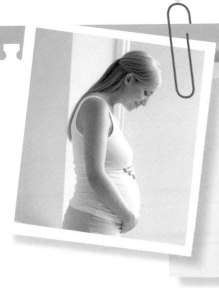

"The majority of tests during pregnancy show that mum and baby are progressing well."

Miscarriage

This occurs in 15 per cent of pregnancies, although after 12 weeks of gestation it is uncommon and affects only 1–2 per cent of women. The risk increases with maternal age. Miscarriage is a process, not a single event, so if you experience vaginal bleeding there are several possible outcomes. Referral to a specialist clinic for investigation will be offered, but often no cause is found.

Obstetric cholestasis

Intense, persistent itching on the palms of the hands and soles of the feet extends up the limbs and is worse at night. This indicates a liver problem, causing a buildup of bile. If you experience these symptoms, consult your doctor. It affects less than 1 per cent of women after 28 weeks, but is linked with premature delivery, bleeding, and fetal demise.

Parvovirus

Symptoms of parvovirus B19 are similar to those of German measles (rubella), but may be so mild they go unnoticed. It can cause late miscarriage, but in most cases pregnancies are followed by healthy live births.

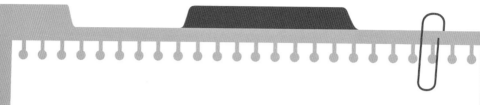

Placenta praevia

The 20-week scan can diagnose a low-lying placenta attached to the uterus, covering the cervix (the exit). Most move up by 32 weeks, but if not there is a risk of bleeding and a C-section maybe required.

Pre-eclampsia

Severe pre-eclampsia affects 0.5 per cent of women and requires immediate medical attention; untreated, it is life-threatening for mum and baby. Symptoms can include high blood pressure, protein in the urine, severe headaches, vision problems, vomiting, heartburn, rib pain, breathlessness, and sudden swelling of the hands, feet, and face. Medical management on medication is the cure, but it may mean early delivery.

Rubella

Catch German measles up to 12 weeks into pregnancy and the baby has a high risk of suffering cataracts, deafness, or heart and brain damage. Ninety per cent of women are immune. Secondary-school-age girls should be offered a vaccination.

Stillbirth and neonatal death

This occurs after 20 weeks. Before that, the loss of the fetus is considered a miscarriage. It may be due to a congenital abnormality, but 50 per cent of stillbirths happen without warning. Stillbirth in labour is now rare (1 in 1,000) and the overall risk in pregnancy has fallen dramatically due to improved maternal health and monitoring.

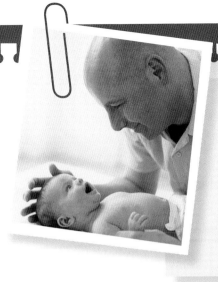

"Very common illnesses, such as colds and flu, are unlikely to cause harm."

Stress incontinence

Women who have a natural delivery sometimes suffer mild, temporary urinary incontinence because the bladder neck has been stretched by the pressure of the baby's head passing through the birth canal. Pelvic floor exercises will help to regain full bladder control.

Symphysis pubis dysfunction

Groin pain can be a sign of SPD, when hormones cause ligaments to relax. Symptoms can appear from week 12 onwards and often feel like a muscle spasm. A "belly belt" will bring some relief. Ask for a physio referral.

Thrush (candidiasis)

Thrush (white curdy discharge and itching) is more common in pregnancy and treatment is less effective, so a long course of antifungal cream may be prescribed. Loose cotton underwear and moisturizing with olive oil help; avoid scented soaps and bath gels.

Toxoplasmosis

This rare infection is transmitted through animal poo and garden soil, and can cause miscarriage and neurological damage during the first trimester. Wear gloves in the garden and don't empty the cat litter.

MATERNITY AND PATERNITY LEAVE

Time off work to look after a new baby is available as official leave for mums and dads in most countries worldwide, but it can vary.

PAID LEAVE gives parents the time to provide great antenatal and postnatal care, allowing a greater sense of bonding. It also lowers accident rates in the work place.

A NEW DAD IN ESTONIA has to wait for three months after the birth of his baby before he is entitled to claim maternity benefit (there is no paternity cover). Only one parent can claim at a time, so if the father takes time off work, the mum has to return to employment.

ONLY FOUR COUNTRIES have no national law requiring paid time off for new parents – Papua New Guinea, Liberia, Swaziland, and the US.

IN GREECE, new dads are entitled to take only two days of paid paternity leave.

IN NORWAY, "parental" leave is given, which includes a quota of 10 weeks paternity leave for dads that can't be transferred to mum; in 2008, 90 per cent of fathers used their quota!

IN THE UK, new mothers are entitled to 52 weeks of maternity leave, 39 weeks of which are paid, though this is set to change in the future. Two weeks of paid paternity leave is also available for dads. Many families choose which parent stays at home according to income – one in seven fathers is currently a stay-at-home dad.

ACCORDING TO A US SURVEY, in 2000 only 12 per cent of companies offered paid maternity leave.

IN THE CZECH REPUBLIC AND SLOVAKIA, new mothers can choose to stay at home on maternity leave for up to three years after each child's birth. However, it is not common for fathers to take any leave.

SWEDEN provides working parents with an entitlement of 16 months paid maternity leave per child, receiving 80 per cent of their wages. The cost is shared between the employer and the state.

ORGANIZATIONS AND HELPLINES

Pregnancy

babycentre.co.uk
The go-to site for a comprehensive look at pregnancy, childbirth, and all things related.

fedant.org
National register of validated professionals in antenatal education.

fitpregnancy.com
Information about diet and exercise during pregnancy, including recipes and workouts.

i-am-pregnant.com
The pregnancy calendar is detailed and has some good clear images of the developing fetus.

midwivesonline.com
Information and advice on preconception, pregnancy, and birth.

mothers35plus.co.uk
Website for older mothers with advice, facts, and forums.

naturalmothering.ca/index. php/pregnancy-a-labour/88-homeopathy-and-pregnancy
Advice on using natural remedies during pregnancy and childbirth.

netmums.com
Netmums is a local network for mums (or dads), offering a wealth of information on both a national and local level. Click on the pregnancy tab for everything from due-date clubs to baby names.

nhs.uk/Planners/ Pregnancycareplanner
Contains all you need for a healthy and happy pregnancy, and to make sure you get the care that's right for you.

TheBump.com
This comprehensive pregnancy website includes tools, such as a due date calculator and pregnancy calendar apps, plus much more.

webmd.com
This family and pregnancy link provides a complete guide to raising a family, with expert advice from doctors and other healthcare professionals.

whattoexpect.com
Pregnancy week by week and much, much more on this great website.

Labour and birth

activebirthcentre.com
Specializes in waterbirths and active birth classes.

aims.org.uk
Association for Improvements in the Maternity Services

caesarean.org.uk
Information about C-sections.

childbirthconnection.org
This is a reliable website that helps mums-to-be make informed choices about maternity care decisions, both before and after the birth.

nct.org.uk/birth
Find out all you need to know here.

tommys.org
Comprehensive website with details on all aspects of pregnancy and giving birth to a healthy baby, as well as a midwife helpline.

Breastfeeding

abm.me.uk
The Association of Breastfeeding Mothers offers help and information about support groups.

breastfeedingnetwork.org.uk
Comprehensive source of information and support for breastfeeding women, and for those involved in their care.

breastfeeding.co.uk
This website is run by breastfeeding counsellors with in-depth articles by a Canadian doctor.

laleche.org.uk
For friendly, mother-to-mother breastfeeding support, from pregnancy through to weaning.

nct.org.uk
The National Childbirth Trust (NCT) is a charitable organization run by and for parents. It organizes local antenatal classes for women with a similar due date, and postnatal classes on breastfeeding. It also runs sales of secondhand baby gear. The classes provide excellent preparation for childbirth and the friends you meet at them can become friends for life. There is a membership fee.

nhs.uk/start4life
NHS website to support breastfeeding mums and advise on healthy living.

thebabycafe.org
Find a café that welcomes breastfeeding mums near you!

Blogs and discussion forums

omyfamilyblog.com/category/pregnancy
There are plenty of mummy blogs online. Here's one of the best.

alifeunexpected-jtm.blogspot.co.uk
A dad's blog on his journey to parenthood.

mama.co.uk
Meet-a-Mum Association offers advice and hosts a forum for new mums.

mumsnet.com
By parents for parents. Every aspect of pregnancy, childbirth, and child rearing is discussed at length with some great resources and tips.

pregnantchicken.com
A funny and irreverent blog about pregnancy; this fun website is full of advice and ideas.

forums.parentingclub.com
Packed with message boards, advice and parenting tips.

For new dads

4newdads.co.uk
All a new dad could want to know with reviews, discount vouchers for baby gear, and solid articles by a selection of dads.

dad.info
Information for expectant and new dads.

fatherhoodinstitute.org
The institute is responsible for collating research on all fatherhood-related issues, as well as offering support services and help.

newdadssurvivalguide.com
Be the best partner you can! Dads' step-by-step guide to labour, birth, and parenting.

General

apec.org.uk
Helpline: 0208 427 4217
Action on Pre-eclampsia provides information and support for sufferers.

apni.org
Helpline: 020 7386 0868
Association for Post-natal Illness supports mothers suffering from postnatal depression.

bcma.co.uk
British Complementary Medicine
Association

The Breastfeeding Network
National breastfeeding helpline:
0300 100 0210

disabledparentsnetwork. org.uk
A national organization offering
information and support for disabled
people who are parents, plus their
families, friends, and supporters.
Disabled Parents Network helpline:
0300 3300 639; e-help@disabled
parentsnetwork.org.uk

fertilityuk.org
National fertility awareness and
natural family planning centre.

gingerbread.org.uk
Advice and support for single
parents, both mums and dads.

gov.uk
Information on work and benefits for
pregnant women and new parents.

iaim.org.uk
Int. Association of Infant Massage

La Leche League
Breastfeeding helpline:
0845 120 2918

multiplebirths.org.uk
The Multiple Births Foundation
Tel: 0208 383 3519

NHS Direct
Helpline: 111 or 0845 4647
Phone for advice if you have any
worries about your pregnancy.

Tommy's
A charity that funds medical research
into miscarriage, stillbirth and
premature birth. Talk to a midwife
about any topic of pregnancy:
0800 0147 800

TAMBA
Twins and Multiple Birth Association
Freephone twinline: 0800 138 0509
tamba.org.uk
TAMBA is a charity set up by parents
of twins, triplets, and higher multiples,
plus interested professionals.

vegsoc.org
Advice on vegetarian and vegan diets
in pregnancy and while breastfeeding.
Tel: 0161 925 2000

workingfamilies.org.uk
Help and advice for working parents.
Helpline: 0300 012 0312

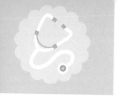

Phrase book
THE A–Z OF PREGNANCY AND CHILDBIRTH

Being pregnant can feel like being in a different country, speaking a different language as parts of your body you hardly knew existed are dropped into everyday conversation. This A–Z of pregnancy and childbirth terminology will help you speak the lingo in no time.

Albumin: Type of protein, which if found in your urine samples may be a sign of pre-eclampsia (see page 232).

Alveoli: Tiny air sacs at the ends of the branches (bronchioles) of your baby's lungs. This is where oxygen is taken up and carbon dioxide passes out, back into your bloodstream.

Amniocentesis: Test to determine genetic abnormalities. A hollow needle is inserted through your abdomen into the amniotic sac, and a tiny amount of amniotic fluid withdrawn for analysis. The test carries a risk of miscarriage.

Amnion: Protective membrane surrounding the sac of amniotic fluid.

Amniotic fluid: Clear, straw-coloured fluid contained within a sac (the amnion). It surrounds your baby, cushioning him, hydrating him, and keeping him at the right temperature.

Apgar test: Your baby's first test! It's a method of evaluating a baby's health immediately after birth. There are five basic indicators: activity level, pulse, response to stimulation, appearance, and respiration. The baby is given a score of 0, 1, or 2 on each and the scores are added up to give an overall mark out of 10.

Areola: Pink or brown area of skin around your nipple, which darkens during pregnancy. If you are

"If you don't understand what is written in your notes, ask your midwife – he or she is there to help."

breastfeeding, your baby needs to latch on to the areola as well as the nipple, as it contains numerous little milk ducts that squirt out milk.

Birth canal: Passage from the cervix that your baby travels through to be born, once known as your vagina!

Blastocyst: Cluster of 100 cells that develops from the fertilized egg and implants itself into the lining of your uterus. The cells develop into all the different parts of your baby, as well as the placenta.

Braxton Hicks contractions:

Practice makes perfect and your uterus warms up with mild contractions as early as the second trimester; so-called because Dr Braxton Hicks was the first person to describe them in 1872. They can cause confusion – is this labour or not? – but these contractions stop; real ones don't until your baby is born. If you aren't sure if these are the real thing, call the midwife.

Breech presentation: Baby is head-up and wants to come out bottom or feet first. A midwife might try to turn the baby in the womb but if this is unsuccessful, you may be advised to have a C-section. It is possible for a baby to turn during contractions, and some are born in a breech position.

Caesarean section (C-section):

When your baby is delivered through an incision in the abdominal and uterine walls. Caesareans can be elective (chosen) or emergency (unplanned but can be life-saving).

Cardiac output: Amount of blood your heart pumps around the body with each heartbeat – this goes into overdrive during pregnancy.

Cephalic position: When the baby is lying vertically in the womb, head-down. An ideal position for labour.

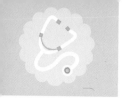

Cervix: Lower portion of the uterus extending into the vagina. Your cervix is sealed during pregnancy to protect the baby from invading bacteria, but when birth is imminent it gradually opens up to let the baby's head through.

Chorion: Outermost membrane around the embryo from which tiny fingers (villi) burrow into the wall of your uterus to tap into your blood circulation and grow the placenta.

Chromosomes: Cellular structures that contain genes.

Circadian rhythm: Internal clock that governs heart rate, breathing, temperature, and hormone levels over 24 hours. It takes your baby a while to sort out which activities are appropriate for day and night.

Colostrum: Thick, yellow liquid secreted by your breasts shortly before and a few days after childbirth, before your milk comes in. It's marvellously rich in nutrients and antibodies and gives breastfed babies a great start.

Corpus luteum: Translates as "yellow body". This is what's left of the ovary follicle that released the egg that was fertilized. It pumps out progesterone to keep the embryo embedded until the placenta takes over.

Crowning: Point in labour when the head of the baby is seen at the vaginal opening. Get ready to meet your baby!

Dilation: Gradual opening of the cervix during the first "latent" stage of labour. Your midwife will check how dilated your cervix is – 10cm (4in) is the target, when your baby can start moving down the birth canal. Then you can begin pushing.

Doppler: A device for listening to a baby's heart or blood-flow through uterine arteries, based on ultrasound.

"Approximately 80 per cent of infants are born with some form of birthmark."

Engaged: When your baby has moved down and two-fifths of his head is in position above your pelvic bone. Usually a sign that labour is imminent.

Engorgement: When your breasts are so full of milk they get hard, hot, and feel like they might explode. This happens when your milk comes in, usually between days two and six post birth. Feeding brings instant relief.

Episiotomy: Cut made in the perineum and wall of the vagina during childbirth to make more space for baby to be born. Surgery is required to repair the cut.

Fontanelle: Gaps where the three bones of a baby's skull meet. The space allows the bones to slide over each other as the skull compresses on its journey through the birth canal.

Human placental lactogen (hPL): Similar to a growth hormone, hPL modifies a pregnant woman's metabolic state to supply sufficient energy to her growing baby.

Lanugo: Fine layer of fluffy hair that covers your baby from about 20 weeks; it falls out by your due date.

Linea nigra: Dark line that develops between your pubic bone and navel thanks to increased numbers of pigment-bearing cells.

Lochia: Post-birth discharge like a period, made up of blood, mucus, tissue, and clots. You will need maternity pads.

Meconium: Buildup of green-black waste in your baby's intestine that emerges as the first poo. Very sticky!

Melasma: Dark, uneven patches of skin on your cheeks, forehead, nose, and chin. Sunbathing makes it worse.

Montgomery's tubercles: Enlarged sebaceous glands around your areola

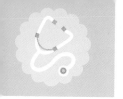

producing antibacterial oil to keep your skin clean and smooth.

Oedema: Swelling caused by water retention and blood pooling in your lower body. In rare cases this can be a sign of pre-eclampsia, so any puffiness should be mentioned to a doctor.

Oestrogen: Hormone, levels of which rise rapidly in the first weeks of pregnancy, thickening the lining of the uterus, swelling breasts, and keeping hair and nails in a growth phase.

Oxytocin: Hormone that triggers the uterus to start contracting in the first stage of labour. If you are very overdue, you may be given an extra dose of synthetic oxytocin via a drip.

Perineum: Area between the opening of your vagina and anus. You contract and release the sling-shaped muscles here when you do pelvic-floor exercises. Helps with bladder control.

Placenta: An organ that grows in the uterus to connect your baby to your bloodstream. It supplies baby with oxygen and nutrients, as well as removing waste.

Progesterone: Hormone that prepares the uterus lining for implantation; it also relaxes your ligaments and blood vessels.

Prolactin: Hormone that stimulates milk production.

Prostaglandin: Hormone that facilitates the contraction of the uterus in labour.

Quickening: The first sensations of your baby moving. Generally felt for the first time at around 20 weeks.

Sonographer: Medical professional who operates ultrasonic imaging devices.

Spider naevi: Tiny new veins noticeable on your cheeks, breasts, and legs, required to help your body disperse the extra heat your growing baby requires.

> *"Many cultures encourage a confinement period after birth, when mum rests and is looked after."*

Startle reflex: Also known as the Moro reflex. Newborns are tested for this reflex to check that the nervous system is working. He will fling his arms outwards, arch backwards, lift his head, and cry.

Striae gravidarum: The official term for stretch marks. Caused by tiny tears in the fibres of the dermis layer as skin expands quickly to accommodate your growing baby, breasts, and butt. Think of them as well-earned stripes.

Surfactant: An important elasticating fluid that coats the walls of the alveoli. It is essential for lung expansion as your baby first breathes in air after birth.

Syntocinon: Synthetic form of oxytocin, given to induce or strengthen contractions if you are overdue.

Tear (in the perineum): Up to 90 per cent of women experience a tear during delivery. First-degree tears in the skin heal naturally, second-degree tears extend into the muscle, requiring stitches. Third- and fourth-degree tears affect the anal canal or rectum and require surgery; this affects around 9 per cent of women.

Transverse position: When a baby is lying sideways in the womb, head on one side and bottom on the other. Usually baby will move of his own accord; however, if he remains transverse a C-section may be needed.

Ultrasound: A scan that produces your baby's first image! A hand-held device (transducer) is applied to your abdomen by a sonographer and the sound waves visualize the baby on a screen. It is used to estimate baby's due date and check for abnormalities.

Vernix caseosa: White, waxy coating that covers your baby from about 18 weeks while in the womb.

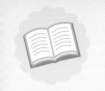

INDEX

C

Caesarean (C-section) births 61, 164, 174–81
bonding after 177
dads and 180–1
elective 174, 177, 181
emergency 174, 176
older mums 63
premature babies 124
reasons for 175
recovery 178–9, 181
stitches and scars 178, 179, 181
caffeine 29, 47, 127, 206, 223
calcium 19, 31, 33, 81, 127, 217
candidiasis 233
cardiac output 17, 46, 83, 128
cardiovascular exercise 78, 210, 211, 213
carpal tunnel syndrome 120, 228
cataracts 185, 205, 232
catecholamines 163
cervix
dilation 145, 160, 161, 162, 164, 165, 167, 169, 172
mucus plug 17, 154
"sweep" 152, 164
chickenpox 228
childcare 99, 206–7
chloasma 67
chromosomes 20, 21
circadian rhythms 102, 135
clothes
baby clothes 23, 136, 150–1

bras 32, 50, 91, 143, 193
during labour 115, 122
maternity clothes 69, 90–1
club foot 185
clumsiness 74
colostrum 143, 190
conception 20–1, 24, 35
constipation 17, 32, 61, 112, 120, 190
contractions 145, 153, 155, 157, 160–3, 164, 167, 172
Braxton Hicks contractions 127, 129, 143, 155
corticotropin-releasing hormone (CRH) 114, 115
cortisol 134, 144
Couvade syndrome 49
cradle cap 186, 198
cramps 33, 113, 126, 127
crowning 161, 225
crying 188, 194–5, 205

D

dads
antenatal classes 140–1
birth partners 141, 172–3
bonding with your baby 173, 206
and C-sections 180–1
financial planning 110–1, 127
getting involved 49, 94, 111, 126, 127, 140–1, 156–7, 206–7
paternity leave 110–1, 207, 234–5
phantom pregnancy 49

worries 126–7
dating scan 12, 58–9, 64, 65
deep vein thrombosis (DVT) 106, 107, 178, 229
dehydration 32, 211, 230
depression 114, 201, 202–3
diabetes 27, 60, 63, 230
diet
breastfeeding 201
calorific requirements 47, 131, 135
food cravings 33, 36
food hazards 28, 29, 222
healthy balanced diet 28–31, 37, 44, 207
dizziness 51, 105
Down's syndrome 58
dropsy 97
due date see Estimated Date of Delivery (EDD)
dysplasia 185, 205

E

early signs of pregnancy 16
ectopic pregnancy 229
eczema 190
eggs 16, 20, 35, 62, 95, 134
eggs in diet 29, 51, 217
embryos 17, 21, 22, 23
endorphins 45, 160, 226
entonox 227
epidurals 138, 139, 167, 180, 227
episiotomy 224
equipment, baby
baby's wardrobe 77, 150–1
basic kit 77, 92–3
big-ticket items 110, 127, 136

Acknowledgments

The authors and consultant on this book include an experienced midwife, as well as writers who specialize in pregnancy and birth. More importantly, they are all mums who have enjoyed happy and healthy pregnancies.

Our consultant

Judith Barac

Judith's belief that a woman's psychological well-being is of equal importance to physical well-being during pregnancy has led her through different areas of midwifery practice. Since 1997 Judith has consolidated her interests in the field of perinatal mental health; she is currently working as a midwife, a private psychotherapist, and a perinatal psychotherapist. Judith lives in London with her husband and youngest son.

Our team of writers

Shaoni Bhattacharya

Shaoni is a consultant for New Scientist magazine and has written for various newspapers and magazines, including Psychologies, and the weekly magazine for family doctors, Pulse. Shaoni has a degree in biology from University College London. She lives in London with her husband, son, and daughter.

Claire Cross

Claire is an editor and copywriter who has worked extensively in the field of health, pregnancy, and child development. During her career she has worked with a wide range of medical professionals. She also co-authored New Mother's Guide. Claire lives in London with her husband and son.

Elinor Duffy

Elinor has been a writer and editor of Dorling Kindersley books for over ten years, working closely with experts in their field. Elinor has three children, born in three different hospitals, and is the alumni of many a baby group! She lives on a farm in rural Hertfordshire with her family.

Kate Ling

Kate has an MA in Creative Writing, and is a regular Mumsnet blogger. She published her first e-book, Bad Roads, in 2012, and also writes, researches, and edits non-fiction and web content. She is married with two daughters.

Susannah Marriott

Susannah is a writer who specializes in pregnancy, babycare, and complementary health. As well as writing over 20 books, her work has appeared in prominent magazines and newspapers, on BBC Radio 4, and on babyexpert.com, mumknowsbest.co.uk, and gather.com. Susannah lives in Cornwall with her husband and daughters.

Dorling Kindersley would also like to thank the following contributors: Proofreader: Angela Baynham and Indexer: Maria Lorimer.

Picture credits

Photography: Claire Cordier for the kind permission to reproduce her photographs: (p.10) Yew Hedge Maze at Longleat House, Wiltshire; (p.17) Bends Ahead road sign and empty road, Valley of Fire State Park, Nevada, USA; and Sadie Thomas for using her 12-week antenatal scan (p.59). All additional photographs © by Dorling Kindersley.

Praise for *The Bees*:

'[A] gripping Cinderella/Arthurian tale with lush Keatsian adjectives'
MARGARET ATWOOD

'Beautifully written and unusual ... a brave and original story that highlights our modern environmental crimes'
LUCY ATKINS, *Sunday Times*

'Ambitious and bold ... told with such rapturously attentive imagination ... few novels create such a singular reading experience. The buzz you will hear surrounding this book and its astonishing author is utterly deserved'
New York Times

'One wild ride. A sensual, visceral mini-epic about timeless rituals and modern environmental disaster. Paull's heart-pounding novel wrenches us into a new world'
EMMA DONOGHUE

'A rich, strange book, utterly convincing in its portrayal of the mindset of a bee and a hive. I finished it feeling I knew exactly how bees think and live. This is what sets us humans apart from other animals, that our imagination can allow us to create a complete, believable world so different from our own'
TRACY CHEVALIER

'An astonishing achievement'
MARTIN CRUZ SMITH

'An extraordinary feat of imagination, conjuring the life of a beehive in gripping, passionate and brilliant detail'
MADELINE MILLER, author of *The Song of Achilles*

'[An] unusual and cunningly imagined thriller ... thought-provoking'
ANGUS CLARKE, *The Times*

'Violent and full of terror, but there are moments of luscious beauty, too'
Telegraph

'There's sex, violence, war, catastrophe, terror, secrets and suspense. A clever and imaginative work'
Independent on Sunday

LALINE PAULL

THE ICE

4th ESTATE • London

4th Estate
An imprint of HarperCollinsPublishers
1 London Bridge Street
London SE1 9GF
www.4thEstate.co.uk

First published in Great Britain in 2017 by 4th Estate

1

With grateful thanks to the following for their permission to reproduce copyright material:
Extracts from Arctic Adventure by Peter Freuchen by permission of Echo Point Books.
Extracts from Farthest North by Fridtjof Nansen by permission of Skyhorse Publishing, Inc.
Extracts from Lost in the Arctic by Einar Mikkelsen, published by William Heinemann. Reprinted by
permission of The Random House Group Ltd. © Einar Mikkelsen 1913. Extract from Polar Bears by
Nikita Ovsyanikov by permission of Quarto Publishing Group. Quote from Judge Rüdiger Wolfrum
courtesy of the International Tribunal for the Law of the Sea. Extract from 'Century of the Wind' from
The Wayfinders: Why Ancient Wisdom Matters in the Modern World, copyright © 2009 by Wade Davis
and the Canadian Broadcasting Corporation. Reprinted by permission of House of Anansi Press,
Toronto, www.houseofanansi.com, and the University of Western Australia Press. Extract from Northern Lights:
The Official Account Of The British Arctic Air-Route Expedition by F. Spencer Chapman, published by
Chatto & Windus. Reprinted by permission of The Random House Group Limited.

Printed and bound in Great Britain by
Clays Ltd, St Ives plc

MIX
Paper from
responsible sources
FSC FSC° C007454
www.fsc.org

FSC™ is a non-profit international organization established to promote
the responsible management of the world's forests. Products carrying the
FSC label are independently certified to assure consumers that they come
from forests that are managed to meet the social, economic and
ecological needs of present and future generations,
and other controlled sources.

Find out more about HarperCollins and the environment at
www.harpercollins.co.uk/green

For my brothers

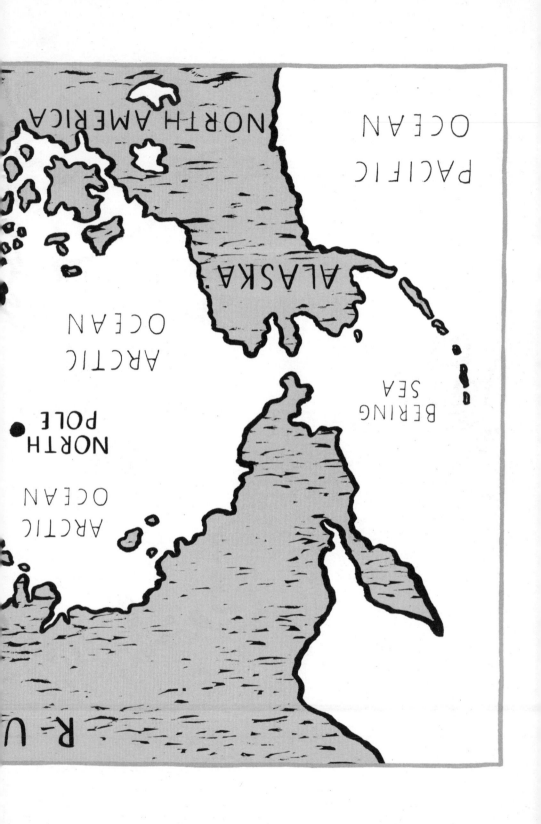

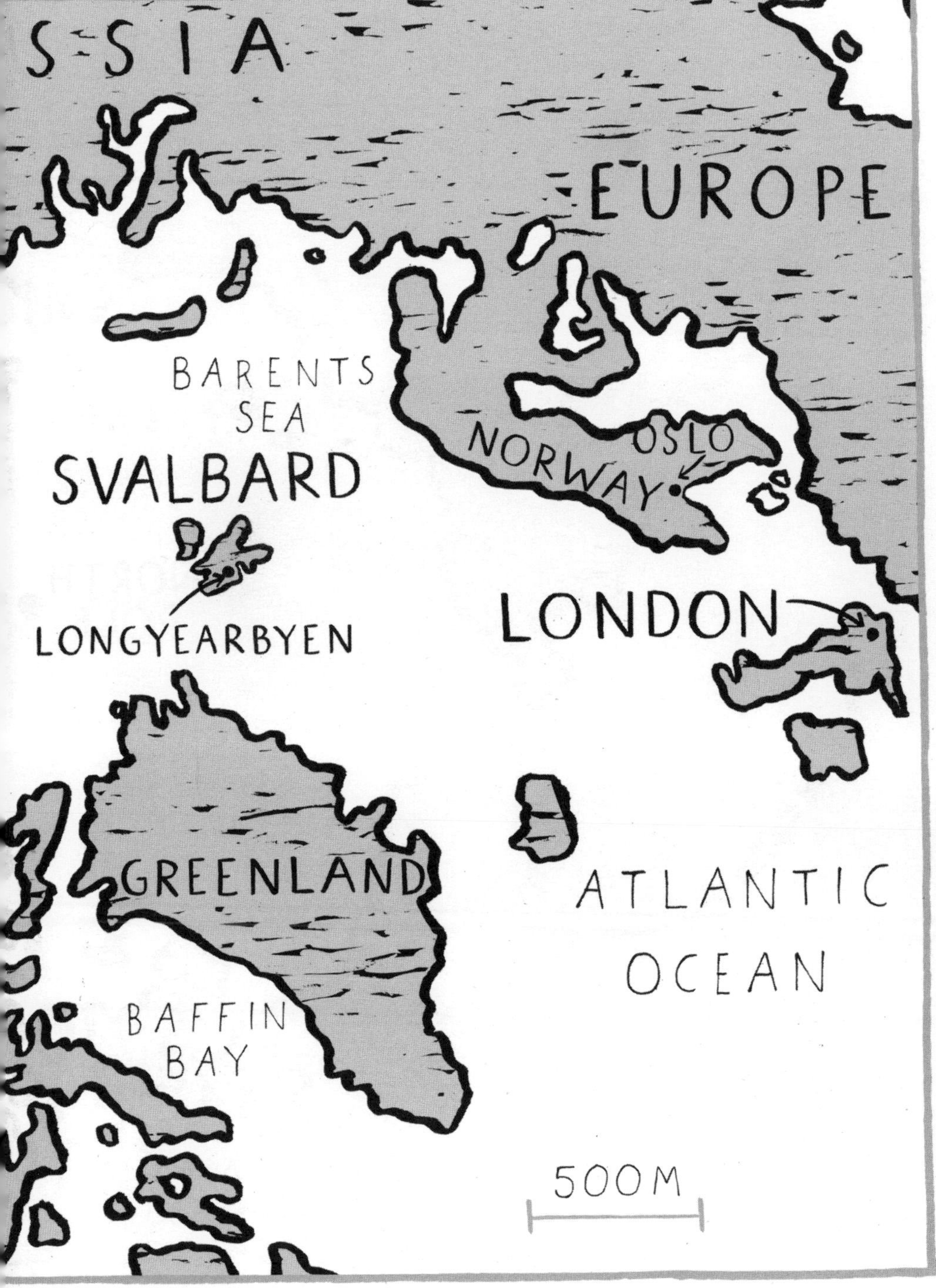

500M

ATLANTIC OCEAN

BAFFIN BAY

GREENLAND

LONDON

LONGYEARBYEN

OSLO

NORWAY

SVALBARD

BARENTS SEA

EUROPE

RUSSIA

Among dogs are found characters almost as various as among men. Some dogs do not give a damn what they eat; some will eat their own mothers, as I have often witnessed, and others will starve to death before touching the bodies of their team-mates. Again, some refuse to eat the meat while it is still warm, but perhaps after it is cold they forget what it is and devour it greedily.

Arctic Adventure: My Life in the Frozen North (1936)
Peter Freuchen

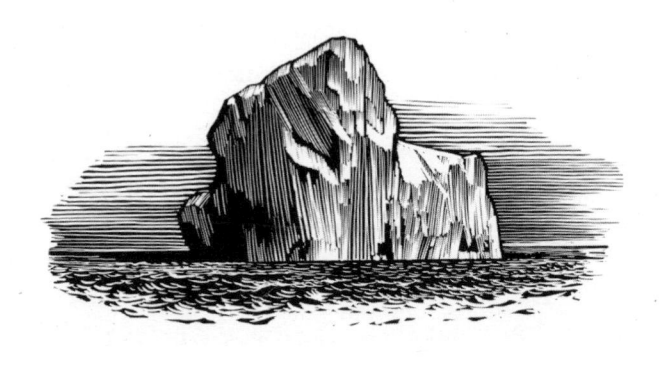

1

They were rich, they were ready, they were ravenous for bear. Nine days into their fourteen-day voyage on the *Vanir*, the most expensive cruise ship in the Arctic, the passengers' initial excitement had turned to patience, then frustration, and now, a creeping sense of defeat. As sophisticated travellers they knew money didn't guarantee polar bear sightings – but they still believed in the natural law that wealth meant entitlement. *Ursus maritimus* sightings very much included.

'Realm of the Ice King' stated the brochure, featuring competition-winning photographs of sparkling ice and polar bears with cubs and kills, taken by recent passengers on this very route. But now instead of high blue heavens, the skies were overcast. Instead of a crisp and exhilarating minus three or even ten degrees (they were eager to test their new clothing), they suffered a vile gusty swelter that turned the Arctic dank as an English summer, and for which no combination of clothing was right. Plus the endless daylight was oppressive – medication schedules went awry and it was always and never time for a coffee to wake up, or a drink to ease down.

There were several lawyers among the passengers. They invited the tour leader to the bar to look at the brochure and hear their formal complaint. The voyage was misrepresented. They had been mis-sold. Enough with the beach landings to stare at derelict huts and piles of whaling junk. Enough birds too, that didn't fob them off. What they'd all paid for were sightings of live ice-obligate mammals. That was the primary focus of the text and image of the brochure, a sales document with a legal duty to accuracy. No icebergs either, just some dirty glaciers. They were considering a class action for compensation of time and money.

The passengers repaired to the salon and put on the compilation film that had become their envious obsession. In this footage, recent and very much more fortunate passengers had seen all the wildlife the Arctic could offer, from vast haul-outs of walrus, to pods of various whales so close you could see the barnacles on the fins. But most of all, they had seen the great apex predator, the polar bear.

With the blinds down to keep out the bullying daylight, the passengers stared avidly at the on-screen polar bears; the one standing on a crimson mat of ice ripping flesh from a red rack of seal carcass, then the mother and her yearling swimming between the floes. Best of all was the large male standing on his hind legs, staring into the camera, his muzzle bright red. *That* was what they wanted.

The tour leader ran to the bridge to confer with the captain and the ice-pilot, who by law they were still required to employ, even though the summer sea ice was two years gone. They stared out at the grey chop of the Barents Sea. All knew, though they would not say for fear of their jobs, that the animals had all but vanished and the footage in the salon was several years old. There was one solution, prohibited, but every tour company knew it as a last resort. Send up a drone and find a bear.

Two miles away around the coast, down a deep M-shaped fjord, a large silvery wood cabin blended with the dark cobble of its beach. Modern extensions at its rear and sides were made of the very rock of the mountain that rose up behind it, and a close look would reveal several windows that reflected sea, sky and rock. But no one did look, in that intrusive unwelcome way, because this was Midgard Lodge in Midgardfjorden, and by direct intervention of Oslo, to the Sysselmann's office in Svalbard, special rules applied.

Most outraging to those who knew of it, was the one which flouted a major conservation regulation and allowed Midgard Lodge occasional helicopter flights between Longyearbyen airport and the tiny beach in front of the Lodge, which was just large enough to land a twelve-person Dauphin.

The second was that no cruise ship penetrate the Wijdefjorden system past a certain point, thereby closing the spectacular rock stratification of Midgardfjord and its peculiar forked glacier Midgardbreen, one side blue, one white, off to tourism.

The third, which caused the autocratic Sysselmann the most disquiet, was that these diktats were verified at the highest level but relayed verbally, via a female assistant defence minister. She refused to confirm them in writing and though the Sysselmann had not heard of her, she was rather too well informed about him. She reassured him that the one occasion when cupidity had got the better of him, was not significant at all. His record was otherwise spotless, his patriotism unquestioned, and he could rely on her appreciation at the end of his tenure. The Sysselmann duly made sure Mrs Larssen's requests were observed, and in consequence, Midgard Lodge was not.

Except for today, when general manager Danny Long, on duty in the cabin office looking down the fjord, felt his instinct tweak him to take another look at the AIS radar screen. He had just checked it at mid-scale, taking in the little coloured arrowheads that showed, variously, pink and purple for fishing and sailing vessels, green for cargo, and god forbid, red for tankers coming in too close. He looked at the screen more closely. He could feel something was off.

He clicked on the green arrows and saw what he expected – Asian cargo ships on the new TransPolar route. He clicked a couple at random: the *Hao Puren*: Rotterdam to Shanghai. The *Zheng He*, going the other way, Dalian to Algiers. A couple of others – everything moving smoothly.

Then he studied the dotted blue arrows of the cruise ships. Now the ice-free and liquid North Pole was just another bit of sea and offered no photo opportunities, Svalbard's stunning coastline was clogged in the summer. All captains tried to stagger their route to minimise bottlenecks, but because of the rarity of animal sightings, the tour operators had an agreement to share the information with each other on Channel 16 – despite this leading to what amounted to a cruise ship race to be second at the kill. The coastguard policed what it could, and was glad of Midgard Lodge's ability to offer search and rescue – but both knew that would be a last resort.

There: he saw it. The tiny blue cursor which had crossed into Midgard's unofficially restricted area. He clicked. Passenger cruise ship *Vanir*, he knew it. High staff-to-passenger ratio, regular circuit – except today. Probably after a bear. There was a huge male passing through, he'd seen it standing in silhouette on the fjord's bone.

He would report the ship's transgression later, but for now the protocol was to ensure front-of-house was neat and clean, everything quiet. Keeping an eye on the *Vanir*'s position, he hit a speed-dial on the iridium phone never far from his hand. A moment later, the phone flashed back at him. Message received, they would stay out until further notice. Then Long called down to reception and was pleased to hear everything was in hand. He returned to the screen, watching the little blue cursor slowly blinking around the headland, coming closer.

When the bear was young and the snow fell clean and white, his fur showed creamy, even pale yellow at times. Now the snow had a grey-ish tinge, causing him to shine even brighter against it. He had grown long yellow guard hairs on his massive forelegs, increasing his appearance of power, and when the sun shone through them it gave him a gold aura. He was following the scented track of a female in oestrus who had passed by, but paused to watch the ship heaving into the narrow mouth of the fjord, its engine thundering the water, its fuel stinking the air.

The deck was crowded with people, bare-skinned faces with shiny black insect eyes turned towards him. Their human body smells mingled with the smell of food from the ship, and metal, and fuel. The engine sound died down and the vibrations slowed then stopped. The voices faded.

The black walls of the fjord held the Arctic silence, until the bear lifted his white anvil of a head, black nostrils flaring for more information. His every move drew clicks and whirrs from the ship, becoming a frenzy as a curl of wind tickled him with a clue, and he lay down and rolled in the female's trail.

On the bridge with the captain, the tour leader looked down at the entranced passengers, and relaxed. The bear was massive by any standards and on the most photogenic port side of the Midgardbreen glacier, where the ice terminus was blue and formed a cliff above the water. On the other side of the black bone of rock, the glacier was younger white ice and debouched in a relatively gentle slope down to the cobbled beach. With a start, the tour operator noticed the silver-grey wood cabin, extending back into the mountain.

'Is this the British guy's place? I heard it'd been sold – what goes on here?' Neither the Norwegian captain nor ice-pilot replied. They had crossed a line to find her passengers their bear. Svalbard had many enigmatic structures. No comment.

Crowded at the rail, excited as schoolchildren and all thoughts of class actions gone from their minds, the passengers of the *Vanir* were busy changing lenses and exclaiming in wonder. The bear was as huge and charismatic a celebrity as they could dream of, they guessed him at eleven or twelve feet, nearly a ton, maybe more. Through powerful telephoto lenses they saw his duelling scars, and the way he stood up on his hind legs, the edge of his pelt shining gold around him. He stared straight back with knowing black eyes, and they felt a euphoric jolt of fear. He could kill them.

Without warning the white god dropped to all fours and changed into a frightened animal, running for the edge of the glacier. In consternation the passengers watched him stagger and clamber to where the jagged peaks threw knives of shadow. They groaned in disappointment, they scanned around for what had scared their bear, but though their hi-mag lenses probed the darkness of the lower crags and pored across the bright rock striations that pulsed strange colours, nothing moved. They stared at the layers of rock and tried to appreciate the earth's history laid bare. But they felt angry and tiny.

Someone shouted out: there! that puff of snow higher up the glacier – surely too far and they had not seen him run – but they focused in hope. They gasped in wonder as a hundred hidden chimneys below the surface puffed out more sparkling ice-smoke. The air clenched and the sea sighed. The *Vanir* lifted as a great pressure wave passed through the water.

And then it started. First a distant boom, a detonation deep inside the glacier. Nothing, for a few long seconds, then a huge tearing, cracking sound that shook the air, before time stretched and the blue snout of the glacier, sliding belly down from the ice cap, moaned and pushed out over the water, a blue bulge of ice filled with energy – and then with thunderous bangs like car-crashes it exploded all along its front, hurling shards of ice into the air and seismic bursts into the water so that the reinforced steel hull of the *Vanir* vibrated with the charge.

Wraiths of glittering ice-dust drifted over the sea. The passengers gripped each other as the *Vanir* lifted and fell again, and the shards of ice so small as they splashed, rolled out into the fjord as icebergs tall as the ship.

And then, as they watched, something happened that made no sense at all.

In front of the still-shuddering glacier, an invisible hand pinched a fold of sea like cloth then pulled it high into the air in a fistful of waterfalls. Out of the dazzling torrent something bright turquoise blue emerged: a great sapphire castle with turrets and minarets, throwing sparkling foam and mist as it cleared the water for one long stupendous second.

All of the passengers on the *Vanir* screamed and shouted as their eyes brimmed with wonders – some saw the streak of gold glowing deep within the frozen blue, some the detail of the minarets, some saw gargoyles' faces in the ice – but their voices were lost in the roaring sound as the vision leaned and fell, making a great bowl of the sea in which it twisted and rolled over, completely inverting itself.

All they saw now was a dark blue ice floe the size of an ice-rink, its pinnacles and spires forever hidden. Like a sentient thing, it glided towards the *Vanir*, a peculiar ridge of water pushing the ship aside as if to clear its way. Unearthly and real, the great dark floe followed the other icebergs out towards the mouth of Midgardfjorden, and the open sea beyond.

The passengers of the *Vanir* had no more words, but one of them, Trudie Burke, was making a convulsive, almost sexual sound. Oh, she kept whispering, still filming everything, the calving ongoing within her. Her lens followed the newborn icebergs, the whirling eddies in the water, and back to the glacier face. She filmed the water slapping and rocking at its base, and the cave of deepening blue ice where the water surged and circled. Something swirled at its centre, making the current waver. Something that had not been there a moment ago.

Without taking her eye from the viewfinder, she reached out a hand for her husband. She pulled him towards her and gave him the camera, still recording. She pointed to the red shape rocking just below the surface.

'John,' she said softly, 'is that a body?'

There is one place on the coast of which they stood in some dread –
the great glacier of Puisortok. Travelling in early summer in their
umiaks, they necessarily hug the coast, and utilize the narrow leads
that exist between the pack-ice and the glacier. The literal meaning
of the name is "the thing that comes up", as this peculiar glacier
often calves by huge pieces breaking off underwater, which come to
the top and shoot like breaching whales into the air. Instant
destruction is the penalty for misjudgement or mere bad luck.

I remember an old hunter saying: "Do not speak, do not eat, until
Puisortok is passed."

Northern Lights: The Official Account of the British Arctic Air-Route
Expedition 1930–31 (1932)
Frederick Spencer Chapman

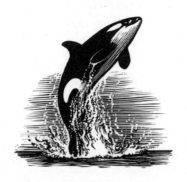

2

The calving of the Midgard glacier was a tiny stitch in a larger pattern. While the male corpse it disgorged was already in Tromsø and under autopsy, all around the Arctic Circle scientists were recording calving events of unprecedented magnitude. This apparently synchronised new behaviour of the ice was strongly active for about seventy hours in Greenland, Nunavut Arctic Canada, Alaska and Russia, before stopping as abruptly as it started.

Twenty-seven degrees south in London, the Saharan dust storm that had blown over Europe for the last three days also ceased, leaving a fine gritty red film on cars smart and shabby, on the window sills of palaces and high-rises and added respiratory patients to overcrowded A&E departments and private surgeries alike. Entrepreneurial Londoners sold white paper masks by tube stations and only the reckless still went running.

Age fifty (but looking younger) and mindful of what happened to his mental state without hard exercise, Sean Cawson was one of them. Although his knees now protested and his thoughts clawed at him for the first two or three miles, afterwards he felt good, and that was rare. He left Martine sleeping, or pretending to, and slipped out of the apartment. He knew last night's conversation was only on pause. He would have to deal with it before long.

He jogged past the neighbour's door, smelling coffee and hearing their new baby crying. His was almost grown up, and hated him. At

11

the beginning, Martine had said she wasn't interested in family life, and he'd been relieved: one failure was enough. Now she'd changed her mind, and he felt slightly betrayed.

He pulled the heavy black door shut and stood for a moment on the empty street while he chose his running music. It was early but muggy, the sky was grey and no birds flew. The white porch pillars of the houses were shaded with the ochre Saharan dust, which also grouted the black and white tiles underfoot and gave an autumnal cast to the plane trees of the communal garden. As he chose a random mix and set off to the park, London looked and felt wrong.

The music matched it – harsh declamatory rap in African-inflected French that fitted the dislocated feel of the city. His feet caught the hard pounding rhythm and as he entered the park by the Kensington Palace gate he felt fierce and strong. The grass was browned with dust as if it had been passed under some great grill, and he left a trail rising behind him. If there was a good gym he might have used it, but the kind of place he had in mind, that stank of effort and crackled with energy – those places belonged to a distant world.

The water of the Serpentine was a dull grey mirror to the June sky. Sean's lungs and muscles were burning, but his will was breaking through his resistance. As if in reward, there ahead of him was one of his favourite sights, one of the privileges of early risers in certain parts of London: a troupe of army horses being exercised. Sometimes he'd pause to watch them cantering on the sand track that ran alongside Park Lane, a powerful river of satiny chestnut and bay muscle. The heavy rhythmic vibration of their hooves into the earth had risen through his feet into his body and connected him to some elusive feeling he could not name – but today he knew it. That lost feeling of wildness inside him, like a wolf hunting.

It was a crazy thought and the horses would easily outstrip him, but he wanted to run alongside them. He pushed himself harder, the punching syllables of the French rap synching with his muscles. He could smell the fragrance of the animals as he cut across the grass, he was straining with the effort but in his mind he was a wolf cutting them off as they turned on the sand track for their canter – he would sprint and burn himself out until they left him behind—

His phone buzzed from his arm holster. There were only two people he set to bypass his Do Not Disturb – his estranged daughter Rosie, who never called, and the other whose name now flashed on the screen, his mentor Joe Kingsmith.

'Joe!' he panted. 'I'll call you back. I'm doing something crazy ...' The riders were gathering up their horses, the animals were stamping, knowing what was coming.

'Don't, Sean, stay: it's an emergency.'

Sean stopped short.

'Joe, I'm here. What's happened? Are you hurt?'

'Me? No. Sean, are you home?'

'I'm in the park – what's happened?'

'Sean boy, I'd have called you at home but no one has a landline any more. I want someone there with you.'

Sean stood still. 'Tell me.'

There was a silence, and by its quality, Sean guessed Kingsmith was airborne. He tried to slow his breathing.

'Sean, I am so, so sorry. I've just spoken with Danny at Midgard. Tom's body washed out of the Midgard glacier two days ago—'

'What?' Sean heard the words clearly, but his mind rejected them.

'They had the positive ID this morning. It's definitely him. I'm so sorry, Sean. I wanted to be the one to tell you.'

The park vanished. Sean's world contracted to the rumble of Kingsmith's voice. 'Out of the glacier?' He felt stupid and slow.

'Shit. I knew I shouldn't have told you on the phone, but how else?'

Sean stared like a blind man. 'No, it's fine. Tell me everything.'

'I don't know that much. There was this huge calving almost in front of Midgard Lodge – that's when his body came out. Some cruise ship was down there and saw it all. Danny got sent away by the coastguard when he went to look, they were holding it as a crime scene—'

'A crime scene?' Sean came back into his body. 'There was no *crime*, everyone knows that!' He was shouting but he couldn't do anything about it.

'Sean boy, I'm trying to tell you, will you please listen? They call it that for protocol when they want to record everything. Of course there was no crime. Now I know you haven't been up there for a while, but Midgard is still a business and this could have a PR effect, so we need to handle it right.'

'They're sure it's Tom?'

'One hundred per cent. They had a good idea it could be and they matched DNA with a family member, apparently.'

'No one told me. No one's rung. They've known for two days?'

'I guess you haven't been in touch so much lately. We knew he was dead but … this is still a big shock.' Kingsmith paused. 'Sean?'

Sean walked away from the people coming towards him, out onto the great grassy plain of the park, the horses forgotten. 'Yes. We knew.' He sank to his knees on the dusty red grass.

'Sean.' Kingsmith's voice was kinder, quieter. 'Without a body to mourn, people are in limbo. They can't move on.'

Sean felt the fingers in his right hand start to burn, as if they still had frostbite. He stuffed them into his left armpit. He was shaking, but not from cold.

'Danny should have called me.'

'I wanted to be the one. I only know because I had to call him about something.'

'What thing?'

'Look: I completely get why you haven't been up there. But you've got a lot of catching up to do, and now isn't the right time. I'm glad you're interested again, but you've got an awesome team taking care of things so don't even worry right now.'

'I should be helping bring him back, I should be there.'

'You can't do anything: it's all in progress. You weren't next of kin, but I guess they'll be in touch with you, they'll be able to have a funeral at last. And an inquest, but that's separate.'

'An *inquest*?' The word was so ugly. 'But we know what happened, I've said it all, we've been through it.'

'I know, but it's what happens when someone's brought home. Same in the States as in the UK – just a formality. I'll be there to support you, I promise … Sean, can you hear me?'

'Yes.' The grey sky pulsed above him.

'You get yourself home, get back to Martine. She's got a good head on her shoulders, she'll know what to do. Sean, say something.'

'What were you talking to Danny about?'

He heard Kingsmith's bark of a laugh.

'Boy, are you persistent! But I've always liked that. OK, mea culpa, I put in a retreat, very small and last minute, a favour for a pal. I saw a void in the schedule and he's paying top dollar. But this is hardly the time—'

'I'm still the CEO. Everything goes through me.'

'And if you are thinking like that at a time like this, you are the right man for the job. Point taken. Sean? You're breaking up but I hope you can still hear me: you need to speak to your friend in Oslo, about keeping traffic away from Midgard – it's important—'

The phone connection dropped out – Kingsmith's signature good-bye – and the French rap blasted back into Sean's skull. He ripped out the earphones and found himself alone on the dusty red plain of Hyde Park, trembling and burning.

Martine was in the wet-room shower when he came in, sweat-soaked like it was raining. Still in his clothes, he walked into the torrent and held her. She smiled, her eyes closed – and then she looked and saw his stricken face.

'Oh my god, what's happened? Tell me – has something happened to Rosie?'

Sean hit his forehead against the streaming wall. 'They've found Tom.'

'Stop! Come here.' She held him to her, keeping them under the streaming hot water, undressing him until he was naked. She kicked the clothes away from the drain and held him until he stopped shaking, then she turned off the water and helped him out and into a robe. As she put on her own, he went into the kitchen. She followed, watching while he took a bottle of vodka from the freezer and poured a big slug into a tumbler.

'Don't,' she said. 'Handle it without that.'

He knocked it back. Then he told her, in the barest detail, about Kingsmith's call, and the facts he knew, including the fact of the inquest. Martine nodded slowly.

'I'm so sorry, my darling. But Joe's absolutely right: this is closure at last, and if there's an inquest we'll get through it. I need to plan how we handle it. First thing is I'll work on a statement on your behalf, and then we've got a bit of time.'

Sean listened to her as she walked around their dressing room preparing for work, thinking aloud. Joe was right, she had a good head on her well-set shoulders, working out which journalists could be trusted, how she would cancel certain invitations so they were not seen out enjoying themselves for a while …

He wished she had burst into tears. He wished she cared more about Tom, and less about damage control. Her voice went on as he stared at the rails of his clothes. Martine had shared her space very fairly, and everything was well spaced, perfectly clean, flatteringly lit like an expensive boutique. She had even had a library built in the hall for all his polar books. Abruptly she pushed her scarf drawer shut.

'What am I doing,' she said, 'dressing for work? I'm staying with you.'

'No,' he said, getting up. 'You go. I'll be OK.' He pulled open a deep drawer and took out his Arctic travelling clothes, now alien with lack of use. 'I'm going to Midgard. I booked a seat on the afternoon flight.'

Martine held his arm. 'That's crazy. You're in shock. Look at yourself.'

He did. The mirror showed him a beautiful young woman standing there half-dressed, her dark hair wet, beside an older man who stared back at him, eyes haunted and dangerous. Sean turned away.

'Joe put in a retreat. Without telling me.'

Martine frowned. 'Really? He shouldn't do that.'

'It's because I haven't been there. I've dumped everything on the team.'

'No. You've delegated. You can't personally run every single one of your clubs, you pick right then you trust people.'

Sean threw some clothes into the bag and zipped it. 'I'm letting everyone down.'

Martine tried again, embracing him and pressing herself into him from behind.

'You're not! Forget about last night, forget all that. Just come back to bed and let me look after you.' She ran her hand down his chest and closed it over him. 'Be sad in my arms. I won't go in today.'

'No, go. I'll be OK.' He kissed her, to deflect the rejection. She stared at him in the mirror as he went out into the bedroom and found his car key. She followed.

'You can't drive, you've just had a huge vodka. And if you're on the afternoon flight you've got plenty of time – where are you going?'

Sean looked out into the square garden.

'It's bad to hear it on the phone.'

'Oh. I see.' She moved away.

'Martine, please, you know how fragile she is.'

'Actually no, I don't think she is, not at all.'

'She loved Tom as well.'

'Fine. But I think she was prepared to pull any stunt to try to stop you leaving. I think she's manipulative and angry and she's turned your own daughter against you, and *me*, and it's totally a mistake to keep being sentimental about a marriage that was over long before I came along.' She sighed. 'I'm sorry. That sounded harsh. I just want to protect you from more pain at a time like this.'

'You're right.'

'Yes, I am. But if you don't want me to stay with you today, or to come with you to Midgard, if you want to just be alone with the bad feelings—'

He pressed her hand to his chest. 'Something's clawing inside me.'

'Maybe the slug of vodka at seven thirty in the morning.'

'Yes! I'm a fucking mess, I told you I was a bad deal—'

'I never make bad deals.' Martine pulled back and looked in his eyes. 'But I do know that if you want healthy boundaries you'll have them, and if you want to put yourself through the wringer, you'll do that too.' She kissed him on the lips. 'So I really care that you're so sad, but as you won't let me help you, I am going to work. Let me know when you're back. I'll be here.'

He listened to her light step down the outer hall, then the click of the front door. He went back to the freezer, but stopped. Martine was right, of course. He was in a terrible state. And if he was going to drive, he should not have another.

The easiest way to learn, of course, was to inquire of an angakoq (wizard), and in the course of my long conversations with Igjugarjuk I learned many interesting things. His theories, however, were so simple and straightforward that they sound strikingly modern; his whole view of life may be summed up in his own words as follows:

'All true wisdom is only to be learned far from the dwellings of men, out in the great solitudes; and is only to be attained through suffering. Privation and suffering are the only things that can open the mind of man to those things which are hidden from others.'

Across Arctic America: Narrative of the Fifth Thule Expedition (1927)
Knud Rasmussen

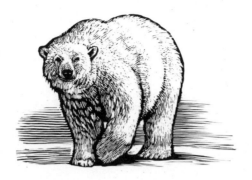

3

Sean once knew the sequence of lights so well that he never got caught on red. Now the route had become as alien as his old home and he misjudged every stretch. To keep his mind away from thoughts of Tom, he focused on driving impeccably and not as if he had gulped three fingers of vodka in the last hour – but the morning rush-hour traffic was infuriatingly slow and he suddenly felt self-conscious in his car.

It was a beautiful Aston Martin Vanquish in a custom missile-bronze colour, and part of its appeal three years ago – the longest he had ever kept a car – were the looks he caught as he flashed past other drivers. But today, passing slowly made him uncomfortable. Was it gaudy? Perhaps he should change it for a Tesla to show what a good, upright, ecologically concerned citizen he was, as well as a flash bastard. Perhaps he should get a personality transplant – but surely that was the point of alcohol.

Perhaps the lights were stuck. The white van alongside him made little feints forward, and he glanced over. Two schoolboys in green uniforms clambered over each other like puppies, waving at him and pointing in admiration of his car. They tugged at their driver dad, a tough-looking young man with a shaven head, who stared straight ahead.

Red-and-amber – the white van surged ahead the very instant the lights changed to green, and Sean saw the boys cheering and goading their father faster.

He drew alongside then fell back a couple of times, pulling faces as if he were striving and failing to overtake, so that the boys screeched with joy and bounced up and down on the bench seat. As he saw the filter lane for his exit, Sean pretended he was giving up, and the boys pumped their fists in triumph as he let the white van surge past him. The tough young dad flashed him a grin and he felt a wave of good feeling. Then he indicated, tipped the wheel and the feeling frayed like a thread as he wound back on the roads of his old life.

He drove slowly for the last few miles, surprised to see it had rained heavily. There was no sign of the red dust of London and the fields were green. The track to the house was badly potholed and he felt irritated – it wasn't as if Gail couldn't afford to get it graded. The thought of the settlement still pricked him. He would have been generous had she let him, instead of taking out her anger against Martine in financial terms. He had not thought her capable of being so petty. But put that aside: he was here to deliver a terrible blow. He knew he was also here to share its impact, with someone who cared.

Gail, I've got some bad news. Gail—

Something on the track ground against the undercarriage and he cursed and slowed down. He would go out the other way. The grading of the lane was not his business and this would be the last time he would come here, so it didn't matter. But still, his eye ran over the orchards in some dismay. The fruit was retarded and the leaves too heavy. All the rain without the sun.

Instead of the old blue Saab in the garage, there was a new silver BMW four-wheel drive. Only now did he consider the possibility that Gail might not have been home, or not been alone. He pulled up, blocking the garage, the way that always made them look out. And there she was, coming to the kitchen window. To his surprise, she waved. He walked down the path, hoping she had not got the wrong idea. No flowers, no bottle, a bad time of day to visit. He brought bad tidings of great pain. *Gail, I've got some bad news ...*

She opened the door before he knocked. One year younger than Sean, the glaze of youth had cracked into a filigree of lines around her

22

eyes. Her face was softening and dropping and she wore her clothes sexlessly loose. But she was still wearing perfume.

'Sean, I'm so sorry,' she said. 'Are you OK?'

'You know?' He stared at his ex-wife. 'How? I only just found out.'

'Ruth called me.' She stood back to let him in. 'Crack of dawn.' She almost smiled. 'Ruth Mott?'

'They told her first.' Sean was assaulted by the smell of home. The old oak floors and stairs, the extortionate beeswax polish. He noticed a bowl of orange roses on the table. 'You cut the Whisky Macs.' They always left them blooming on the path, for visitors to enjoy their scent.

'Saves them from the rain. Someone called her from Svalbard: Tom named her next of kin, apparently. But you already knew that.'

Sean touched a rose and its petals dropped. 'I don't remember every single detail of that time.'

'I do ... But they saw each other, didn't they? That one last time.'

'Yes, but I didn't realise she was officially ... next of kin.'

Sean disliked the idea of Ruth Mott relating her version of that last night. But that was the only way Gail could know, because at the time they were in the final throes of *nisi* to *absolute*, and only their lawyers were speaking. He looked up the stairs. Someone else was in the house, he could feel it.

'Whose silver car is that out there?'

'The colour's called mineral white. And it's mine.'

'You said you wanted to keep the Saab forever.'

'If it kept working I would have. But: it didn't. Apparently this new one's attached to a satellite, so I'm tracked from space if I want and even if I don't, unless I sit down online for hours and work out how to switch it off. It's got this inbuilt ...'

She tailed off because Sean wasn't listening. His attention was caught by all the changes in his old home that he could feel but not quite identify. He stared at the cut roses then looked away. It didn't matter any more.

'I'm glad you've got yourself a good car.'

'I took advice.'

She'd moved the pictures around. There was a new light on a table. Tom was dead, that was why he'd come. So that Gail could express his grief. She wasn't doing that properly.

'You and Ruth have made up then.'

'I hope so. I – I was unfair to her.'

'She shouldn't have meddled.'

'She knows. And I should have listened.'

Alarmed by the tremble in her voice, he went into the kitchen. A muscle memory prompted him: dump the coat, dump the bag – he looked down at the settle. The newspapers and the big tabby cat that slept there were gone.

'Where's Harold?' He looked around, making the sound that called him.

'He died too. Last year. Tea? Coffee?' Gail filled the kettle, her back to him.

'You didn't tell me.' He couldn't help himself, he looked around. Each thing he recognised was like an accusation. 'Isn't this place too big for you now?'

Gail turned. 'Sean, why did you come? You could have phoned.'

'That's what Martine said.'

'Ah. She's so thoughtful.'

'You don't even seem upset about Tom. Aren't you upset? You could have called—' He stopped. It was obvious she was upset.

'Yes it's a shock and yes I'm upset, but I don't call you any more, about anything, unless it's Rosie. I assumed you knew.' She did not cry. 'So, there'll be a funeral, what else? Your knighthood's finally arrived?'

'Not yet, but it will.' He felt bewildered. Gail wasn't like this. She was soft.

'Your services to British business. One in the eye for my father.'

'Here's hoping.' He looked away, feeling the trembling ghosts of parties and dinners, the familiar plates he'd eaten off, the cupboards that held them. The bunches of herbs hanging up. 'The lane,' he said abruptly. 'It's in a shocking state, do you want me to make a call? You'll never get round to it and it'll just get worse. I don't mind.' He wished he hadn't said that. He hoped she would decline.

'I know you're a master of the universe and all that—'

'Those are bankers, I've never been a banker—'

'—but in case you hadn't noticed, it's been raining solidly for a month.'

'It hasn't rained a drop in London.'

'I don't care what happens in London! You can't grade a flooded lane, you have to wait for it to drain. It's all organised. But thank you for pointing it out.'

'So you're OK then. Not – clinically depressed.'

'Sorry to tell you, I'm absolutely fine.' She wiped her eyes, her back to him.

'Is that Sean?' His daughter Rosie swerved round the kitchen door in a long T-shirt that said OCCUPY, and her honey brown hair ruined into dreadlocks. Her ears were multiply pierced, and to his dismay, he noticed another tribal tattoo on her upper arm.

'Rosie,' he groaned. 'What have you done to yourself?'

'Grown up without you? Why is Mum crying? Sean, why are you even here?' Rosie put her arm around her mother and glared at him.

'I'm fine,' said Gail, 'really. We're just talking.'

'And I don't like you calling me that,' he said. 'I'm still your father.'

'Uh-uh, you sacked yourself. A father is someone you're supposed to be able to trust, who gives his word and keeps it, who doesn't cheat and lie again and again, when they've promised not to. Mum cries every day you know.'

'Oh for goodness sake, I do not—'

'My god! Why does *everybody lie* the whole time?'

'Some day, Rosie,' he said, 'you might understand that things are not always black and—'

'White,' she finished for him, 'I know. They're in the *grey*, and in the *grey*, Rosie, is where people like me make their money and tell their lies and generally screw up other people's lives. In the grey. I've got it. Sean.'

'She doesn't know,' Gail said quietly.

'Know what? Ugh: you're expecting a little bébé with *her*. Well it's never going to have anything to do with me.'

'No, that's not why I've come, and I didn't know you were here, I thought it was term time. I came to tell your mother that Tom's body has been found. And in person, Rosie, not to be insulted by you but to break it gently to her. Except she already knew.'

Rosie stared at her mother in shock.

'Ruth called me this morning.' Gail put her arm round her daughter. 'I'll tell you all about it.' She looked at Sean over Rosie's shoulder. 'Thank you for coming. I appreciate it.'

He stared at his crying daughter, and his stranger of an ex-wife. He was being dismissed from his own home. Ex-home.

'Rosie,' he said gently, 'if you ever wanted to see me—'

'Why would I want to do that?' She didn't look at him.

'Because you're my daughter and I love you.'

'Don't hold your breath.' She ducked out from under her mother's arm and ran upstairs, her face crumpling.

The Vanquish blinked an electronic greeting. Sean drove carefully down the rutted, waterlogged private lane, then into the long single-lane road. The numbness was definitely gone, the encounter with his ex-wife and his daughter left him raw with failure. He had wanted to comfort them—

A short sharp blast of a horn ahead returned his attention to the narrow road, where a battered red Land Rover pulling a trailer was upon him. A man and a woman in matching jackets – James and Emma Goring. OK, he could do this. He'd only just gone by a passing place so he waved then reversed, shaking himself out of his funk, ready to greet them. The shattered bones of the past, knitting back together. He would tell them what had happened.

James and Emma – he couldn't remember their children's names – but over nearly a decade they had eaten at each other's houses, bought rounds at the Acorn, gone to firework parties, shared New Year – the stuff of life that slowly accretes into friendship. He felt better for seeing them, but they did not appear to recognise him. In fact, James raised a casual finger of thanks and was about to drive on, until Sean called out.

James did a double-take, and stopped. 'Sean!' he said. Emma lowered the phone she had been checking, and just that second also officially recognised him too, with a bright smile.

Engines running, they exchanged enthusiastic concerns about the weather and the state of the lanes, and Sean told them about the dust storm, which they'd seen on TV but only got a little of here, weren't they lucky with their microclimate? And then the awkward pause.

Sean knew they wanted to go. He felt angry, he kept them talking, anything, about the vineyards, the farm, while he absorbed the fact they hadn't wanted to stop. Pretending they hadn't recognised him. People got divorced, people moved on – he looked pointedly at their trailer, where big sound speakers were covered with a tarp.

'Of course!' he said. 'Your solstice party – here's hoping for sunshine!'

'Oh,' James said quickly, 'very small this year.'

'Big speakers, for a small party.'

'Not really.'

They looked at each other, their smiles fading. They were not going to invite him.

'I came down to tell Gail a dear friend of ours died.' Sean had to look up at them from his lower vehicle. 'You should know we're still friends.'

'Best way,' said James. 'Sorry for your loss.'

'Absolutely,' Emma said. 'So sorry. Take care, Sean.'

James put the Land Rover in gear and the loaded trailer rattled dangerously close to the Aston as they passed, attention fixed on the lane ahead. Then they were gone.

Sean stared after them in the rear-view mirror, his heart pounding like he'd been in a fight. He'd thought of them as friends – he'd brought out his best wine and put up with their tedious company in the hope that they would surely reveal themselves at some point – he presumed it was just that English reserve—

No. They had never been friends; they had always been cold to him. It was Gail they'd liked, he knew they thought she'd married down. The loss of Tom burned through him again: Tom who had been a true friend and a gentleman, always showing the same kindness and self-respect whether he was talking to a tramp or a billionaire. Sean heard Kingsmith's voice in his head, from the old days, when he'd taken a business loss. *Learn, and don't look back.* He checked the time, and told the satnav Heathrow.

There is a power that we call Sila, which is not to be explained in simple words. A great spirit, supporting the world and the weather and all life on earth, a spirit so mighty that his utterance to mankind is not through common words, but by storm and snow and rain and the fury of the sea; all the forces of nature that men fear.

When all is well, Sila sends no message to mankind, but withdraws into his own endless nothingness, apart. So he remains as long as men do not abuse life, but act with reverence towards their daily food.

No one has seen Sila; his place of being is a mystery, in that he is at once among us and unspeakably far away.

Across Arctic America: Narrative of the Fifth Thule Expedition (1927)
Knud Rasmussen

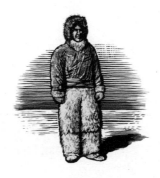

4

Sitting in 1F, crammed against the plastic wall, the smell of his neighbour's duty-free aftershave in his nose, Sean remembered Tom's grim
prediction that Svalbard would become the Ibiza of the north. The
midnight sun, exotic locale, and public awareness of the fragility of
the region had created the strongest driver for tourism the Arctic had
ever seen. Now Longyearbyen even had its own club scene, the most
popular being the dance bar Extinction, a Mecca for outward-bound
hen and stag parties and rich kids bored of skiing.

Sean watched the stewardess and her cart coming closer. The clink
of ice made him swallow in anticipation. A shocking event, but with
it, closure. A stone – a literal heavy headstone, could be laid on Tom's
recovered body in its grave, and on the hope he would return. Or if he
were cremated, maybe a cairn, a rough and enduring memorial. He
grimaced at the stupid thought. The Arctic could not be
transplanted.

'Sir, any drinks or snacks?' the stewardess repeated, with an econ-
omy-class smile. She passed him his two miniature vodkas, tin of tonic
and a plastic cup with a single ice cube and moved on quickly before
he could ask for more. He didn't bother with the tonic, just poured in
both vodkas and knocked it back, staring out at the clouds. No. No
matter what Kingsmith and Martine said, in his heart he knew this
was anything but closure. He'd learned to live with the idea of Tom
lost in pristine obscurity – that was how many Arctic heroes ended

their story. His reappearance was unscripted, as if the glacier itself had moved against him.

Another shadow fell on his thoughts, provoked by Gail's reference to his still-imminent knighthood. The New Year and Birthday honours had come and gone three times, but there was always a good reason he had to wait – bit of a backlog, wheels within wheels, don't worry—

No no, he didn't worry, he was patient. He knew how to be a good chap not a chippy upstart, how to keep his eyes on the prize – there was a verbal deal and he had more than fulfilled his side of it – but that didn't mean he wasn't getting impatient and resentful that he was being strung along, even while he put on a good face, and waited. He didn't even know when he'd started wanting it, but now he'd been promised—

He guessed why it hadn't yet materialised: there were questions about the accident. Two men go into the glacier, only one comes out. He twisted around to see where the stewardess had got to – he needed his fighting spirit. All right then, let the inquest lance that boil of suspicion, which had been far worse than any outright accusation he could refute. What happened? In detail? He'd tell them whatever they wanted to know and as he publicly cleared his name, he would also remind the world that risk and danger were at the very heart of exploration and even to this day the fittest and best-prepared polar adventurers still sometimes died. Surviving was not a crime.

But Sean had done more than just survive; he was making a fine living from Midgard Lodge, where the beloved Tom Harding had died. An aggrieved journalist, turned down for membership at Sean's other clubs, had written about Midgard and called it 'Dirty Davos'. This was not entirely untrue. Sean Cawson's group of membership clubs around the world catered to a global elite, but Midgard Lodge was different. The northernmost hostelry in the world and converted from an old whaling station, it was inaccessible to all but its guests, and provided for those who valued discretion, whose reputations were perhaps not the holiest, but who wanted to improve their standing in the world as well as their profits. These were the people about whom the World Economic Forum felt squeamish, who would never be invited to actual Davos, but whose decisions were of great economic and political import. If they were excluded from the best business society – publicly, at least – they were welcome to meet, and talk, and explore different business models in the stunning environment of Midgard Lodge. Sean believed and Tom had agreed that it was pointless preaching to the converted; also that honey caught more flies than vinegar. A luxury retreat in a uniquely inspiring location, security assured, was part of the realpolitik of environmental progress.

The stewardess was at the rear of the plane. Sean turned back to the dull white clouds. A delicate thing, for a CEO to re-establish the chain of command after so long an absence – but Danny Long was clearly slipping up as general manager if he was reporting to Kingsmith first. Kingsmith might have recommended him, but he was only Sean's sleeping partner in Midgard, not an official shareholder like Martine and her clean-tech investors, or Radiance Young and her friends in Hong Kong. Sean always smiled at the thought of Radiance and her bare-faced insistence she was investing all her own renminbis, not those of the People's Republic behind her. Fine, if that was what she needed to say. But she certainly brought the Party with her.

It would probably be a few days before details were released to the press and then the news cycle and the eulogising would start up again. 'Glacier gives up the ghost', or more soberly, 'Body of missing British environmentalist discovered'. As if Tom Harding were Franklin's lost expedition, the subject of national mourning for decades. And then, of course, there would be the pictures. Tom shaking hands with indigenous protestors at the line of jungle they had saved. Tom swimming with that bloody whale shark, as if he were the only person in the world ever to do that. Tom with actors draped on his shoulders, celebrity trading for rugged moral virtue.

The prospect of reliving the cult of Tom was as irritating now as it had been while he was alive, but the worst of it was, Tom had disliked it too. Sean couldn't even call him on his ego – or his looks, which were not his fault. Women adored him, men admired him, and this idolisation was a large part of why Sean had so doggedly courted him for Midgard, refusing to take no for an answer. But it wasn't the whole of it. Despite their years of distance, Sean knew that if Tom believed in Midgard, then he had truly created something of real value to this world. His old friend's approval had really mattered – and

Kingsmith was right, he must get out in front of all this. He must gather up all his energy and use the drama positively.

In the aftermath of the accident Sean had given interviews, written his own account of it and set up a foundation in Tom's name that gave far more generously than most corporate social responsibility departments of far larger organisations. Now he must do it all again, but instead of telling the truth: No More Sea Ice! The Arctic Open for Business! Governments form an orderly queue! – he would have to deliver environmental pieties that made even his interviewer's eyes glaze over.

'Don't make people feel guilty,' Tom had insisted. 'It's not fair and it shuts them down. That's the big trick of the all-deniers: make it *your* fault, not the governments that won't stand up to business and the bullshitting politicians sitting on the boards of fossil fuel companies.' And Sean had listened to Tom go on for a while, amazed at how his friend had changed. He was impassioned and unstoppable.

'Learned it from you,' Tom used to say. 'I don't stop for arseholes.'

'Up in our country we are human! And since we are human we help each other. We don't like to hear anybody say thanks for that. If I get something today, you may get it tomorrow. Some men never kill anything because they are seldom lucky or they may not be able to run or row as fast as others. Therefore they would feel unhappy to have to be thankful to their fellows all the time. And it would not be fun for the big hunter to feel that other men were constantly humbled by him. Then his pleasure would die. Up here we say that by gifts one makes slaves, and by whips one makes dogs.'

A hunter, to Peter Freuchen
Arctic Adventure: My Life in the Frozen North (1936)
Peter Freuchen

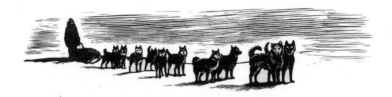

5

Fourteen nations signed the Svalbard Treaty of 1920, giving each of them the right to settle, purchase property and conduct business on the archipelago, provided that, in the words of the legislation, it was 'not for war-like purposes'. By the time Sean Cawson was writing draft after draft of his purchase proposal for the old whaling station, the Treaty had forty-three signatories and seven new-formed states seeking approval. But treaties and laws are as subject to ageing as the hands that wrote them and the times to which they applied.

Family firms likewise. The derelict structures he bought by consortium and rechristened Midgard Lodge, were built and owned for two hundred years by a wealthy Norwegian family: the Pedersens. The oldest members lived in fossilised grandeur in Oslo but had devolved power two decades previously to their children, now themselves in late middle age and dispersed all over the world. They avoided each other in person, but each sensational headline about 'the race for the High North', or the 'Arctic Cold Rush', stirred their conscience, or their greed.

The youngest generation of adult Pedersens rejected their elders' pride in their whaling past, instead feeling shame that their family fortune was built on the near-genocide of several cetacean and pinniped species. It was like inherited wealth from slavery – no bar to public office, as Great Britain proved, but something they felt a debt to repay. In karmic offset, they embraced diverse environmental causes to distance themselves from the documented accounts of their fore-bears, of the joyful slaughter of pregnant beluga whales in Midgardfjorden, and the flensing of live walruses on the beach they still owned. The surviving elders, who still used the candelabra made of narwhal horn on Sunday nights: they wanted the whales to come back to be hunted again, and mourned many aspects of the past under the safe code word: Tradition. The middle generation just wanted the money, and so in strictest confidentiality, in Doha, Wellington, Manhattan and Johannesburg, they made discreet inquiries about the old lodge on the shores of Midgardfjorden. The price it might fetch, the complications.

In strictest reciprocity in Svalbard, Oslo, Bergen and Tromsø, each realtor charged with this investigation broke into a lubricious sweat at the prospect of the Pedersen family reuniting for one last spectacu-lar kill: private property for sale in Svalbard, demesne to encompass landing beach, deepwater access, and a plot reaching right back to the mountain. Of course all land permanently belonged to the Crown of Norway – but that was a matter of casuistry to vendor and purchaser alike. Numbers were crunched, their bones sucked for all associative commissions. Chins were wiped of slaver at the prospect of selling a piece of the last frontier the world had to offer, before Space. Because the most demurely conservative estimate of the value was stratospheric.

For once the family agreed: it was time to let Midgard go. They chose a single agent, Mr Mogens Hadbold. Very discreetly, he dropped a hint of that possibility into international waters. The feeding frenzy was almost instantaneous. First came the Norwegian government itself, who brought much patriotic pressure to bear on the family agent, who duly passed it on – noting that two Russian oligarchs (bitter rivals) had more than doubled the government's best offer. Both were ready for a bidding war, but one was ruled out for his rapacious extrac-tive activities in the Laptev Sea, albeit carried out by a Romanian proxy company. The other, a prominent Siberian landowner, had airlifted every polar bear within three hundred square kilometres to create a private reservation close to Moscow 'for conservation' where he was reputedly breeding cubs for sale as pets. He too was ineligible.

The still-patriotic Pedersens paused to consider. The property was worth far more than the Norwegian government was willing to offer;

why did they did not understand? Their agent explained: if the government paid the premium the Midgard property commanded, they might then find themselves hostage to any Norwegian landowner north of 66 degrees, keen to leverage large amounts of cash. This sad truth caused the Pedersens' patriotism to somewhat fade.

But other bidders – from the US, Canada, Russia, China (the most) and India, were numerous. Seventy-five per cent were ruled out in the first round of investigations, but then the British-led consortium returned, demanding ('begging really,' said the family agent) to be reconsidered. This was because of the new involvement of one Tom Harding – a name that rang discordant bells (Greenpeace?) for the older Pedersens, but chimed most harmoniously (Greenpeace!) for the younger. The young petitioned the old: Tom Harding had led the charge to clear the Plastic Sargasso and driven the public outcry leading to the investigation into clinical trials corruption at Lynch-Ziegler and the collapse of that besmirched chemicals giant. The older generation, privately unconvinced but emotionally blackmailed by their children, allowed that the British consortium could re-submit its proposal – so long as they knew that the odds were against its success.

Long odds were what Sean Cawson had beaten all his life. The sale went through, Midgard Lodge was built and still running despite the terrible accident that had marred its birth – and three and a half years later, here he was disembarking into the sharp mineral air of Longyearbyen once more.

It was good to see Danny Long standing waiting on the tarmac. Behind him was the familiar yellow and blue Dauphin helicopter in which they would fly to Midgard, and standing by his general manager's side, a Longyearbyen airport official ready to conclude the briefest of passport formalities.

He and Danny greeted each other warmly. There was no difference in Long's appearance, or his comfortable quiet manner. He was everything you wanted in a pilot, and though Sean had intended to broach the difficult matters straight away – as they rose up over the slopes of the coal mine behind the airport then veered away from the town, he silently absorbed Svalbard's stark beauty. This time he beheld it without the churning panic of his last visit, unwisely made too soon after the accident, when being there again had jammed his brain with fear and made decisions impossible. He was here to put that failure behind him and lead with confidence again.

Not until they had left the black peaks and steely water of Adventfjord behind them, and were beating their way over the whiteness of the von Postbreen glacier, up to the razor-tipped ice plateau of King Olav's Land, did he clear his throat. He heard the tiny answering click as Danny Long turned up the sound in readiness. To Sean's surprise, the pilot spoke first.

'I'm sorry I didn't call you, sir, about Mr Harding. But Mr Kingsmith called, so I told him – then he wanted to tell you himself.'

'Yes. He told me he'd put a retreat in. You know that—'

'Yes, sir. Everything to go through London, he set me straight on that earlier today. If you don't mind my saying, Mr Cawson, it's good to see you again.'

Sean smiled. 'And you, Danny. It's been far too long. But I'm back.'

The pilot looked straight ahead. 'I still feel very bad about—'

'Not your fault, Danny.' Sean looked down at the ice. 'A true accident.'

'But if I'd been in there with you ...'

'You were needed on watch. But thank you.'

He remembered how much he liked Danny Long. In his late forties, he was blunt-featured, of average height and stocky build, and his modest manner belied his high competence – but that was probably part of the protocol of close protection. Kingsmith had told him he had saved his life on two occasions, but the details were private. Sean admired both of them for not turning it into a drinking anecdote.

He stared down at the ice cap, filling up on its peculiar charge of beauty and fear. Today it was glittering white velvet, strewn with lozenges of emerald and turquoise lakes. He did not remember so many of them.

'Danny – are we going a different route?'

'No, Mr Cawson, but there are probably some changes that are new to you.' He veered away, then Sean saw a line of five white radomes on a plateau of tundra. They had not been there the last time he was here.

'Indian,' said Danny Long, in answer to his unspoken question. 'In the last year. Over on Barentsoya there's another new construction going on. Telecom, or meteorology.' Danny Long's eyes crinkled. 'Improving our broadband.'

'Good broadband is a valuable asset.'

'Indeed, sir.'

Sean did not speak again until they were over Hinlopenstreten, where a convoy of cruise ships made white dashes on the dark water. He remembered Kingsmith's admonition about his friend in Oslo.

'Have there been many ships in Midgardfjorden? Before that one?'

Danny Long shook his head.

'Sometimes they stop at the mouth – for photographs, I believe. Then they go round the other way. But the *Vanir* came right down deep. When it all went off on the radio – not the calving, when they went out and confirmed it was a body – the coastguard were close across at Freyasundet, in that new fast boat of theirs.'

'Joe said they held it as a crime scene.' He kept his tone neutral.

'They did, sir, but they told me and Terry not to worry about the words, it was just so they could take all the phones and such from the passengers.'

'What then?'

'I'm not sure. We were ordered to stand down – return to the Lodge – by the coastguard. That's what we did.' He paused. 'We had Mr Kingsmith's guests to look after.'

'And what did you tell them?'

'Basic facts, sir: a body had been recovered from the water. They didn't know anything until they came down for breakfast. The coastguard had gone by then.'

'How were they? The coastguard.'

'Very polite, sir, as always. It was Inspector Brovang, he was out on their new boat, that's why he was in the area.'

They were silent for a while, in which Sean imagined the heavy medevac cradle swinging in the air, trails of water falling behind. Tom's dead body netted and trussed beneath a helicopter, as high as he was now. Less than forty-eight hours ago.

He put his right hand under his left armpit and pressed down on it. The tingling had come back. Nothing physically wrong with his hand, no nerve damage. Brovang had saved it, with his own body heat. He had taken Sean's statement as he recovered in the Sickehaus in Longyearbyen, but they had not spoken since that time. Nor had

Brovang taken up the standing invitation to either visit Midgard Lodge with guests, or any of Sean Cawson's other clubs around the world, though he had declined courteously. Sean cancelled out the obscure bad feeling that gave him, with a large annual donation to the children's charity which Brovang supported and mentioned on his Facebook page. Brovang had never accepted his Friend request.

'Well, at least he had all the details. He didn't want to speak to the visitors?'

'No, he was keen to get going. I said they were asleep. They had nothing to do with it.'

'Who exactly are they?'

'Excuse me, sir, I'm not good at names, especially foreign ones. Faces, I never forget. But you can meet them, they're still at the Lodge.' He banked the Dauphin over the great crumpled blue-white sweep of a glacier – that stopped short of where Sean's eye expected it to turn.

He must have misremembered the glacier, it could not have retreated so far in a year and a half. Everything seemed different, but he still trusted Danny Long not just because Kingsmith did, but by his own instinct. He wanted to get things on a good footing again. 'Danny,' he said, 'remember something: Midgard Lodge is my company and *I* am your CEO. Not Joe. You report to me.'

'Yes, sir. I know. I made a mistake. I should have informed you first.' Danny Long's voice did not change, but Sean remembered Kingsmith telling him that Long held himself to higher standards than anyone else, and took criticism hard.

'Good, then we're sorted. How's everything else?'

'All good, sir. I was in town a week before the Tata-Tesla retreat, and there were some Russian boys from the new place.'

'The Pyramiden hotel? Or the one in Barentsburg?'

'Oh those are long finished, and two more as well. This new one's called the Arktik Dacha. They were joking with us about it, but in a friendly way. I reckon they've had a look at us.'

'How would they do that?' Sean's stomach lurched as they suddenly rose up over the last peaks that pierced the ice cap.

Danny Long grinned. 'Same way we don't, at them.'

Although I had joined the Royal Geographical Society some years earlier, under the misapprehension that by so doing I would obtain Sunday tickets for the Zoo, I had only the haziest idea as to what a glacier was. I did not know at what temperature water froze. I had no head for heights, was not used to handling large, fierce dogs, could not row or ski or splice, and knew nothing of the working of an internal-combustion engine, or even a Primus stove.

But none of these considerations sobered my high spirits. I had enlisted for Adventure, and that was all I asked for. I had no responsibilities or misgivings and was as carefree as a kitten.

Sledge: The British Trans-Greenland Expedition 1934 (1935)
Martin Lindsay

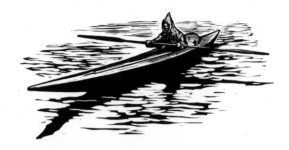

6

They landed on the narrow strip of cobbled beach. He saw that the boathouse doors were ajar but all was quiet. The Lodge itself looked better than Sean remembered, the wood more weathered, the structure even more camouflaged. He waited for the bear all-clear signal then went in to greet the mystery guests. The discretion of Midgard Lodge did not extend to its founder and CEO, and absent or not, and no matter how much he delegated to others, he had a right to know who he was hosting.

Two men were waiting in the lobby and jumped up to greet him. The first of Kingsmith's pals turned out to be the businessman Benoit, from the Central African Republic. He was tall and broad with a winning open smile, and he pumped Sean's hand warmly.

'You don't remember me? I came to all your parties on Spring Street!' He looked to his companion, a young elegantly dressed Asian man who was also smiling politely. 'Jiaq, our host gave the best parties in Manhattan, didn't you?'

'You're very kind.' Sean smiled over his confusion. He had no memory of Benoit, but he had indeed lived in a loft on Spring Street in New York, owned by Kingsmith, in his first year after graduation. Kingsmith had him running errands and apprenticing for him, while he learned what he called 'housekeeping'. Spring Street marked his first experience of making real money through his mentor's generous guidance, and he had never looked back.

If Benoit said they'd met, they probably had. Now he looked at him more closely he saw he wasn't young at all, but something exuberant and vigorous about him gave that impression. The other man, in his early forties, introduced himself simply as Jiaq, from Shanghai. He complimented Sean on Midgard Lodge and apologised for not personally knowing Miss Radiance Young, though he had certainly heard of her.

'Your men are a credit to you,' Benoit smiled. 'We feel very safe!'

'Excellent. I'm glad it's all going well for you.' Only when he politely declined Benoit's offer to call down 'the girls' from upstairs, did they recall the tragic reason for Sean's visit. Benoit apologised for their own unscheduled one – the result of a chance call to Joe, who suggested that if they were in the neighbourhood …

'The neighbourhood?'

'Of Iceland.' They broke into peals of laughter. They explained they had been showing off their new ice-class yachts to each other, comparing anti-pirate protocols. Now the Arctic was open for business it was good to be prepared, like boy scouts!

Their high spirits grated. Sean said he was very pleased to have them there, and excused himself. Part of him was glad that Midgard was apparently running so well without him, but the larger part resented their presence, and the profane tone of commerce that erased everything else he wanted to feel.

He pulled on waterproofs and went back down to the beach. The Dauphin rested at one end, facing down the fjord in readiness for their return. At the other, Danny Long had pulled one of the smallest Zodiacs from the boathouse, alongside the single kayak Sean had requested. This was his manager's mute comment on the safety infraction of Sean's stated intention to go out alone. A breeze glittered the water of the fjord – and carried the faint beat of rock music. He looked around. It came from the building beside the boathouse.

Sean looked at Danny Long in question, then walked towards it. His manager came with him.

'I'll tell them to keep it down, sir. But now might be a good time for them to meet you, if you're happy with that?' He hurried alongside as Sean pushed through the vestibule doors, then into the barrack room.

Twenty men jumped to attention off their bunks, their eyes down. Sean stared in surprise. No one said anything. He had never seen any of them before, and did not remember there being so many of them on his last trip. But everything about that visit was confused. He would check when he got back.

'The new detail, Mr Cawson – they've only been in a week, but they're all good.' Danny Long's voice changed as he addressed the men. 'This is your CEO, Mr Cawson.'

The men looked at Sean and saluted. They wore dark clothing and looked very fit.

'At ease.' Sean had no military training, but apparently it worked because the men sat back down and resumed looking at their screens, or lying on their bunks. Danny Long seemed to be waiting for him to say something.

'Good,' he said, to cover his surprise. He went out into the open air. A retreat was in place he knew nothing about and a new detail of men – he had forgotten that part of the arrangement – were gathered in that dark cavernous room, at ease. 'So everything's all right.'

'All good, sir.' Danny Long was watching him. Sean felt he would answer any question, but he did not want to ask. 'Line of command is clear, Mr Cawson.'

'Good.' He stood on the beach, a stranger to his own business. Too long away, avoiding this moment. He felt he'd returned not a moment too soon. He took out his own binoculars and stood back to back with his manager, sweeping the rocks and peaks of the bay with hi-mag scrutiny.

Danny Long's radio crackled from the upper lookout in the Lodge, where his second in command Terry Bjornsen was also scanning for bears. All clear.

'Waiting,' Long said into his collar, as he completed his own slow survey. He raised his arm to the Lodge. 'All clear below.'

Sean lowered his kayak into the water, climbed down the steel ladder and slid into the seat. He took the paddle from Long, coiled the red tethering rope into the cockpit and pushed off with a long slow glide. There was no wind. Midgardfjorden was a black mirror, the only movement was the undulating wake behind Sean's kayak, and the slow rise and fall of his paddle, hissing softly as it cut the water.

He skimmed out towards the centre, the rising shimmer of light around him showing that the sky was drying as the sun burned through. His consciousness fused with the subtle motion of the kayak and the long ripples of sunlight. He kept his eye on the jutting inner point of the M. He knew the current that circled the inlets and made a little area of turbulence close to the shore that could capsize the unwary – but here it was now, all the way out in the centre.

Dipping his blade, he felt the pull from the water, the tug all the way up into his arm, as if it had caught on something. The current swirled like a water snake but Sean had good upper body strength and kept his head. He judged its velocity and angle, then twisted his paddle blade into its force. He felt the energy from deep in the water travel up his paddle, his hand, his arm, into his shoulder, neck, and face. He held the strain – and the hook of the current released him in the right direction. Only five or six seconds – but long enough to go in if he'd panicked. But he hadn't – and in that instant of instinctive reaction, in that correct response, his feeling of power came flooding back – and he was embracing that beautiful and terrifying lover once again: the Arctic.

His heart pounding with joy, he glanced back. Danny Long stood on the jetty, a tiny figure beneath the rearing mountain, his rifle above his shoulder like a tribesman's spear. Sean rounded the point and moved out of sight.

From the air the glacier was one thing, but approached in humility by kayak, she revealed another nature. Sean lifted his paddle and slowed, poised in the water. The towering blue and white face of the ice filled his vision, the Arctic silence his ears and mind. Sometimes it was so intense it almost formed into a sound; sometimes he had heard the bumping and scraping of the pack ice form abstract fragments like music.

The silence gathered around him so that he could almost hear the squeeze and suck of his heart in his chest. He felt his sweat blot his base layer, and the bracing of his tendons far away inside the kayak shell. Below him the dark depth of the water; above, a thread of breeze that dried the molecules of sweat. His vision filled with the deep blue strata of the most ancient compressed ice, forty thousand years old.

*

When Sean Cawson was eleven and in the care home while his mother was recovering from yet another attempt, he saw a huge oil painting of icebergs on one of the off-limits staff landings. It was so beautiful he started using this longer route, despite the threat of punishment if he were caught, just to gaze at the space and the colours of this pristine frozen world. While he stood before it, he forgot the misery of every waking moment of this new life, and threw his consciousness into the ice.

There was a mast from a shipwreck in the foreground, and he imagined himself the sole survivor. Everyone else was dead but he must find a way to keep going. As he gazed at it one day it came to him like a truth – his father was on that ship, or one like it – he had gone exploring and been shipwrecked, that was why he'd never known him, why his mother was dying of grief. The ice had taken his family and he must go there to get them back.

The iceberg painting grew in his imagination, even when his mother returned from the hospital and reclaimed him to the ugly council house where she struggled on in depression and drinking. Sean fixated on his lost explorer father, who was noble, clean and far better lost in the ice than occasionally passing through the house like the other men who visited his mother. By the time Sean was thirteen, the Arctic was his obsession and he had bolstered his fantasy father with such authentic details, and backed it up with angry fists for doubters, that it became fact.

His fighting was a problem until a social worker intervened. Sean was in danger of serious delinquency but clearly bright, and the social worker goaded him into agreeing to sit the scholarship exam for The Abbott's School.

This was the grand, grey-stone public school where Sean had often joined the townie gang in attacking boys who wore the strange uniform – but now he was to be one of them. He'd listened outside the door after his interview – 'Oh, the poor boy, think of what he's gone through, yes, yes let's extend a helping hand.'

So Sean Cawson received the academic scholarship and the sports bursary and the charity award that topped up the rest and meant he could go for free. By the age of fifteen, he had become a chameleon at Abbott's, sloughing off the misfits who would have been his natural friends and gravitating instead to the leaders of the pack, in sport and academic excellence. There he worked out the answer to the question he'd always pondered, about fairness and beauty and ugliness and justice. It was wealth.

Sean blinked. Not eleven in the care home, not in the dorm at Abbott's. In the kayak, frozen. The current had taken him closer to the ice face – how long had he been zoned out, thinking of the past? A few seconds – a couple of minutes? The temperature had dropped and the light was that milky veil that can suddenly appear in Arctic air like a spell, blanking out contours, hiding crevasses, wiping out direction.

His heart slammed. In the few seconds he had mentally drifted, the current had taken him directly in front of the mouth of the cave into the glacier from which Tom's body emerged. It was deep; the ice was the darkest blue he had ever seen, and as he paddled backwards, he could hear the echo of his blade striking the water. His ears blocked as if he were airborne and his mouth was dry. The new cave was the source of the pull in the water, it had changed the current pattern of the fjord.

He felt a terrible urge to go in, but he knew that was crazy, like standing on a high cliff and thinking of jumping. Of course he would not do it. He braced his feet and bladed back, admiring the cobalt twists in the ice, the darkest sapphire catching flashes from the water. There was nothing more beautiful than Arctic ice.

Something touched him. Not physically – but he felt it in the prickling of his scalp – something was there, around him or under him. He stared into the cave but saw nothing; he looked down and the water was grey-green translucent. Then he looked up.

Standing on the lip of the glacier, staring down from directly above him, was an enormous male polar bear. It was close enough for Sean to see the duelling scar that twisted his black lip, giving the impression of a cynical smile. It must have stalked him while he was years away, and now they had come together.

Sean dug his paddle to move away from the cave but caught another current that pushed him closer to the ice face. The bear watched with interest and slowly walked along the edge above him, keeping pace.

Sean knew not to take his eyes from it. He felt it most distinctly – the bear was pondering leaping in now, or waiting a little longer. If he came closer, if he lost control and capsized, it would take the chance and jump. Bears had been known to go for kayakers before, but always from the shore.

This glacier was high – but the bear was enormous and highly intelligent; it knew the currents – it was standing waiting for him. When he met its gaze, he felt it willing him to panic and make a mistake. He stared back with equal force and ignored the jolt of fear down both legs.

The current was a muscle of water writhing around his paddle, tugging it under the kayak. The light glittered and the mountains reared up black and strobing around him, locking him in. The bear lowered its head, looking for where to jump. He wanted a knife – why had he not brought a knife with him? He might have done something with a knife …

As the bear gathered itself, a sharp growl bounced against the granite walls of the fjord, and it looked up in irritation. The vibration of the Zodiac engine came through the water. Sean did not take his eyes away – the bear would still strike, even now. Man and animal felt each other's stare. Advantage animal – but man was lucky. The bear turned and loped away up the glacier and out of sight.

Danny Long slowed the Zodiac as he approached, his rifle on his back. Benoit, Jiaq, and two young blonde women were his passengers, all wearing bright orange survival suits and busy photographing the scenery. They had not seen it.

'Excuse me, sir: the guests wished to come out.'

Sean reached down into himself for human speech again.

'Of course.'

Long carefully circled the Zodiac around behind Sean, giving him the benefit of the wake to help him out of the current. 'How is it, in the kayak?'

'Great,' Sean said over his shoulder. 'But no one else out alone. The current.' He scanned the slopes. The bear had vanished and he was glad.

'Yes, sir. It's changed, I noticed as well.'

Sean left Kingsmith's guests exclaiming over the colour of the glacier and paddled back. Only as he boarded the plane that evening did he realise he had not thought about Tom for a moment out there. He had gone to see where he'd died, and mourn, but instead the confrontation with the bear had made him feel more alive than he had done in years. And now he wanted sex.

As I raised my rifle, again I felt clutching at my heart that terrible sensation of life hanging on the accuracy of my aim; again in my bones I felt that gnawing hunger of the past; that aching lust for red, warm, dripping meat – the feeling that the wolf has when he pulls down his quarry. He who has ever been really hungry, either in the Arctic or elsewhere, will understand this feeling. Sometimes the memory of it rushes over me in unexpected places. I have felt it after a hearty dinner, in the streets of a great city, when a lean-faced beggar has held out his hand for alms.

The North Pole (1910)
Robert E. Peary

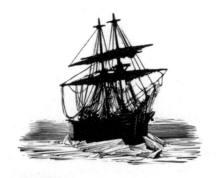

7

Sean recognised Economy Smile greeting passengers as they boarded the return flight to the UK. When she saw him, she switched up to First Class wattage and her posture changed.

'Welcome back on board, sir! My name is Lisa, please do let me know if there's anything you need.' She escorted him the three feet to his seat. 'We have plenty of ice this time, and I'll make sure I save you extra. Are you staying over in London?'

'I live there.'

'So do I!'

His heart sank. She had clearly been told who he was.

He sat down, thinking that at least he didn't have to worry about whether Martine's interest in him was financial. Almost sixteen years younger than he was, she was highly successful and could buy herself whatever she wanted – and therefore appreciated gifts even more: so long as they were exquisite, expensive, and very hard to source. Otherwise she considered them 'high street'.

He watched the cabin crew getting everyone in. Lisa's pretty colleague glanced over and gave him a special smile as well. He looked away.

Once it would have felt almost wasteful not to invite them both out to dinner in London, and let his lower nature take its course. *Kill the hunter, kill the man*, Kingsmith had once said to him, and he had even tried that justification with Gail.

It had not worked. In fact, it might have been the beginning of the end, or at least the point at which she refused to accept his lies any more. She didn't want to hear about those times he'd succumbed to temptation, or chased a woman too beautiful to ignore, not so much for the sex, but for that magical time when he saw himself reflected in her eyes: a hero, an explorer, a powerful man. That fleeting feeling of acceptance. He never actually managed to say all that to Gail, because she was too angry and upset – and because he hadn't known how.

The stewardesses were talking about him. When he asked for a vodka tonic, Lisa made it herself in the galley and brought it to him, very strong and with plenty of ice. When he went to use the lavatory – he had learned to call it this, despite the illuminated sign that said Toilet – she brushed against him, her eyes merry with promise. He locked the door and looked in his pocket. She had given him her card. He'd joined the Mile High Club a number of times – Lisa too, he guessed.

As the flush roared in the tiny cubicle he washed his hands and looked at himself in the mirror. He wanted to be back with Martine, and he wanted her a certain way – not frazzled and exhausted from her own day, but ready to look after him. In his fantasy, he would walk through the door, smell something fabulous to eat that she had made, and she would be wearing something beautiful and revealing, and be joyful to see him.

Martine had a car waiting for him at Heathrow, and was at home with a decanted bottle of Margaux 1966, and if not the lengthily slaved-over meal of his dreams, had at least bought good steaks. She was wearing a black dress she knew he liked her in, and dressed the set with candles and flowers. She was also a clever woman who knew the times when sex must precede talk, and that this was one. Only afterwards, when she propped herself up so she could see his face, did he remember their unfinished conversation.

'I want to know what it's like,' she said. 'As a woman I want that experience. I don't want to miss out.'

He pulled her back down and held her, his face angled away. 'It changes everything.'

'But it's what I want. I don't know why we haven't, yet.'

'You've got an implant.'

'Not for six months. But still nothing.'

He closed his eyes, to hide what might show. Six months of him not knowing, and her not saying. He felt her lean over, then kiss him on the lips.

'But now is not the right time. Sorry, darling.'

He lay still as she got up to use the bathroom. When he heard the water running, he jumped up and dressed. He poured himself two fingers of frozen vodka and downed it, then decided to get on with the cooking himself. Steaks were within his repertoire. He opened a second bottle of wine while the skillet heated.

Sean didn't want another child. The one he had hated him, and he couldn't bear to look back to when she hadn't. To that naïve and innocent time when he thought he could do marriage, fatherhood and commitment—

'Burning ...' Martine retrieved the skillet from him and took over, sleek, scented and in charge. 'Don't worry,' she said, 'we'll park all that. Let's just enjoy the evening.' She refilled his glass and took one for herself, and Sean watched her cook, and she must have put music on, and then they were sitting eating together and that was what he focused on, the here and now, and the beautiful young woman opposite, his partner in business and life, who had helped bring Midgard Lodge into being.

Martine listened carefully as he told her of Benoit and Jiaq, and their new ice-class yachts. 'Joe's not used to asking you for anything. If you're back in charge—'

'I am. I'm going to get back up to speed on everything.'

'Good! I'd like to take a group of investors – could we plan that?'

'Sure.' Sean smiled, the second bottle at last warming away his tension. He listened and made the right sounds as Martine relaxed and told him of all her new triumphs at work, but his mind was back in the kayak, staring at the bear that had seized him in its black gaze. It had wanted to kill him. He leaped up.

'What is it?'

He took her by the hand and pulled her from the table back to the bedroom. The bear had wanted to kill him but instead had made him feel alive. Flashes of other women invaded his mind and drove him on

– the two stewardesses – and Martine thrilled to his ferocity as Sean shoved her back the way she liked and poured wine over her dark tanned body with its pale triangles. Extravagantly ruined, the white sheets soaked red around them, like a kill.

'Svarten,' alias 'Johansen's Friend,' looked bad in the lantern-light. Flesh and skin and entrails were gone; there was nothing to be seen but a bare breast and backbone, with some stumps of ribs. It was a pity that such a fine strong dog should come to such an end. He had just one fault: he was rather bad-tempered. He had a special dislike to Johansen; barked and showed his teeth whenever he came on deck, or even opened a door, and when he sat whistling in the top, or in the crow's nest these dark winter days, the 'Friend' would answer with a howl of rage from far out on the ice. Johansen bent down with the lantern to look at the remains.

'Are you glad, Johansen, that your enemy is done for?'

'No, I am sorry.'

'Why?'

'Because we did not make it up before he died.'

And we went on to look for more bear-tracks, but found none; so we took the dead dogs on our backs and turned homewards.

Tuesday, 12 December 1893
Farthest North: The Norwegian Polar Expedition 1893–1896 (1897)
Fridtjof Nansen

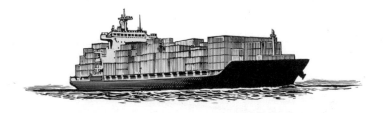

8

London, four years earlier

Sean and Tom were not exactly estranged, but they had neither seen nor spoken to each other in over two years. But now he needed Tom and, though Tom didn't yet know it, he needed Sean. Because here, in his old friend's gift, was a golden, global opportunity that he could not possibly pass up. A chance to protect the Arctic – and for once, get handsomely paid.

Sean rang Tom rather than emailing, catching him in high spirits in a cab back to Richmond from Heathrow after a long-haul trip to a sunken Pacific nation whose name Sean pretended to know. Tom was surprised but genuinely pleased to hear from him, and very interested that the rumour of the Svalbard land for sale was true. Not land, Sean corrected, just property. It's Midgardfjorden.

'Seriously? Are you buying it?'

'When are you home? I want to send you something to read.'

'Email it now, I can't wait.'

'I want to send a hard copy.'

Sean wanted to send something else as well. While he waited for the courier, he took a small framed photograph down from his home office wall. It was from his Oxford days, and had gone with him everywhere since then, even during his two peripatetic years apprenticing with Kingsmith, when all he had was his suitcase.

The sepia faces of best friends and polar explorers Knud Rasmussen and Peter Freuchen looked out at him from somewhere in Arctic Greenland, circa 1925. As a student, he'd found it in a junk shop and intended to give it to Tom, who was obsessed with the pair at the time. But as soon as Sean tried it out on his own wall he wanted to keep it, even though he himself was more interested in the British Arctic Air Expedition of 1930, led by the glamorous and tragic Gino Watkins and his band of bright young men. But Rasmussen and Freuchen felt totemic, so he kept it.

'Must have been in Greenland,' Tom had murmured in envious admiration when he'd peered at Sean's new treasure. 'On their way to Thule. If you ever don't want it ...' Twenty years later, Sean tucked it into the document case with the proposal, and the courier took it away.

Their time at Oxford had been the high-water mark of their friendship, but without physical proximity, the gap between them widened with each career decision. Now they were no longer posturing: Tom really did want to save the world and Sean really did want to put his name on the map and become phenomenally wealthy. Both were articles of faith.

Sean served his apprenticeship with Joe Kingsmith, proving himself humble and energetic in the service of whatever his mentor required – back-office support with administration, proxy purchases of properties, and occasionally, holding large amounts of money in his own name – which he scrupulously and instantly returned the moment he was asked. He had no criminal bent, he wanted wealth by the straightest possible road, and Kingsmith applauded him for it, and helped him towards his goal with pearls of advice Sean was quick to act on. His investments prospered, and Kingsmith increased his protégé's line of credit.

Soon Sean was able to buy and renovate a small unfashionable hotel, which he turned into a home away from home for people like Kingsmith. Though his mentor never used it, he put business Sean's way, and then he was able to buy another. He consolidated. He expanded. He raised prices, and standards, and prices again. It was extraordinary – the more expensive he made it, the harder it became to join the elite membership, the more people wanted to stay and to play there.

Tom declined membership of Sean's clubs, even as a gift. They were not his crowd. They weren't Sean's either, but now he was far wealthier than Tom and the line had blurred. He could no longer switch his chameleon-like abilities on and off, but automatically took on the colour of every surrounding. When he saw Tom, he was struck by his old friend's unfamiliar bolshiness – as if they had exchanged some part of themselves. But Tom was still sweet-natured at his core, and Sean was still amazed by his own good fortune, and for a while, they managed to ignore the new differences, but the ease was missing. So the friendship became historic, and then, when Tom embraced Greenpeace – and to Sean, an uncompromising attitude about how the world should be run – they both let it gently ebb away.

The last time Sean and Tom had spoken had been the night Martine dragged him to the opening of an exhibition painted by one of her new investment clients. It was in a small gallery in St James's, and the white Kenyan artist painted cheetahs in all their forms. A manifesto on her price sheet declared her family's love for all African wildlife, and their longstanding commitment to teaching the native people how to better steward their land. Sean couldn't believe it was really Tom, adrift in a sea of booming-voiced striped shirts and tidy women, one of whom was talking incessantly at him, drunkenly clinking her glass on his as if to get him moving. Her hand flashed with diamonds. Tom saw Sean, grinned and excused himself. He came straight over and bear-hugged him.

'Strange crowd for you,' Sean said, awkward and moved by Tom's affection.

'I've become a whore.' Tom looked furtively over his shoulder. 'She thought I still worked for Greenpeace and said she'd donate ten grand if I'd come. So I came, even though I don't.' He noticed Martine, and his expression changed as Sean brought her forward, her hand in his.

'Tom's reputation and annoyingly handsome face precede him, and Martine runs the Linnaeus fund, which is—'

'I've heard. Clean energy tech.' Tom nodded but did not smile. 'Hello.'

Martine's smile dared him. 'Please think of us as a new force for good.'

Tom turned to Sean. 'Does Gail know?'

A flash went off and the photographer saluted his thanks. Sean darted after him, and Martine and Tom heard his low urgent tone, asking him not to use the picture. The photographer shrugged and nodded, then two women greeted Sean and he paused to exchange pleasantries.

Tom and Martine sized each other up.

'He's talked about you a lot. He misses you.'

'Here I am, we're still friends.' He looked at her. 'You should probably know I'm Gail's friend too. Sean's wife.'

'What a thankless job that always sounds.'

'Perhaps you've never been offered the position.'

'You think?'

'No. I don't. It's none of my business.'

'I couldn't agree with you more.'

'Are they still married? They have a child.'

'For now. And she's a very independent-minded young woman.'

'Ah yes. She dropped in on you at work, didn't she?'

'It was a very unpleasant and immature thing to do.'

'I thought it was courageous.'

Sean returned and felt the freeze. 'What?'

'Sean,' Martine said. 'I'm tired of hiding. I'm not a bad person, but your friend Tom seems to think I am. I don't deserve to be shamed like this.'

'That's not what I intended.' Tom put down his glass. 'Sorry, Sean, but I don't know how to talk to your mistress when I'm friends with your wife. And I won't be learning.' He walked out.

Sean had not spoken to Tom since that night, until the Midgard Lodge tender came up. Then they talked, but only about the business in hand. Tom had gone through everything, he understood the stakes. His credibility plus Sean's money. A vulnerable piece of the Arctic on the block. He could hardly refuse.

This snowless ice-plain is like a life without love – nothing to soften it. The marks of all the battles and pressures of the ice stand forth just as when they were made, rugged and difficult to move among. Love is life's snow. It falls deepest and softest into the gashes left by the fight – whiter and purer than snow itself. What is life without love? It is like this ice – a cold, bare, rugged mass, the wind driving it and rending it and then forcing it together again, nothing to cover open rifts, nothing to break the violence of the collisions, nothing to round away the sharp corners of the broken floes – nothing, nothing but bare, rugged drift-ice.

Friday, 15 December 1893
Farthest North: The Norwegian Polar Expedition 1893–1896 (1897)
Fridtjof Nansen

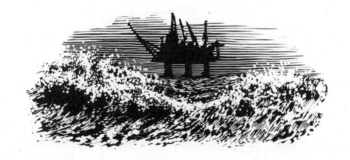

9

'I don't want to do this.' Tom didn't even wait for the meeting to officially start. The Pedersen family agent, Mogens Hadbold, their lawyer and their accountant, stared at Sean in confusion.

'Wait.' Sean felt like he was in a bad dream. 'Tom, what is this?' They were in a penthouse suite at Claridge's in the final round of the bidding for Midgard Lodge, and Tom was destroying everything. Now he was holding up Sean's bid proposal in its embossed leather cover.

'I do not want the Pedersen family to sell their property,' Tom said, 'because it's in such an environmentally sensitive location. All change is disruptive, and the Arctic ecosystem is already massively stressed by warming seas. There *is* no more summer ice. Politicians pay lip-service to bringing the temperature down while quietly drawing dividends from their fossil fuel investments. We've got government ministers on the boards of oil companies. I don't want that either, but that's reality.'

Sean consciously relaxed his hands so they did not make fists. What an absolute fucker, telling him one thing and waiting until now—

'But,' Tom continued, 'we're here because someone is going to be chosen as the new owner. Someone is going to become responsible for that corner of the Arctic, at a most critical moment for its safety. I'm here to tell you that, if this sale is going to happen, I stand with this man to buy it. We're here because the numbers are right.'

'Certainly in the correct area,' confirmed the family agent. 'But above a particular threshold that Mr Cawson has passed, the family are even more concerned to select the correct buyer.'

'I led Greenpeace for two years,' Tom said. 'I've been involved in environmental issues my whole life and I will continue to be. I've known Sean since we were at college together. I've learned a lot from him, and as I'm now in this room, I hope it's become a two-way street. I used to turn my nose up at people whose main interest was money, because they didn't seem to care how they made it. Now I'm less naïve. The only way the world will change for the better is if it is precisely those people who start thinking differently about profit.' He looked at each of them in turn.

'Last year's coup in the Maldives cost every hotel group there untold sums as well as several lives. Many people saw it coming, the hotels were warned, they absolutely knew what was going on, but profit blinded them. Climate change means the poorest people suffer first – people who don't buy organic or vote for liberal democracy. The Maldives is happening all over the world, in every poor country where the sea level is rising and the land is flooding.'

'Mr Harding,' Mogens Hadbold smiled patiently, 'we all care—'

'Caring is meaningless without action. We must stop the economic apartheid that is killing this planet.'

'Tom, for pity's sake!' Sean was on his feet too. It was appalling, Tom was like a mad man, he hadn't seen him like this before.

'Sit down, Sean. You wanted me here, you wanted me on board, so let me continue. I'm nearly finished. Look at the world – a great big band of drought or flood that just happens to coincide with mineral resources, with political instability and then with foreign intervention by the very powers that benefit from the extractive rights. Powers that do not give a shit about the cost, human or natural, of that resource exploitation. What we're looking at is a global environmental *sacrifice zone* – and the Arctic is just the latest part of it.'

Sean sat there, his face burning. Tom's ego was out of control. How could he not have seen it? What was he doing now, with the mineral water? Holding it up to the big mirror on the mantelpiece. He looked mad, speaking to the flowers.

'Bottled at source in the Alps. Where the shrinking snowline means only the highest resorts still exist, and their prices make even the rich feel poor. And if *they're* starting to think about climate change, you know we're in the last-chance saloon.' He turned and came back to them. 'When that chunk of Venice collapsed into the lagoon, the dead included guests at the Cipriani, as well as refugees.'

He drank again.

'So if you're not worried, you're not paying attention. And if you are, then it is your moral and civic and patriotic duty to either keep your property and be vigilant stewards of the Arctic, or, ensure that you only sell to a buyer who will use it to be a vigilant pain in the arse to any and everyone who is trying to make a killing up there. I don't know, you might be those people yourselves. I don't know you, but I do know this man.' He pointed to Sean.

'Arctic obsession started our friendship. We've gone our separate ways, but that's still our bond. He's the capitalist pig in a great suit and I'm the pain in the arse in jeans. He's clever or crazy enough to invite me to be a board member, and if there's one thing I've learned it's that people hear you better if you're in the room, not yelling through a loudhailer from the street. That's why I'm in with Sean: he knows the very people I want to reach, the brokers between governments and mining companies, the shipping people, the people who make things happen, or make things disappear. I'll be in the room with them on this.'

He laid down the bid proposal on the table. 'How can people say what they really think at places like Davos? It's about being seen to do good, and someone with a vested interest in the outcome is always playing the host. Sean's plan takes that layer away. A luxurious private retreat in Arctic grandeur – who doesn't want to go there? Who wouldn't be affected by those surroundings?'

Sean stared at Tom. He was selling it better than Sean had ever been able to. Such a showman, Sean had to admire him. No – not a showman, every word felt genuine. Tom had made protecting the environment his life's work, he had the broken bones, scars and jail time to show for it – as well as the adulation of thousands of people. He'd put all his money into it too, though his family had tried to stop him; Sean remembered hearing that.

'Enough with the bleeding-heart liberals crying over the polar bears. I want the greediest, ugliest-thinking, most short-sighted, ego-crazed politicians and plutocrats we can find to stay in the place

Sean will build on the shore of Midgardfjorden. There's a reason men have risked their lives again and again for the Arctic; it shows you your soul, even if you think you don't have one.

'I'm naïve: I still believe you can reach people through their hearts. But I'm battle-scarred: profit speaks louder. Sean's plan combines both those things. So that's why I say that my first position is still no more development in the Arctic. But as it *is* happening, from all sides, as the summer ice has gone – twenty years ahead of government projections, and as it *is* a free-for-all, no matter what people say, then let us be there, let us try to guide development to do the minimum harm, and protect the life of this fragile, sublime, vulnerable environment. You can only lose it once.'

Tom walked round behind Sean and put his hands on his shoulders. 'I know my friend and I trust him. So if you can't beat 'em, join 'em.' He took his seat again.

No one spoke for a long moment. The atmosphere had shifted. The lawyer and the accountant were staring at Tom with that star-struck look Sean had seen on people's faces before. Mogens Hadbold's laptop pinged, two, three, four times, breaking the spell. Hadbold looked across to the mantelpiece and waved. Only then did Sean spot the tiny camera in the flower arrangement.

'Yes,' said Mogens Hadbold. 'I'm sorry that I did not tell you the meeting was streaming live. They wanted to be present, but discreetly.' He started laughing. 'Sometimes I wonder if they really trust me! No no, it is to make sure that they could form their own opinion.'

He turned his laptop to face Sean and Tom, and the quartered screen showed different Pedersens on Skype.

'That was very impressive,' a female voice said, out of the screen. 'We will let you know. *Tak*, Mogens.'

He replied in a rapid burst of Norwegian, and closed the laptop.

'Mr Harding is something of a hero to the younger generation, you know this. They are the ones making all the big noise about the right buyer. The older ones – well, you know how we are as we get old. We like security. And money! But the young have the power.' He stood up, as did the lawyer and accountant. 'Thank you very much for returning.' The meeting was over. Sean stood too.

'You don't want to ask me anything?' He looked from one to the other. Mogens Hadbold shook his head. 'We have looked into your partners, Miss Martine Delaroche and Miss Radiance Young. We are satisfied of your financial commitment. And of course we know Mr Harding's environmental work. And you know Midgardfjorden, so there is no more to say on that. Everyone is clear what is on the table. You are the last presentation, and I hope the family will not keep us waiting for their decision.' The old man winked at Sean as he walked them to the door. 'I too long to know the future.'

They were both silent in the lift going down. Tom was buoyant, Sean furious. Only when they were out on the street did he explode.

'You knew there was a camera!'

'Yep. Want a drink?' Tom grinned. 'I'm gasping.'

They went into the first place that smelled of beer. It was the middle of the afternoon, a strange time to be in a pub, but everything was strange. Sean had taken Tom to the presentation as his mascot; Tom had taken the meeting. Sean had said almost nothing. Tom put his arm round his shoulder.

'I wasn't so bad, was I?'

'You were an utter, utter, bastard. They loved you.'

'Didn't overdo it?'

'You chewed the furniture – I wanted to throttle you.'

'Result.' Tom ordered two pints without asking what Sean wanted. Sean wasn't a pubbish sort any more, certainly not any old boozer on a midweek afternoon. Not that he was in any state to do business – he was fizzing with energy and outrage at Tom's hijacking of his event.

'You are the most egotistical fucker I have ever met, Tom, you know that?'

'You're very welcome. If I'd gone in there all mealy-mouthed, you'd be dead in the water.' Their pints came. They clinked.

'Bastard.'

'Bastard.'

They drank hard and talked lightly of current affairs, excluding the one with Martine. Tom thanked Sean for the picture. They discussed the latest closure of the Suez Canal, the skinhead revival, and remembered a mutual friend from college, recently killed reporting from Ukraine.

'We underestimated him,' Tom agreed. 'A hero in our midst.'

'Like you,' Sean said. 'You're a hero.'

Tom drained his pint. 'Win Midgard, you will be too.'

Sean felt a glow that was more than the beer, and the afternoon sun coming in through the sand-etched windows. Putting the world to rights with Tom, boozing an afternoon away. What a rare pleasure. He was about to tell him that; he might even have been about to tell him how much he'd missed him, after ordering another pair of pints, when the door opened and a beautiful girl walked in.

She was about twenty-five, fresh-faced, casually dressed. Without realising, Sean pulled in his belly and sat up straighter. She looked across and walked over. Her smile was lovely. Perhaps she'd been in one of his clubs, and recognised him. He prepared himself. Tom put his arm round her. They kissed.

'I'm ready,' he said.

'Then hello and goodbye.' She smiled at Sean, playful and polite.

'You look so familiar,' he said to her. 'Have we met?'

'I live in Berlin. Do you go there?'

'Christ,' he said. 'Tom, she's the image of Ruth.'

'Rubbish.'

'Is that a good thing?' The girl looked from face to face. 'Who is Ruth?

'Mutual friend,' Tom said. 'A brilliant woman.'

The girl's smile lit her up. 'Then I don't mind at all.'

Sean gazed at her until Tom punched him lightly on the shoulder.

'Let me know how much they hated me.'

Sean smiled automatically and watched them disappear out onto the street, and into their shared afternoon. He found himself alone, quite drunk and acutely bereft.

The lovely German girl was young enough to be Tom's daughter, if he'd had one. This brought the image of his own sharply to Sean's mind. Rosie, the angry sad child who could not understand how her father needed to feel like a man more than a husband. How her mother had changed into a woman who saw him as he really was, instead of who he wanted to be. It was Gail who had caused him to fail, with her impossible standards.

Sean knew he was drunk, but maybe that was the best way to tell Rosie how he felt. He wanted to say sorry, for so much. There at the bar he took out his phone. The call went straight through to her voice-mail. At least it didn't ring several times, as often happened, before going dead. That meant she knew it was him, and didn't want to talk. This time, she was just busy. Then he called Martine, and the same thing happened.

Why did they not pick up? And Tom, the shit, hadn't even told him he had plans, yet he must have had that arrangement in place all along. As if he might try to muscle in, or something. Sean left his pint unfinished. Only sad old men drank pints on their own in daylight. Tom had done this to him.

A bright burst of laughter seemed aimed at him and he turned. Two girls sat at a corner table, they looked away when he caught their eye – but not before flashing him a quick smile. He did not know what to do with himself; it was that awkward time when the pub was just filling up with the early after-work crowd, the low earners who couldn't wait to get away. One minute he was enjoying a liberating freedom with Tom, drinking pints in an unfashionable pub at the hour they felt like doing it – and the next he was beached on the shores of other people's lives – like some loser.

The girls sent arcs of laughter up through the air, they were lassoing him and drawing him over, they wanted to play. He looked in the mirror behind the bar, where he could see them angling their thighs towards him, rearranging their shiny hanks of hair.

Before he left, he spoke to the barman and bought a bottle of champagne to be sent over when he'd gone. Their faces fell as he went out, and he felt a grim satisfaction that he had not fallen for it, drunk as he was. He could have gone over and within a couple of drinks – maybe not even that – adjourned to somewhere more comfortable. A hotel. *An* hotel. He had learned to always use that weirdness, to demonstrate his adherence to the right set of rules. Inviting people for 'a kitchen supper', never 'dinner'. Repeating 'how do you do,' instead of ever answering the question. In English society, nobody cared – that was something he learned too – and they would be horrified if you told them. He did however draw the line at eating soup backwards; that was just madness.

Standing outside, Sean watched the girls receive the champagne. They were suitably over-excited and he drew back as they scanned the pub for him. What a strange thing to have done. It gave him no pleasure, he was just acting out the anxiety of waiting, of being compared and judged after the presentation. He should have just said that to Tom, but he'd been too busy struggling with the feeling of inadequacy because of how brilliant Tom had been. If they'd only had longer, and more to drink, he would have blurted it all out, they could have talked again like they used to – he could have told him about how it had gone wrong with Gail. Tom was kind, he was always kind, he would have known what to say. Instead, he'd gone off with Miss Berlin, who did look like a young Ruth.

Sean slammed into the wall of the pub, drunker than he'd thought. When he and Tom had been drinking together, he'd been happy in a way he had forgotten, relaxing into that feeling of comradeship and solidarity that was peculiar to their friendship. Only now did he realise he'd been looking forward to talking about their Greenland trip again, to indulging in a full-blown nostalgia fest, to drinking more, to calling Martine drunkenly to say he was having dinner – supper – with Tom, that it didn't fucking matter what happened with the Midgard deal, at least they'd reconnected.

He peered through the pub window. To feel so disappointed was pathetic. Nostalgia was for people whose lives were over. Tom had a date, and those girls in there had been joined by two meaty-looking boyfriends. Sean watched some animated talk about the bottle and the boys jerked their necks and squared their shoulders in ritual male display for the rich sod who'd undercut them.

Aimlessly drunk, emotionally disorderly, he decided to clear his head and walk back to Devon Square through Hyde Park and Kensington Gardens, in the hope of seeing the cavalry.

But it was too late in the day for the horses, and Sean sat on a bench with a coffee from one of the kiosks, trying to sober up. Vodka he could skilfully calibrate, but pints of beer somehow sidestepped that control and made him too emotional. From deciding as he walked away from the pub that he would park the whole Greenland nostalgia trip, he was now flooding with memories of it. He'd been there on three separate expeditions, the first with Tom, on the Lost Explorers' Expedition when they were twenty. They had been racing partners on the ten-dog sled, and both had imagined that reading about it was tantamount to expertise. They had made complete fools of themselves and had never had a better time. The next couple of times had been for Kingsmith, investigating some mining tender that came to nothing; he had spent time in the capital Nuuk – but it had still been Greenland, still the Arctic.

The first time was the best, despite their incompetence. Because of it, perhaps. He and Tom sweating and stumbling about in the snow, desperately trying to wrestle ten dogs into their harnesses, the air snapping and flashing with the frenzy of excited barking, the dogs fully aware they had novices to deal with. One by one they got them in, resorting to both of them grabbing one dog and managing at last to work out which leg went through which bit of harness – exhausted before they even set off, but the dogs howling and leaping with the thrill of it, as if they'd never done it before either.

It was a shock when his phone rang, in Hyde Park. It was Mogens Hadbold, and he had good news.

One is often asked what is the attraction and what are the joys of Polar exploration. The answer is – Adventure – going where man has never gone before. Achievement – discovering something of value to mankind, such as the whale-fishery of South Georgia; or ramming your way through ice or any difficulties under steam or sail. The wonderful pure beauty of these regions, the healthy invigorating life; and last but not least – comradeship – the comradeship of men. Men who fight alongside you, toil with you, laugh with you, and chaff you. Pals who rack their brains for abuse and epithets to hurl at each other, and who fight for their absent chums. Pals who stand by each other through thick and thin; who share trials, hardships, joys, dangers and food, and are determined, at all hazards, to 'see it through' together. For such men you feel a great affection, and the results are teamwork and loyalty of the finest, highest quality, with joy of memory that never fades away.

Under Sail in the Frozen North: The Log of the 1926 British Arctic
    Expedition (1927)
Frank Arthur Worsley

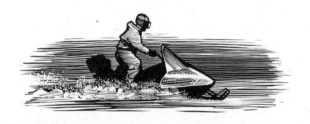

10

From his park bench, Sean sent emails to Kingsmith, Radiance and Tom. He phoned Martine and said he would be over soon, then he called Gail, to say he wouldn't. He told her the news and first she congratulated him then asked for a divorce. She knew that Martine was part of the consortium and not one of his silly little girls, and she understood that now his relationship with her would become paramount. Gail wanted the dignity of immediate separation. She told him her lawyer's name and hung up. Sean was both relieved and shocked that she was so prepared.

When he arrived at Martine's apartment she had a spare key and a bottle of chilled Krug waiting. This was the moment they had imagined, and though he enjoyed seeing her blaze with their triumph, he felt oddly detached. Perhaps he just no longer liked champagne. Perhaps this was a sign of success; when vintage Krug became a fizzy drink. Not a noble pint in a fuggy all-comers pub, with a mate who kept you level.

Martine slid down onto her knees in front of him and smiled, in the way he understood. He closed his eyes. The effort was over, success was his. The strain of living a lie with Gail was also gone. And Tom had come in and done exactly what Sean had brought him in to do: make him the winner. But he did not feel happy. After a while Martine looked up, concerned. He wound her hair in his hands and nodded, his eyes still closed. She resumed, and he focused on her skill. He tried harder to respond, thinking of the two girls in the pub, of recent porn – an appetite no woman would ever wean him from, even if she knew about it, which Martine did not. Still nothing. Gently he lifted her back up to him. He held her.

'Why am I not happy?'

'You got what you wanted. Now you feel empty.'

He nodded. It was true, and her insight made him feel tender. He stroked her hair, in silent consolation for their first erotic non-event. Later they watched television together, also for the first time.

'A decent man's content with profit,' Kingsmith used to say to him, in the early days. 'Only fools want more – and fools are tools but never partners.' And Sean, or *Sean boy* as Kingsmith called him, had laughed and watched the money rolling in, and worked seven days a week if necessary, as it often was, learning his mentor's particular ways, travelling with him, growing familiar with the Russian dolls of his financial habits, and Kingsmith's migratory routes: the Caymans to Panama, Monaco to Jersey, to Zurich – to thin air. Very often a scrap of a percentage point of profit fell under the table to Sean, sometimes as a cash bonus, but more often as a last-minute allocation of some IPO, some hitherto obscure company Kingsmith had carefully cultivated up to its stock market debut, usually but not always connected with mining, one of his major interests. Sean proved himself an excellent steward of his financial good fortune, using part of his profit to grow his property portfolio, and always reinvesting in something else Kingsmith recommended.

Both knew Sean would never be in the same league, but he was a quick study and had become personally wealthy beyond the dreams of his twelve-year-old, or even twenty-year-old self. Wealthy enough to acknowledge that money was not enough. What he'd always dreamed of was his name on the map. Literally. Like Barentsz or Bering or – well, OK, not like Cecil Rhodes – but to be a man of daring and discovery and honour, whose explorations could name mountains and seas.

Now, after the Pedersen deal, that secret glory-seeking part of him rejoiced like never before. He, Sean Cawson, had pulled himself up by his bootstraps and at this most critical moment in its history, owned a tiny piece of the Arctic. The ice was receding and the TransPolar sea route was busier every day, moving global markets from supermarket checkouts to construction contracts as the price of goods went down. Untold mineral wealth was newly unprotected and within reach. There was something magical in the air; it *was* a new golden age of trade and opportunity, and he was a very modern buccaneer, in it for influence, not plunder. He was known for bringing people together, and now he was about to do this in the Arctic, the new business arena where trade and logistics rubbed up against the environment. Surely that was worthy of some sort of recognition?

Midgard was his biggest coup, but somewhere deep inside he had always known he would succeed. Several months ago, and in the face of the heavy odds against him winning the bid, he had placed a large retainer on the services of his chosen Norwegian architect, in order to capitalise on the narrow time window for the work. The morning after the Pedersen decision, and after Martine had left for work, he made that call from her apartment, and the sound of jubilation in the Oslo office buoyed him in happiness all the way across Kensington Gardens.

He was walking towards Selfridges, to kill a bit of time before meeting Joe Kingsmith for lunch. As yet he did not know the venue or the hour – but that was typical. Sean hadn't even known he was in London but found the email when he woke, saying he'd be at the Wallace Collection just behind Selfridges, and then they could grab a bite. He liked to look at the old weapons collection, Sean remembered. It was the older man's indulgence to himself, and usually meant things were going well. He lived in hope of owning something connected with the Roman general Crassus; Sean always meant to look him up, so he could talk knowledgeably about him – but he had never got round to it.

The sky was an empty blue and it was so hot for February that although the trees were bare the joggers were dressed for summer. Sean walked across the park, repressing a feeling of irritation at how his mentor, affectionately though he felt towards him, still seemed to think of him as the callow and grateful undergraduate, willing to dance attendance on his whims. That was a lifetime ago – but Kingsmith didn't seem to age the way other people did.

Sean passed the top of the Serpentine, watching a pair of swans gliding down to land on the water. If Kingsmith still treated him like a kid, then that was the price of access to his capital. One hundred and fifty million dollars in this case, which, along with Tom's participation, had got him Midgard Lodge. Once he'd referred to him as 'the old man' and people had thought Kingsmith was his actual father. He had not corrected them; he felt much more Kingsmith's son than his own unknown father's. And though wild horses wouldn't have dragged it out of him, because Kingsmith was awkward around emotion, in Sean's heart he was sure the old man had some paternal affection for him too. So Kingsmith had good credit. Sean would kill some time in the Watch Room at Selfridges, and wait for his call.

This was a place long soothing to Sean's spirit, and he had visited it many times before he could afford the things he wanted. It was always the same, the dawdling wealthy shoppers, sparkling vitrines and his own enhanced reflection in the tall apricot-lit mirrors.

He should commemorate his journey from staring at the painting of the icebergs on the care-home staff landing, to standing here, the legal owner of a piece of the Arctic, with – of course – a watch. A new time in his life, something that fitted his new role of merchant prince and environmental champion. A watch of subtlety, with a rugged outdoor quality, its high value only apparent to the cognoscenti. Nothing vulgar. Sean had no idea which that would be. It amused him that as he went from case to case, the glittering dials, exotic straps and satin-draped plinths jostling for his attention, he gathered sales assistants like iron filings to a magnet. There was a new display case since he had last come in, 'The Hall of Fame' case. And in it, a platinum Rolex Cosmograph Daytona gleamed at him, with its ice-blue dial the colour of a glacier. He tried it on and looked at his reflection. He didn't want to take it off so he bought it and slipped his Patek Philippe into his pocket. Collecting beautiful watches went with his idea of himself.

Perhaps he should buy a watch for Martine too. No more philandering. Marriage to Gail had not worked, but he still wanted a mate

– not to be like Kingsmith, who for all his wealth and rosters of willing beauties around the world, seemed to lack the centre of gravity that a relationship gave. He had no children, no regular partner, but a different gorgeous woman was always available, wherever he was. Once Sean had thought this highly desirable, but now it seemed increasingly sad, though that was one emotion he'd never seen Kingsmith display.

Sean browsed the women's watches. He also wanted to buy something for Rosie, but the idea of calling her and saying where he was, and her being vile to him on this day of triumph – this was not the time to do that. What about Radiance Young then? This was also her triumph. She had brought China to the table and he wanted to show his appreciation – but she was so eccentric. Who knew what sort of inappropriate behaviour a gift from him might trigger? She kept her Facebook page frequently updated and either referred to herself as 'Bi-Polar Babe' due to her extraordinary feats of endurance at both Poles, or, 'Simple Girl Looking For Love'. Sean had yet to meet another thirty-four-year-old single Chinese woman with hundreds of millions of dollars at her disposal. Or a chain of specifically Chinese-friendly hotels in hitherto untapped markets (most of Europe), a portfolio of interests in several African countries, and her own shipping line, a wharf in the port of Dalian included. Radiance was bumptious, exuberant in her appetites, driven, tactless and generous: but simple she was not.

'That's so pretty, would you like to see?'

A smiling sales consultant was already unlocking the case before him, and lifting out a black ceramic watch with a diamond bevel. Sean took it from her. Yes, it would look good on Martine. The sales consultant cocked her head.

'Someone special?'

'Is it waterproof?' He imagined it dripping on Martine's wrist when she wore a black bikini. He knew she wanted to be invited onto Kingsmith's beloved yacht *Brisingamen*, the nearest place he had to a home. He would ask him about it over lunch, and Kingsmith would say yes or no, or more likely not even acknowledge the request, but he would definitely remember. As if by telepathy, his phone trembled in his pocket and he grabbed it at once – Joe never let it ring more than three times before hanging up.

The name Rupert Parch flashed on the screen. Sean knew him vaguely, he was not quite sure how, but apparently he had given him his number.

'Rupert.'

'Is that the famous polar explorer?' said an enthusiastic voice. 'I said I'd get you. I'm testing this amazeballs app from the MoD, locates your contacts. Asymmetric intel, heard it here first. Probably not though, you're well clued up. DQM, though.' Which in Parch-speak meant: don't quote me. 'That's a nice watch, by the way, you should get it.'

Sean spun round. Parch's voice was in his ear, and also coming up behind him in person, a big smile on his beaming face, his hand out-thrust. Sean took it and Parch pumped enthusiastically.

'You – are – the coming man! Massive congrats!' He looked around conspiratorially. 'Ah, but maybe you're still keeping the schtum-pow-der on it? Shouldn't bother, everyone's talking about you. Sean Cawson has never been so sexy. True dat.'

Somewhere in his early forties, Parch still looked like a naughty schoolboy, with bright colourless eyes that sparkled, pale brown hair he wore to one side, a slim frame and a rapid, confident delivery. Sean was never quite sure what Parch actually did; he seemed to move around a lot, like some kind of cleaning fish, his exuberance commen-surate with the status of his current host. Large, by his manner.

'Have you just traced me, illegally?'

'Illegally? As if! I just happened to be in the area. Although sadly not dropping sixty grand on man-candy like the plutocrat I'll never be, hashtag sighs. No, definitely not illegally. But you have correctly sussed that Parch has gone up in the world. And my master is terribly impressed with your latest news.'

'What news?'

'Don't freeze me out.' Parch looked even more innocent. 'Anyway, he desires me fetch you to him for a spot of luncheon, were you avail-able at such short notice.'

'And your master is?'

'Philip Stowe. I'm his new private secretary. Proud to say I've already outlasted my predecessor. Very talented man.'

Sean had heard many other things too. Stowe had seized the post of Defence Secretary after a vicious and decimating Westminster rumble of his own creation. Sean waited for his payment to be processed. Stowe had sent for him? He felt Parch's eyes on his back and smelled his soapy cologne.

'Might you be free? Offers like this don't tend to repeat. Unlike my master, but I shall never mention that. By the way, there's a car waiting outside, on a double yellow. Only if you had no other plans. I'll run along if you do.'

Sean's phone buzzed again, this time Kingsmith. He had never before dropped his call. But the money was banked, the deal done, and Midgard Lodge was his. The buzzing stopped, and Parch turned from the display case over which he'd busied himself.

'Nothing vital?'

'I'm free.'

'Good man! Hope Indian's OK? One of those pop-ups, all the rage. And if you don't mind my saying, you look like you could kill a Cobra.'

Inouarfigssouak, Grand Massacre Bay
Grand Massacre? Kratoutsiak explained it in a few words. The story,
though old, is worth telling. It remains in all memories.

Two boys were fighting on the shore of an island – the island
where we were. A little brutally perhaps, like most children. One of
them fell over. He shouted. The other, to keep him quiet, pummelled
him with feet and fist. By chance, the grandfather of the fallen boy
saw him. He ran up and joined them as he ought. There was a battle.
Full of anger he hit so hard that one of the boys fell dead upon the
rock. The other grandfather was furious and intervened. So did
fathers, shrieking mothers, mothers-in-law, uncles, aunts, cousins,
nephews and nieces. The whole camp was fighting. Injuries,
invectives, horrors. All were in a state of unspeakable fury. They
threw stones and bones at one another's heads. Someone pursued a
woman with a bloodstained harpoon. They destroyed themselves.
Of the whole village only one person was left.

The story does not say how the survivor died.

The Last Kings of Thule (1956)
Jean Malaurie

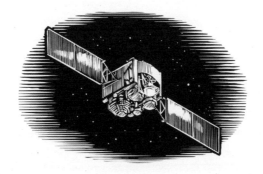

11

As the ministerial car with darkened windows headed south, Sean assumed he was meeting Stowe at Westminster, and all this cloak-and-dagger stuff was Parch's misplaced sense of drama, intended to impress Sean with his own command of perks. But they skirted Parliament Square and sped east along the Thames, and Parch begged Sean's forgiveness in not saying more.

By the time they were passing the Tower of London, Sean guessed they were en route to Docklands, and by Canning Town and the highly visible police presence on the streets, he remembered seeing some protest on the news about the bi-annual arms fair, held at ExCel Centre. Parch rolled his eyes.

'Word to the wise: we say Defence Expo.' They looked out. A dense crowd of respectable-looking businessmen, and a few women, waited at the main entrance. Many had flight cases. 'The British Government would not dream of sponsoring something as mercenary as an arms fair. Oops, don't say that word either.'

'What, mercenary?' Sean enjoyed his temporary Whitehall gravitas, reflected in the faces of the armed police waving their car through security.

'I'm serious. I can't tell you why you're here because all I know is that Stowe's keen to meet you, so I crow-barred some daylight in his diary then chased you down, like the good dog I am. I'm guessing it's a one-shot opportunity, but who for I don't know. DQM, or poor Parch will be thrown off the gravy train.'

The car passed through tall steel gates and into the shadow of a line of battleships, moored outside the conference centre. As they got out they paused with a small crowd, watching a black-clad commando team demonstrate how they would take a ship, from a rigid inflatable boat several storeys below on the brown water of the Thames. Six men in balaclavas shot lines that attached to the freeboard of the ship, which they then scaled with extraordinary strength and dexterity. Watching them, Sean felt soft and inadequate.

'Here' – Parch slipped a lanyard over his head – 'you're an MoD consultant for the day. Anyone asks if you're a journalist, leave them in no doubt. One weaselled in yesterday under false pretences, then refused to leave. Started shouting about freedom of information. Like he'd know what to do with it. Come on, I'm starving.'

Parch's 'super-cool pop-up' was in the Officers' Mess of the Indian naval destroyer *Kali*. At the top of the gangplank a phalanx of dazzlingly starched Indian naval officers waited to welcome them and Parch was as airy in his greetings as if he were the British Defence Secretary himself. He led Sean through to the source of the delicious aromas – a buffet hidden behind a wall of tall and broad khaki, navy and black backs, gold braid abundant on their shoulders. There was no getting through for a while, so he and Parch accepted samosas and bottled Cobra beer from passing waiters. Parch looked wistful.

'We did one on ours, yesterday. A lunch. Friends, allies and countrymen, poached salmon and Coronation effing chicken, who thought of that? I wouldn't say the tumbleweed blew, but it was nothing like this. Waft a bit of curry around, et voilà! Prey and predator at the watering hole. Spend on the catering, that's the motto. A beast with a full belly is safer.' He dropped his voice. 'Problem with old Team GB is, their tastes were formed at public school. No gristle in the custard, they send it back.'

Sean tried not to stare. The mess looked like a fancy-dress party before people had had enough to drink. The bristling moustaches did not look real, and the braid and ribbons were comically bright. Out of a porthole he could see a golf-buggy full of men in Arab robes stopping at the bottom of the gangplank. One had a large hooded bird on his wrist.

At that moment, a volley of laughter burst from a nearby group and Sean saw the face of the British Defence Secretary, animated at its centre. The Indian commodores and generals around him were vastly amused.

'Probably just mentioned Coronation Chicken,' Parch murmured, smiling deferentially at his boss. Stowe nodded to Sean and held up his finger. Like Kingsmith, he thought. Sit, stay, up for a biscuit. But ... good biscuits.

'Before I go,' Parch said in a low voice, 'he's very pro your price. For what you've pulled off, everyone thinks you deserve it.'

Sean took a slow pull at his Cobra. Stowe could have arranged a meeting in London at any time. Why here, why now? Whatever he wanted must be important.

'My price?'

'Come on.' Parch looked at him sideways. 'A Special K. You said you wanted one.'

'Wasn't that some kind of old nightclub drug?' Sean knew exactly what it was, slang for a knighthood. But how on earth did Parch know he wanted that?

'I believe it might have been. Didn't you mention it at that brilliant party after Wimbledon last year? Or was it Royal Ascot? Land of Hope and Glory ring any bells?'

'Not really.' Sean looked at his watch.

'Five minutes,' Parch pleaded.

Sean drank his beer. He remembered all too well. It was at a post-racing party in Berkshire held on the Last Night of the Proms. Things had been very bad with Gail – or rather, he had behaved extremely badly yet again and only a massive bender could anaesthetise his shame.

It had all culminated at this party. At first all was well – he liked the beautiful horses in their stables and the Union Jack bunting, he liked the strangers who shared their coke, he liked the cocktails – and then out of nowhere he was talking about his marriage, any marriage, surely everyone knew marriage was hard, surely everyone needed help?

The coke grabbed him by the lapels and announced through his drunken mouth that he didn't mean to be such a shit, he was going to fix that just like he'd fixed himself his whole life, he wasn't finished yet, and one day it was his ambition – he was up on a table by this stage – his ambition to serve his country and do something that mattered. He would show the world that he was a man of honour and the proof would be that he, Sean Cawson from nowhere, would win a fucking knighthood. For his country. He loved his country even if it didn't love him. People had clapped, someone had helped him down. No. He had fallen.

'I was totally fucked up too,' Parch confided, '*much* worse than you, don't even worry. I only remember it because it was such a rousing speech. You were like Russell Crowe in *Gladiator* when he's going to kill the one with the twisty face. I knew you meant every word and I thought, aha now, there's a man to watch. And wasn't I right? By the way, I even heard you mentioned at Chatham House the other day, in the same breath as the words: paradigm shift. *Before* you won the bid. Certain people have been watching you very closely. Obviously I can't reveal who.'

'Obviously.' Sean felt his heart beating faster at that terrible memory. He had never taken coke again, nor seen those people again. While Parch wittered on, name-dropping the latest world leaders and giving the impression he was almost on sleepover terms, Sean kept an eye on Philip Stowe. One more minute, then he would leave. The new Defence Secretary ensured he paid smiling and intent attention to each of the Indians in the circle. Sean could not decide which way the interview was going – or if it were a circle of wolves deciding whether they would eat the creature in the middle. As he looked at his watch, Stowe disengaged from the group. He put down his beer and wiped his hands.

'Go away, Parch.' Philip Stowe had a pleasant voice and twinkly eyes, which he kept on Sean. He offered his hand. 'Good of you to come.'

'And you to ask.' Sean shook with equal brevity and firmness. Stowe had asked for the date, let him lead.

'How'd you do it?' Stowe didn't mess around. 'Midgardfjorden. Not the biggest, not the prettiest, ruled out weeks ago – but suddenly you've got the ring on your finger.'

'Charm?' Sean picked up his beer again. Parch was already on the far side of the mess, hooting with laughter at someone's joke. Stowe didn't smile.

'Well done. However you did it. Wanted to congratulate you in person, not bloody email. How many do you get a day? Don't tell me – I don't care. Give me a proper problem, that's my pleasure.' His smile flashed. 'So, the Midgard Consortium—'

'Trust. It's a trust.'

Stowe's eyes flickered at his misinformation.

'A trust. Registered in Tortola, administrated through Jersey?'

Stowe was guessing. He had no legal power to compel Sean to shed more light, and was himself known for many obscure directorships. He knew all the routes. Sean smiled. Stowe looked irritated for a second.

'So that's your management company for the consortium. Private British equity with some foreign partners, correct?'

'Correct, sir.' Sean intuitively added the sir, not from respect but because he'd sized up Stowe as not nearly as rich as he was grand – and therefore likely to resent the far greater wealth of the self-made man. Whatever deal was on the table, Sean wanted him to feel superior. That was when people revealed themselves.

Stowe's eyes were also recording Sean. 'You got, what? Forty, forty-five per cent majority?'

'Fifty-one.' That much Stowe could discover; he would save him the trouble. 'The balance shared between my foreign partners, one of whom has dual Swiss-American citizenship. But in both law and cultural perception, Midgard Lodge will be a British enterprise.'

'You're the CEO. Buck stops with you.'

'One hundred per cent. The work has begun and should be completed next year. The season is very short.'

'So soon?'

'I commissioned the plans when I made the proposal to the vendors. I've had the architect and contractors on retainer.'

Stowe raised an eyebrow and Sean knew what he was thinking. How expensive. But instead the Defence Secretary looked thoughtful.

'Midgard. Norse mythology. The world of men.'

'That's the name of the fjord, since whaling days. Maybe because the mountains are in the shape of—'

'Fascinating political environment, Svalbard.' Stowe looked up as the Middle Eastern golf-buggy passengers with the hawk entered. He paused to catch their eye and raise his hand, before turning back to Sean.

'Our Norwegian friends are relieved it was bought by a British citizen.'

'Rather than ...?'

Stowe twitched a smile. 'The Russians still believe Svalbard is theirs. Svalbard and a large part of the Arctic up to and including the North Pole.'

'Because of the Lomonosov Ridge.'

'Exactly. We'd do exactly the same if we could. Shetland doesn't quite cut it.'

'But don't Norway and Russia have an amicable relationship on Svalbard?'

'Amicable is a word that only ever implies tension.'

Sean thought of the email from Gail's lawyer, waiting in his inbox first thing that morning. The word 'amicable' had been used. The Arab group were moving closer, the bird now unhooded and staring around with fierce golden eyes. A nervous waiter came up with a saucer of raw meat. The bird turned away.

'Don't worry about them,' Stowe didn't look. 'They're early. Bringing the falcon's a good sign. We've got too many pigeons. Tell me the real reason they chose you.'

'Tell me why I'm here.'

'You're attracted to power. You're curious.'

Sean decided he liked Stowe after all.

'OK: the money was right, but we're small, British, environmentally committed – we're not a threat.'

Stowe leaned forward.

'Bullseye. No flags on the seabed, no subs turning up unannounced with two hundred men for an unscheduled sleepover, no new settlements under construction. You're a legitimate British business with an environmental champion at your helm, a clean tech hedge fund filling in, and a Chinese partner bringing stability and responsible investment to Guinea Bissau and the DRC.' The eyes twinkled again. 'Or do I mean the Central African Republic?'

'Both.' Sean didn't smile. 'It's like you've read the confidential bid proposal. It's like you can see my emails.'

Stowe waved that away. 'You'll offer different security details for each retreat?'

'I'm anticipating we'll have VIPs, I hope political as well as corporate.'

'Bit of a faff, isn't it? All that bureaucracy with the Sysselmann's office each time, all those different permits?'

'We'll manage.'

'And you trust all your partners.'

'Of course.'

'Even though you know Greenpeace does more to ruin brand GB than—'

'That's contentious. Anyway, Tom left Greenpeace over five years ago. I trust him with my life and his participation is the reason we closed the deal.'

'And in so doing, created a unique opportunity to serve your country.'

Time slowed for Sean. The great door was opening at last – to what, he didn't know. But the Defence Secretary of Great Britain was definitely offering him something.

'To serve would be the highest honour, sir.' This time the sir was unforced.

Stowe held his eyes.

'And an honour, your fitting reward.' Stowe's tone became casual again. 'Lot of interesting stuff at the fair, especially the Scandinavian pavilion. Care to take a look?'

Sean felt the impatience of the Arab contingent, waiting close behind. 'Don't you—'

'Oh no, not with me. Completely under your own steam.' And with a quick nod, Stowe pivoted into his next meeting.

As Sean came down the bright gangplank, his sense of surreality was heightened by the sight of fighter jets and Chinooks parked as close as space permitted outside the vast hangar of the ExCel. The little boy and kit fetishist in him very much wanted to go and have a look, but he understood Stowe had given a cryptic instruction, and he went directly in search of the Scandinavian pavilion.

At least, he intended to – but there was simply too much to look at. Each of the four sections of the conference centre was designated a compass direction, and each was the size of a sports stadium. Presentation arenas were cordoned off for military speakers of distinction, and military men and associated suits were crammed in, standing-room only.

The sound in the halls had a curious booming underwater quality, and the ambience evoked something of a cross between Selfridges and a souk of death, with all the bright display cases holding bullets, pistols, rifles, RPG launchers and missiles. If Sean looked too long at the carpeted seating areas, the huddles of men would pause in their discussion and look up with undisguised hostility. But the vendors avoided his eye. He was not their customer, they would not waste time.

Like all trade shows, the best pitches were bought by the big companies, and the independents who could afford it, lined the edges. Sean avoided the village-hall-style cheap tables featuring 'non-lethal crowd control' utilities and rubber bullets, and gravitated towards the massive gleaming rocket launchers at the centre. Here was space to breathe, amidst pleasingly designed and spotless military hardware. Some looked familiar from news broadcasts in war zones, others were of exotically futurist design.

Sean picked up a programme and located the Scandinavian pavilions – on the far side. He paused to take a complimentary orange juice from the stand of an upright British company whose earth-moving equipment was unremarkable on any building site – except here, where large mounted photographs featured it demolishing settlements on what looked like the West Bank. Sean pocketed an exact miniature of a digger from the give-away bowl and moved on into the crush.

The crowd looked either military or business, and seemed to consist of small groups that flowed around a dominant individual who carried nothing. Sean continued through the tanks of the Land Arena, where he was barged aside by meaty men in tight-fitting uniforms and contemptuously sidestepped by brisk-paced officers of the upper echelons. Only the unhealthy middle-management types lugging flight-cases scanned him with cold eyes and he instinctively disliked them. He should have been at the Scandinavian pavilion by now, but he must have taken a wrong turn, because he found himself in the Medical Arena. He stopped short.

Under a big sign that read 'Follow the Care Path!' a young soldier lay on the ground, his bleeding shattered legs stretched out in front of him. Sean could not look away from the obscene sight of the bloody white cartilage and spikes of bone, and the dark clotted gore between them. Then a nurse with a tool box sat down on a stool by his side, and began reapplying the gore. She pulled at a bone shard to make it more prominent. Sean felt faint.

'Lovely,' the soldier said admiringly. He looked up at Sean. 'Just like it was, you can see it over there.' Sean looked where he directed, and saw a body on an operating table. A theatre nurse in a Union Jack mouth-and-nose mask went through the motions of the field-hospital operation, footage of what he assumed to be the real event, playing on a large HD screen to one side.

'There I am,' the soldier on the ground called out. 'Lucky or what? That's me on the table too, up close and personal, and this is me here on the ground – still waiting for my Equity card. Job for life – travel the world, legless!' He looked very pleased with himself. 'What's it with you then, PTSD? No shame, mate – all in it together, aren't we? Sometimes you find yourself right where you need to be. Just admit it. You'll feel better.'

'I don't,' Sean said. 'I don't have PTSD.'

A large man in a white coat loomed up beside him, his smile deep and cold.

'Can we offer you support? It can be hard to accept. Denial is the first stage.'

'Nah, you muppet,' called the legless soldier. 'It's the bloody injury!'

'I'm looking for the Scandinavian pavilion.' His mouth was dry.

'I can show you.'

Sean turned at the friendly female voice, with its faint Norwegian accent. A tall blonde woman, her beauty plain as new bread, smiled at him with white teeth and pink gums.

He followed her past the disappointed pastor of the Medical Arena, and into the frenzy of the Scandinavian pavilion, where thrash metal deafened from the Finnish stand. This was inadequate to contain the colossal green-and-black tank jutting out into the walkway, which also starred in its own wall-mounted music video.

Sean and his new friend paused to watch for a moment, as, to the apocalyptic soundtrack, the tank crashed through a pine forest, breaking trees like matchsticks, before the film cut to an urban setting where it rumbled down a deserted city street, raising clouds of white dust. It pivoted with amazing dexterity before ploughing into, then over, a row of shops. The largely shaven-headed crowd roared approval.

The woman smiled wryly. 'Finland is not in fact in Scandinavia, but is a Nordic country. I am surprised the Expo did not differentiate.'

'Me too.' Sean said it knowledgeably, though this was also news to him. He walked on with her and they entered a serene and spacious area marked Dronningsberg, the centrepiece of which was a snowy missile launcher whose base was the size of a large tractor, and whose barrel protruded so high over the surrounding stands, that Sean had seen it from halfway down the huge hall, but assumed it was part of the building. The name Dronningsberg rang a bell – yes, it was in his architect's plans – they were the provider of broadband on Svalbard. They also did missiles.

The woman indicated a couple of chairs. As Sean sat, an aide drew a screen across, concealing them from the rest of the stand. She poured them both some water, drank deeply, then offered her hand.

'Mrs Skadi Larssen, Assistant Defence Minister of the Kingdom of Norway. I am so pleased to congratulate you, Mr Cawson, on your success at Midgardfjorden in Svalbard. We are extremely happy to welcome you as our newest neighbour, and this is a wonderful chance to say hello, and take the opportunity to discuss your plans!' She looked at him with great warmth. 'If you have five minutes?'

Sean had as long as Mrs Larssen needed.

'In Svalbard we have something of an open house, as you know.' He nodded, absorbing her provocative combination of size, strength, and femininity. 'A lot of friends,' she went on, 'can mean a lot of different values. It is very enriching – but sometimes, like now, we feel somewhat anxious about one of our neighbours.' She looked at him directly. 'Sometimes we feel quite threatened, but to discuss such things might make us seem weak, and maybe even encourage a lack of respect. And increasing our home security would almost certainly be seen as antagonistic. Then maybe our neighbour would want to do the same.'

'And you would feel even more threatened.'

He heard the strain in her laugh. 'How can I help?'

She leaned forward. 'It would be very good to think we had a new friend in Svalbard, who would understand our concerns and keep an eye out for us. Who would be there for us, in an emergency.' She paused, and they both listened to the rowdy shouts passing nearby, hidden by the partitions. Sean didn't know the language.

'Is that Russian?'

'Danish. The bear next door has been too boisterous to be invited this year.' Her clear blue eyes met his. Sean felt she wanted him to say something.

'Ah. In Ukraine.'

'In quite a few places.' She held him in her gaze, silently prompting him.

'I try to be well informed, Mrs Larssen, but most of us only know what we're told by the news, don't we?'

'Mr Cawson, Philip tells me you are an explorer, and you have a deep and longstanding love of the Arctic.'

'That's true.' Sean felt incredibly gratified that Stowe had passed this on, that he had even known it in the first place.

'Our two nations share historic loyalty and friendship.'

'Now you don't come raiding any more.' Sean's attempt to lighten the mood fell flat.

'Those were the Danes.' Mrs Larssen paused. 'Now. Do we trust each other?'

Philip Stowe, Defence Secretary of Great Britain, thought of him as a noble explorer. Sean unconsciously added in that word to the compliment.

'Yes, we do.'

'I think so too.' Mrs Larssen leaned forward, and Sean kept his eyes above the glimpse of lace under her jacket. 'Mr Cawson, it would be wonderful to be able to count on your friendship in Svalbard. In return, we will do all we can to assist you in establishing Midgard Lodge. Philip tells me you will be hosting a variety of security details for your guests? I hope you don't mind that I know this; the security of Svalbard is my business.'

'How can I help? I'm all yours.' He wasn't sure of that, but it sounded right to say it, and he wanted to see where Mrs Larssen was taking him.

'I would very much like to think so.' And she explained her idea. Midgard Lodge would host a private standing security detail, which could also be an emergency resource of the Sysselmann's department – mainly for Search and Rescue – if required. Very unlikely it ever would be. But so comforting for her to think of it. And Midgard Lodge must benefit too, in ways they would devise.

Sean thought for a while. 'Mrs Larssen, I'd love to help, but Midgard Lodge is necessarily small and discreet. We couldn't make a difference in terms of strength.'

'But knowledge is power.' She smiled. 'Observing the beauties of Svalbard, the ever-changing conditions.'

'As in, spying?'

'Such an old-fashioned word! But romantic.' She stood up; the meeting was evidently over. She seemed to be offering her cheek, so Sean kissed it. She laughed.

'A charming gesture!'

'Sorry – I didn't mean – I didn't mean to offend you.'

'I am not offended if you find me attractive. Thank you so much for your visit, Mr Cawson, and once again on behalf of the Kingdom of Norway, welcome to Svalbard. Looking after Midgard Lodge will be my pleasure.'

90 N LAT., NORTH POLE
April 6, 1909

I have to-day hoisted the national ensign of the United States of America at this place, which my observations indicate to be the North Polar Axis of the earth, and I have formally taken possession of the entire region, and adjacent, for and in the name of the President of the United States of America.

I leave this record and United States flag in possession.

The North Pole (1910)
Robert E. Peary

3 May 2007: Vladimir Putin makes a speech on a nuclear icebreaker *urging greater efforts to secure Russia's 'strategic, economic, scientific and defence interests' in the Arctic.*

2 August 2007: Russian expedition Arktika 2007, *led by Artur Chilingarov and employing MIR submersibles, descended to the seabed at the North Pole, where they planted the Russian flag. They took water and soil samples for analysis, continuing a mission to provide additional evidence related to the Russian claim to the mineral riches of the Arctic. Several other countries wish to extend their rights over sections of the Arctic Ocean floor. Both Norway and Denmark are carrying out surveys to this end.*

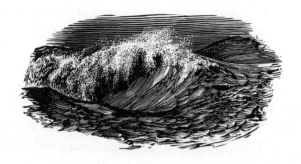

12

Martine was in Paris for the night, so for the first time Sean was alone in the apartment. It was not their habit to call each other for the sake of contact and he was glad of a night alone to absorb the tumult of the week. In particular, today's visit to the Defence Expo (not arms fair) where he had been tapped to provide a standing security detail (not mercenaries) by not one, but two actual defence ministers. And mentioned, if Parch was to be believed, in glowing terms at Chatham House.

Life was certainly getting very interesting. Sean felt as though some brake had been removed, and this time it had happened through his own individual striving rather than a hint or handout from Kingsmith. He tried to think if they'd actually had a plan to meet for lunch, or if it were just contingent on Kingsmith's last-minute availability – the usual dynamic. He worked his way through the last few numbers he had for him, none of which took messages, then rang the Carrington and asked to be put through. They apologised; they could only take a message. Sean smiled – he must point out to Joe that for someone who valued discretion so highly, his favourite hotel always gave the game away when he was staying. He left word he'd be there for breakfast.

It felt good, setting the agenda for once. A healthy levelling of their relationship, long overdue. He owed so much to Joe – he always would – but now they were operating together as equals, not squire and lord. With nothing urgent to deal with on the clubs, and only one missed call from Parch – no doubt for a chummy debrief – Sean disconnected from the outside world.

Bell ringers were practising from some nearby church as he opened a half-bottle of claret and looked for something to eat. The fridge held mysterious bottles and vials of things he didn't understand, and suspected were skincare. He left them alone and made himself spaghetti with parmesan and olive oil, then sat down on one of the elegant white leather sofas to watch the news.

More coastal towns uninhabitable after the floods. Record deaths this month both sides of the Schengen Fences. The riot belt still burning in the US, Japan finally ceding the Kuril islands to Russia, bewailing its lack of international support. Then the usual footage of interchangeable street battles somewhere in the Middle East, a Kevlar-vested reporter shouting to camera as behind her young men ran for cover. Compared to what he'd seen earlier today, the weapons looked ancient. With a bizarre sense of decorum he waited until a big explosion had finished, then switched off.

Without Martine's animating presence, the apartment was passive as a hotel suite. His minimal possessions were all neatly berthed where she had made space for him, but it would take time to feel like home. Opening another half-bottle, he turned off the lights and sat on the window seat in the dark, listening to bell-ringing practice and watching his new neighbours move about in their golden rectangles of light, magic lantern shows through the bare branches. He had emerged from what Martine called his 'ten-year burial in the leaves' and London had changed. It was shinier, richer, and colder.

He wondered what Tom was doing – but to call him at this hour on a Friday night would be strange, and over-emotional. He'd have plans, probably with the pretty German Ruth-alike girl. Perhaps they were in his tiny Richmond flat, its 'river view' only visible while standing at the kitchen sink. The last time he'd been there was for Tom's flat-warming party, when he was still with the original Ruth, and Gail was pregnant. When a magnum of champagne was still a rare excitement, and fatherhood another chance for Sean to excel.

Ironic, Sean thought, that for all his aplomb in creating congenial environments for others, and with two of his own clubs a short cab ride away, where he would be greeted and feted and surrounded by people, he hesitated to call one old friend. It wasn't just the possibility of Tom being with the girl. It was that, even if he weren't, Sean didn't want to say what he'd done today. He had a good idea of what Tom's reaction would be.

With an almost monk-like sense of self-denial, he resolutely avoided going online, just to fill up his anxiety at being alone. He wanted a real pint in a real place with a real friend, or for Martine to come back so he could lose himself in sex. Instead he took a sleeping pill and went to bed alone, intending to enjoy the travesty of thinking of Mrs Larssen and her pink and white smile, but he was asleep before he could summon her to play.

In his grey joggers and hoodie, Joe Kingsmith looked like a conscientiously fit American retiree, braced by some early morning exercise in the Royal Park, and now tucking into eggs Benedict in his regular suite at the Carrington. He waved away Sean's apologies about yesterday's lunch plan, also his opening gambit of laying out the schedule of works for Midgard Lodge.

'I'll leave all the details to you, Sean boy,' he said. 'Complete confidence. Coffee?' He picked up the silver pot to pour but it was empty.

'I'm good thanks.'

'I'm not.' Kingsmith looked around. 'There. They don't stick properly.' He retrieved a large silver button from the carpet, clicked it and dropped it on the breakfast cart. 'You want to ask me something big, but you're nervous. Spit it out.'

'I've been asked to host a permanent security detail at Midgard.'

'Have you indeed.'

Ignoring Kingsmith's slightly irritating look of amusement at this revelation, Sean had just begun explaining Mrs Larssen's suggestion when the door buzzer sounded.

Kingsmith went to the door and looked through the spyhole before opening it. Followed by a butler bearing a tray with another silver pot, he came back to the table. 'Go on. Don't mind him.'

The butler laid down the new coffee. 'Will there be anything else, sir?'

Kingsmith pointed at Sean.

'A dinky private army for my friend. Very discreet.'

'Not quite like that.' Sean pushed down his irritation. At what point was Joe going to take him seriously? And revealing it in front of just anyone—

'Our only army is of butlers, sir.'

'Then we're good.'

Sean waited until the door had closed behind him. Kingsmith was watching him.

'You're frowning. You didn't like my little joke.'

'I just wondered – how did he know you wanted coffee?'

'Oh, that button thing. I'm not sure I like it.' Kingsmith's smile faded. 'So who's this anxious pal of yours, and what does he want? Boots on the ground, eyes in the sky?'

'She's a woman. And she specifically doesn't want it to look like that. She – thank you' – Sean accepted a coffee he did not want – 'she wants us to offer top-level security to our guests that is flexible and vigilant on Norway's behalf.' Kingsmith drank his almost scalding. He chuckled.

'A private military on Svalbard, with a fluffy green eco-front.'

'Joe, you're mocking me.'

'I'm not. OK, maybe I am, but you are so deadly serious, and this is not the big deal you think it is. But go on.'

'It's important to her it's genuinely our own in-house security. We were going to let clients bring theirs in, with all the bureaucratic hassle that rotating in and out meant – surely this is better.' Sean watched Kingsmith absorb this. 'Everything's more streamlined, it makes our life easier and it adds value to what we offer. Plus we can offer twenty-four seven emergency response and search and rescue.'

Kingsmith chuckled.

'She's worried about the Russians.'

'She calls them the bear next door. Have you ever worked there?'

'I have pals there, sure. Pals everywhere. But you know me, I like to do things my own way. I'm happy with my patch.' Kingsmith rubbed his hand over his bald head, gleaming and smooth. 'So what are they offering you?'

'Offering?'

'We don't spend our own money.'

'Oh. Flight permits, for a start. Cuts the transport time, makes it much more practical to attend for a day or two. And naturally I build it all into the retreat costs so that everyone saves. From landing at Longyearbyen, all the way through, to airborne en route to wherever next. Midgard handles every detail.'

Kingsmith held a pot of marmalade up to the light.

'A bitter jelly full of twigs. It's perverse.'

Sean knew what this was about – Kingsmith wanted him to plead. And if he refused, then later changed his mind, it would mean locating him wherever else he was in the world and doing the whole dance all over again.

'Joe,' he said, 'one of the first things I learned with you is that you can't work from a place of insecurity. I know it's not one size fits all; every private military company is different.'

'Sean boy, that's not the side of things you've ever been interested in. It's not your strong suit, you're on the sunny side of the street. You should stay there.'

'I'm not a kid, Joe. I've been asked to do something very important, and yes, it's a stretch, but not for you. This is what you do, you make places safe. You did it for the *New York Times* in Basra, you do it for telecom companies in Africa – it's how the world does business now.'

'If they can afford it. So, what sort of size are we talking about? What sort of anxieties does your pal have? Maybe she could get in touch—'

'No. Please don't take this the wrong way, but it specifically has to come through me, as the British CEO of Midgard Lodge. That's crucial.'

'Crucial. I see.'

Sean bore Kingsmith's long look, willing himself silent. If Kingsmith wouldn't help him, there were other sources he could tap. But none he trusted so much. 'Attaboy. But why does your special friend, or friends, trust that you know a single thing about private contracting in the Arctic environment?'

'I won the bid, I'm having breakfast with you, so I guess I'm qualified.'

'Hah! Are you taking some kind of supplement I should know about? I've never seen you like this.'

'Carpe diem.' As Sean said it, he knew it was true. 'Midgard Lodge is my great opportunity to not only be in the Arctic whenever I want, but also help protect it. And make money. From the time we met—'

'I know. Obsessed with the ice. But, just to be quite clear: you're offering me more risk and more work, for nothing?'

'For the stake you already have, in Midgard. And for honour. To do something worthwhile in this world.'

'Tell me what they've dangled at you. It must be something special.'
Sean said it as casually as he could. 'A knighthood. I think.'

'A what? Some bit of ribbon and a fancy name? I hope it comes
with a side of real estate. Come on, I thought you hated all that inherited privilege crap.'

'I do. But you know where I come from. I've worked, I'm talented,
I pay my taxes and create jobs and wealth – and I want my place at
the table. Money's not enough in this country. Money alone doesn't
get you respect.'

'You think a bit of ribbon will?' Kingsmith shook his head. 'Sean
boy, let me tell you something. When I was last in Dallas, I went to
that art museum and I saw your painting. *The Icebergs*, Frederic
Church. Saw it with my own eyes, stood in front of it, and imagined
you looking at it as a kid. How old?'

'Twelve.' Sean felt choked at the thought of Kingsmith doing that.

'I asked if I could buy it, so I could give it to you.' Kingsmith looked
at him. 'You know, it is literally priceless – they wouldn't sell, at any
figure. Come on now, don't get emotional, you know I can't cope.'

'Of course I'm not.'

'Good. I only mention it so that you know, I truly do recognise how
far you've come. My favourite people come from nothing and you're
one of them. You're a rich man. But if that's not enough, if you want
to bust a gut for a bit of ribbon – OK, to you it's more than that.'

'It's the fitting reward for answering the call. And helping protect
the Arctic.'

'Fine. Each man has his demons or grail or whatever. So if you say you
want my help on this, but the rest is all on you, then you've got it. OK?'

'Thank you, Joe. Thank you very much.'

'Told Tom about this little detail?'

'Not yet.' Sean said it easily, but he did not want to meet Kingsmith's
eyes. He hadn't told him yet; he could do it later.

'Here's what I'll do.' Kingsmith was looking at his phone. 'I'll hook
you up with Danny Long. Countryman of yours, but really a global
citizen. A very safe pair of hands. Tell him I recommended him.'

Sean's phone buzzed with the contact. The mention of Tom made
him uncomfortable. He would have to find the right moment to
explain things to him, but first, he must get things moving.

In 1867, the United States paid the Russian Empire $7.2 million for Alaska (US$123.5 million in 2016), officially ending Russia's reign over the area. Of this sum, a reputed US$165,000 was supposedly used to bribe senators opposing the purchase, to vote for it regardless. The purchase, made by Secretary of State William H. Seward, was initially ridiculed as 'Seward's Folly', but in 1880 gold was discovered, and in 1890, oil.

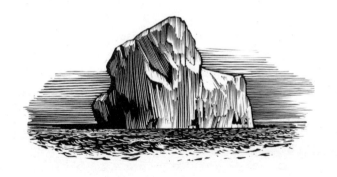

13

The plane trees of London form a scattered forest. Pollutant-resistant, their tall deep trunks shed scales of gold, green and grey. Normally they came into leaf in May, but later that February evening as Sean hurried along the South Bank to meet Martine, he noticed they were already tipping green. They were attending a private screening of the 1927 documentary *Nanuq of the North*, hosted by the Canadian Embassy. He'd seen it a long time ago, when the Lost Explorers' Society had screened it as a backdrop to a party – but been so drunk he couldn't remember a thing. Tonight it was the official main event, before the actual one of Arctic networking at the post-show reception.

The audience was seated and the house lights dimmed as Sean apologised and bumped his way along to his seat with Martine. She squeezed his thigh in greeting and kissed him. Parch craned round from a seat three rows ahead, and waved to Sean. He mimed a drinking gesture then pointed at his watch. He'd come for gossip from the arms fair.

A woman and three men came on stage. Tanya Tagaq introduced her band, then the big screen flared with sepia light, and the Arctic of 1927 came back to life. Sean jumped as the woman began to sing – if that was what her unearthly keening and grunting sounds could be called.

The Inuit people on the big screen moved in quick jerky movements, familiar in Charlie Chaplin films but disconcerting in an anthropology documentary. Wearing clothes of skin and fur, they bent down to the camera and waved out at the twenty-first century. Sean couldn't concentrate, because of the noise the singer was making. He vaguely remembered on the invitation that it was with live musical accompaniment, and had expected something worthy in the orchestra pit – not this twisting fury in a long bronze dress clinging to her like fish skin, and whose bizarre sounds agitated him to his core.

The band followed every swoop and dive of her voice. Sean focused on their sound instead of hers – it was human at least, even if its abstraction and runs of sound were not what he would call music, exactly. But the woman's voice had him pinned back in his seat like an Arctic gale, her body now in spasms so violent he was sure her dress would split any second. One moment she sounded like a bird wheeling in the air, the next, some underwater devil gurgling obscenities.

Her vitality seized his full attention, it was the only way to bear the experience and sit through the film that she prevented him from watching. Sean gave up and stared at her – her strong female shape, her pale flesh gleaming in the stage lights. Her face was broad, her eyes slanted above high round cheekbones. Her long dark hair, which began pinned up, was now coming loose and her performance was more a case of public possession with an audience.

As he stared at her and surrendered to her sound, the singer and the band disappeared, and Sean was with Nanuq the hunter, smelling the mineral scent of snow, narrowing his eyes against the needling wind. His body stayed in its deep leather seat in the Queen Elizabeth Hall, but he was on the great walrus hunt.

Her voice hovered in pent-up excitement with the hunters as they spied the great prey hauled out and resting on the ice, and the drums sizzled their restraint. Tanya Tagaq slid inside her dress as her voice dropped down, coming in to ambush the walrus, closer and closer as the camera inched forward to where the walrus families rest unwitting.

One beast, a big male, is singled out. Nanuq's spear is pure hunger as he crawls towards the animal, the rest of the hunt behind, crafty and low on many bellies towards the walrus, still blissful on the ice.

A couple of animals raise their heads on lookout, but the hunters freeze faster – and the walrus return to their grooming and nuzzling and rolling together. Sean does not know how tense he is, leaning forward as Nanuq the brave edges forward with his spear, kneels up and in one fluent move buries his harpoon deep into the creature's flank. It bellows in pain.

On stage, Tanya Tagaq channels the terror and panic of the walrus herd as they stampede into the water for safety, but once there they do not abandon their stricken fellow. He tries to plunge in after them, but the tearing barb in his flesh holds him back, and the hunters come out like wolves. Mindful of his tusks and strength, they too hurl their harpoons into his body – a big bull walrus full of meat and warm blood. They close in on him as he struggles to reach the water, his big eyes rolling in terror. They haul on their lines to drag him away, back from the sea where the herd have all turned and are bellowing to him and watching in horror.

The sweat shines on the singer's white flesh as she roars the walrus bull's agony, the drums thunder the passion of the kill as the hunters twist the lines of the harpoons around an axe head buried in the hard ice and four, five, six, seven men strain to pull him in as he roars and struggles for his life. Their numbers bring him down and they drag him back towards the edge of the floe to finish him off. But in the water one cow walrus comes in closer than the rest, at risk of her own life, her eyes wild and riveted on the stricken bull, and Tanya Tagaq channels her too, as the merciless camera goes closer on her face as she watches her mate butchered on the ice floe.

The audience stayed stunned in their seats until *Nanuq of the North* had finished. Then they found themselves on their feet, roaring in praise and relief, stricken and thrilled by their part in the kill. When it was over, they rushed for the reception, and the drinks.

News of Sean's Midgard victory had spread. The Canadians greeted him warmly, and Sean inquired after the health of their new ice-breakers. Then as a group of Chinese businessmen approached, the cultural attaché took Martine's arm and they segued away to greet them. Rupert Parch materialised in her place.

'Obvs one doesn't actually *enjoy* something like that, but dear me, you know you've been out. Enjoy the curry, the other day?'

'Delicious, thank you,' said Sean.

'Must have been, as I'm told rather gracelessly to keep my nose out of it now.'

'So you're stalking me?'

'Oh, you know me, I go to as many openings, closings, commemorations, launches, memorials, bar and/or bat mitzvahs, Diwalis, festivals of Eid, Speed – you name it. Protracted throat-singing combined with a very long silent documentary is just another top night out. Look around – this is a Who's Who of the new Arctic! Listen to that buzz. It's a blizzard of business cards: each one's worth tens of millions of pounds.'

Sean saw Tanya Tagaq come in with her band. She was still in the bronze dress, but had wiped off most of her stage makeup. She was immediately surrounded by admirers. He jumped as Martine slipped her arm through his.

'She's so intense. But come with me now, and meet my new friends.'

They were as useful as Martine hinted, they knew and admired Radiance, they had been to the Yellow River research base in Ny-Ålesund, they invited Sean and Martine to visit them in China. They had more feeling for Iceland than Norway and more still for the opportunities of Africa – the Arctic was busy and crowded – but they were very keen to be among the first retreatees at Midgard Lodge. In fact, they had bid for it themselves. And then all conversations foundered, because of what was going on in the night sky beyond the glass wall of their reception room.

Three days earlier and ninety-three million miles away, an eruption through the surface of the sun caused a colossal cloud of magnetically charged plasma to burst into the solar system, travelling at a million miles an hour. The cloud spread out into many charged particle streams. Around the time Tanya Tagaq's shell-shocked audience began colliding with alcohol, one of those cosmic currents discovered the atoms of the earth's atmosphere.

The smokers outside on the terrace of the Queen Elizabeth Hall shouted out to attract the attention of guests inside, urging them to hurry out. In London's night sky huge veils of Auroral light rippled green and violet over the city. Cries of delight in several languages went up as a curtain of gold fluttered through the heavens, over the UK and unprecedentedly low latitudes of Europe. The news reported it lasting just over eleven minutes; its like had not been seen since the Carrington Event of 1859. Meteorologists cautioned it was not cause for celebration, but Sean took it as a most auspicious blessing on his new venture.

Why did you take this voyage? ... Could I do otherwise? Can the river arrest its course and run up hill? My plan has come to nothing. That palace of theory, which I reared in pride and self-confidence, high above all silly objections, has fallen like a house of cards at the first breath of wind. Build up the most ingenious theories, and you may be sure of one thing – that fact will defy them all. Was I so very sure? Yes, at times; but that was self-deception, intoxication. A secret doubt lurked behind all the reasoning. It seemed as though the longer I defended my theory, the nearer I came to doubting it. But no, there is no getting over the evidence of that Siberian drift-wood.

Sunday, 5 November 1893
Farthest North: The Norwegian Polar Expedition 1893–1896 (1897)
Fridtjof Nansen

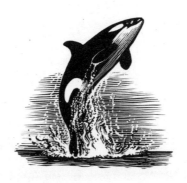

14

Four years later, in Kent, the parish church in the village of Wickton was hosting Tom's funeral. It was a tiny Saxon structure with an already overflowing graveyard that had taken over a neighbouring field. The car park was on the other side of a fence, and as Sean got out he saw the raw earth pit waiting. *Tom's grave*, he forced himself to think, though the words seemed ludicrous. He hurried in to beat the undertakers unloading the coffin, which also seemed completely unconnected with Tom. At least it was proper solid-looking wood, not some frail, terrible wicker thing.

The cold church smelled of stone and tuberose and dusty kneelers. He had come without Martine, glad to plead its small capacity. There were Gail and Rosie at the front, and without thinking, he went up to join them. He saw they had both been crying and wished he had too. They looked at him in surprise as the entrance hymn began, and made room.

On the other side of the aisle, across from him, were Tom's family – Angela his mother, Granny Ruby, and he presumed, some other relatives, weeping unashamedly as the coffin was brought in and placed on the stand in front of the altar. They did not appear to notice as he came in, and his mind tumbled with how to speak to them afterwards.

I'm sorry I didn't visit more – I thought it would make it worse to see me – when the truth was that it was unbearable to see them. After the accident, he had gone back to Wickton once, and endured an agonising tea with Angela and her mother-in-law, Granny Ruby, reminiscing about his student days with Tom, Greenland … They had taken out photographs, they had wept – their raw grief tore at his, it ripped at his mind and heart all over again until he knew that all he wanted to do was move on past the pain. That was survival.

Sean stared at the coffin, gleaming and dark and conventional with its brass handles. *Tom's body is in there.* He repeated it to himself, hoping he would be overcome with emotion. *Behind that wood, under that lid. Is it screwed down? It must be, by now.* The priest was speaking; he couldn't focus on a single word but he could feel the frigid two inches Gail was keeping between them and hear someone sobbing. He needed to see Tom's body for proof, and now it was impossible.

The priest was small and business-like, Sean doubted he had a clue what Tom was like. He had been agnostic, which hurt his devout mother, he'd said that once. Surely he'd rather have had a Viking burial on a burning ship, out in Midgardfjorden. Or remain lost in the depths of the glacier. That was as pure a burial as anyone could wish for.

The service went on, dreamlike, a lot of standing and sitting, the coffin filling his vision until he could see every screw in the plates of its handles, the grain of the wood, the details of the corners. Sean let the green clothbound covers of the hymnal fall open, because he could not open his mouth, let alone read or sing. He felt a tap on his arm – Gail – and he realised everyone had sat down. Quickly he did too, and as he did, looked directly into the eyes of Ruth Mott, getting up out of the pew and walking to the front to make a speech. Even in her funeral black, she looked vaguely hippyish. To his horror, she didn't go up to the altar, but stood beside the coffin, resting her hand on it.

'Tom, our truly beloved Tom' – and she stopped for a moment – 'is not really inside this box.' Sean stared in amazement. Her eyes hurled him back as if by force.

'Tom is still alive, in everyone's heart who ever loved him, in the passion he communicated to us all about how to look after our world. Tom won't die, while we continue his work. And I'm sorry, but this building is no closer to god than the Arctic that he loved. The natural world was his true cathedral, it's mine and it's everyone's, it's where we can all feel something sacred.' She looked at the priest. 'But what's also true is that Tom's family take great comfort in the Church, so I think he'd be happy to know they took comfort – in this ceremony.'

Ruth Mott gathered herself for a moment, and in the silence, Sean heard Gail make a sound, her eyes fixed on Ruth, as if urging her to be strong. Ruth met her eyes and nodded.

Friends again, Sean thought. *And I wasn't even asked to speak.* He kept his eyes on Ruth Mott's hand, its bitten nails, its firm contact with the coffin. She said Angela and the family would be organising a bigger memorial in London later this year, for all those who wanted to come today but could not. People could put their details in the book at the back of the church. Then she made her way to her seat, and her hand left an aura of moisture on the wood.

Sean sensed Gail weeping silently beside him. He felt paralysed. If she turned to him, he would have to put his arm round her, but she didn't. The service finished, and the bearers took up the coffin. He got up first, but allowed Gail and Rosie out ahead. They walked arm in arm, and though both were civil to him – Rosie managing a tearful hello but keeping her distance – he let them go on. Tom's family went out, comforting each other, Ruth Mott with them. It was like he did not exist.

It was a relief to be out in the fresh air and sunshine after the tomb-like church; and after the ponderous organ music, the birdsong was bright as jazz. The mourners became human beings wearing black, revived to conversation and mutual consolation. Sean watched them hugging each other in bursts of laughter and crying, but he remained alone, no one took his arm.

It hit him: no one wanted to be near him, and he had not been invited to speak because he was the reason Tom had died. His venture, that he had called Tom into. His fault. He wanted to laugh in sheer tension at how awful it all was – he wanted to shout at them to turn around, all of them, and acknowledge that he was Tom's friend, he loved him too, the reason he'd kept himself away was that it hurt too much …

He caught up with the group and positioned himself closer to Angela and the family. They didn't seem to notice him. He began to pulse with self-consciousness. He heard someone mention the wake

– to which he had not been invited. The email from the funeral director only mentioned details of the service, and he had just presumed –
he wished he'd let Martine come with him, as she'd first wanted. If
this was how they were going to treat him, what did it matter what
anyone thought?

The coffin was lowered into the pit. Sean watched the faces of the
men who did it, not the pall-bearers, but gravediggers who had
appeared from nowhere. No chance to see the body. No one speaking
to him, though the priest included him in his gaze. He stood in his
black linen suit, a force-field of repulsion around him. The mourners
processed past, those who wanted to throwing handfuls of earth,
flowers, messages on pieces of paper.

Sean walked away from the terrible sound of the mud on the coffin.
That's what it was, mud, on a wooden box, that held what was left of
his friendship with Tom. They didn't want him there. But he was
Tom's friend, he had a right to pay his respects. He watched Ruth
Mott comforting Angela Harding, and went over.

'Angela,' he said, 'Ruth. I'm am so, so, sorry.'

Angela Harding took his hand. Ruth Mott looked like she would
shatter if someone touched her.

'You mentioned a memorial,' he said, 'later in the year. If you haven't
already planned it, perhaps I could help? At our annual fund-raising
dinner, we could make a new award in his name, we could come up
with something together.' Sean imagined it whole and complete: the
huge bequest, the warmth of the big ballroom at the Carrington,
hundreds of guests rising to applaud Tom's memory, Angela and her
family hosting their own table, restored, not broken like this.

'Sean, thank you,' said Angela. 'We've missed you. Haven't we?' She
turned to the small white-haired woman whose hand Ruth Mott was
now holding.

'Granny Ruby,' Sean said. He was going to kiss her, but she held
herself back. Her old blue eyes were wet, but she was no longer crying.

'Sean,' she said. 'You've been a stranger.'

'I thought I gave you more pain to see me.'

'It's as if you were hiding.' The old lady turned away. 'Excuse me.'

She went with her daughter to the embrace of other mourners. Sean
and Ruth Mott stood stranded together. The thuds of earth on the
casket fell slow and hard.

'How's Midgard?' she asked. 'Making you a fortune?'

'Please, Ruth,' he said. 'Not now.'

'Do you even know what's happening in the Arctic any more?'

Even here, at Tom's funeral, he thought, she's ready for a fight. Especially here. Unless it was the way she coped with pain, like an animal.

'It's changing, we all know—'

'Some of us know more than others though.' Her eyes were very bright.

No, he thought, right the first time. She's ready for a fight.

'What are you talking about?'

She shook her head. 'I'll say more at the inquest.'

'Don't wait. Say it to my face.'

'All right, I will: Tom was the love of my life and you took him from me.'

Sean recoiled as if she'd physically hit him.

'I didn't. It was an accident.'

'Then I wish it had been you instead of him.'

'So do I!' He didn't realise he shouted it until he saw all the horrified faces turned towards him. Gail was coming to them, for a moment he thought to help him, but she went to Ruth and took her away, quieting her in the soft voice he remembered. He watched Ruth crumple into her arms, Gail held her, and he couldn't hear what she said.

He felt a soft touch on his arm – it was Rosie. He looked at her in gratitude, but she went past and put her arms around her mother and Ruth. Sean watched transfixed as Ruth realised who it was, and held Rosie at arm's length to admire her. He hadn't seen his daughter's smile in so long, and now he could see the beautiful pagan maiden she had grown into.

'Forgive me,' Ruth said to Gail. 'Forgive my big stupid mouth.'

'What's to forgive?' She and Ruth hugged fiercely, and then they laughed. Rosie laughed too, burrowing in between them and slipping back to childhood for a moment. Sean stood riven with pain and happiness at the sight. No one called him over.

*

He was in his car before he knew it, driving the blind green bends of the country lanes without really seeing anything, until the broad grey monotony of the M20 clicked into focus at ninety miles an hour. He slowed down. He did not remember leaving the funeral, but he was glad he had. The last hymn went round in his head like static.

All things bright and beau-ti-ful, all crea-tures great and sma-all ...

It could only have been Angela's choice. Tom would have gone for something like Joni Mitchell. They paved paradise blah blah. A cliché, but it would work at the Carrington fund-raiser, if he could persuade Angela to agree. It was the least he could do. And Martine would goad and seduce the business community into embracing its corporate social responsibility – they only ever scheduled those meetings at 5 p.m. on Fridays, they bloody knew it wasn't enough.

All things wise and won-der-ful ...

He switched on the radio, anything to rid his brain of the plodding infantile rhythm. Old Kylie, *Newsbeat*, Shostakovich, Gordon Busbridge Furniture will enhance your home – he clicked through the stations searching for anything with a decent signal. A scratchy white noise disrupted all of them.

It must be all the pylons. Wickton was a forgotten pocket of rural beauty in Kent, no longer en route to anywhere but itself, saved by its uselessness, but here on the M20, a swathe of industrial developments were broken by a few thistled fields, on which grazed scatterings of doomed sheep and occasionally, a few raw-boned shaggy horses. The miles of desolate development below either side of the sweeping motorway gave Sean an idea for the speech he would make at the benefit.

All around us is evidence. Greedy piecemeal interests. Now all anyone wants is investment in the US-Russian Arctic Agreement ...

Sean put his foot down. Now was not the time to compose a speech. The radio hissed white noise from every station and he slammed the wheel in irritation. The CD player had broken too, the magazine whirring but refusing to load. And now the day which had been so bright and blue was whitely overcast. It looked like smoke from somewhere, drifting thick across the four lanes of traffic, forcing everything to a crawl. Probably from one of the industrial estates – Sean opened the window a crack to sniff for chemicals.

To his surprise, the air was freezing cold and damp, like sea fog. A hard wind whirled around the cabin and he pressed the button to close the window – but the electrics jammed and it stuck open an inch from the top. When he pressed the button again he heard a whining sound inside the door, and then a crack as if something broke. He switched on the seat heater and all the cabin heating, so that warm air whirled out from several ports. Then that too cut out.

Sean stared out, into what was now a mere fifteen feet of visibility. He could just make out the double red glows ahead of him as the traffic moved on into the fog. It was July – this was freezing fog. Shivering in his lightweight black suit he remembered the travel blanket in the boot, unused and still in its leather bands – but he couldn't see to pull over.

The fog lights shone cones of swirling whiteness. Tiny pale specks formed on the windscreen – snow, or ash from some volcanic cloud? The lights ahead melted into the milky gloom and disappeared. Sean stared out into the pale shape-shifting glow, his muscles clenched in the cold. Some primal part of his brain took over. Pull over. Get the blanket. Get information. Something must have happened – maybe a factory accident at one of those massive complexes a couple of miles back. A fast-moving front from the North Sea.

He indicated and moved cautiously across what he judged to be one, two, three lanes. There was nothing to gauge where he was, no bumps in the road he could feel – but no collision either. Instead, he had a sense of vast space around him. Perhaps this part of the motorway had been newly widened, and he didn't notice on the way down because he was so fixated on getting there in time. Perhaps he had strayed into a marked-off area. Perhaps there was a great drop he couldn't see, and he was at the edge. He had that sense.

He stopped where he was, his heart going fast. There was no sound coming from outside, only the swirling white. He already knew before he looked at his phone that there would be no signal.

As he opened the door the wind yanked it back so that the heavy panel almost banged against the chassis. The wind was freezing cold as he climbed out, and there was something in it that stung his eyes. He had to almost close them as he felt his way around to the boot of his car. Too late he felt ice underfoot and slipped – and found the ground around him soft with snow. He touched it in amazement. The blizzard whirled around him as he stood back up, reaching for the car to steady himself.

It was gone.

Not possible. He had just got out of it, not taken two steps from it.

But there was something in the whiteness, a familiar sound: the ting-ting of metal traces jingling – the sound of a dog team in harness. He shouted, but the wind took the sound. He could feel the vibration, the distant rhythm of the dogs' trot, too fast for a man to walk alongside, too slow for him to run. That funny pace you had to use – two steps run, one step walk. A big team, eight or ten pairs, coming closer – he tried to shout again but he couldn't make a sound. The traces sounded wrong, a metronomic clicking, or some harsh drum. The drum took over.

Sean jerked awake to the sight of a police officer's face outside his window. Blue lights flashed beyond the windscreen where two highway patrol cars were stopped. The repetitive clicking was the sound of his own hazard lights. The Vanquish was parked nose-first, inches from the concrete wall of the hard shoulder, at a crazed angle. His key was still in the ignition.

Sir, the officer was saying. Sir, please open the window.

Sean did. His head hurt, he felt pain in his chest and throat, where the seatbelt was tight against them. He looked around in dismay. Sunshine, motorway traffic, though it slowed to see what was going on. The police officers stared in at him.

'I pulled over,' he said hoarsely. 'In the blizzard. Or whatever it was. Has there been an accident?'

'Sir, have you been drinking?'

Sean hauled his mind back down to walking pace.

'No,' he said emphatically, giving himself more time to think. 'Definitely not. I've been at a funeral, but I haven't been drinking.'

They breathalysed him anyway, and he waited in silence, stunned by the hallucination. Surreptitiously, carefully, he looked around. Everything was dry. There was no sign of snow. He wanted to kneel down and check the ground, but instinct told him not to.

'Mr Cawson,' said the first officer. 'You show no alcohol in your bloodstream, but could you tell us what happened? You mentioned a blizzard.'

Sean made himself stretch, so his watch came into view: 2.50 p.m., said the ice-blue face. The funeral was at 11 a.m., he must have left the churchyard by 1 p.m., and been on the M20 within half an hour.

He put his fingers to his temples and massaged circles, thinking fast. Blizzard.

'That's the easiest way to describe how it feels,' he said. 'The migraines, they're like a white-out in the snow. I was at a funeral in Wickton and I hadn't eaten. Perfect storm: high stress, no food. I should have known. Usually I keep biscuits or something in the car, but—'

'Tom Harding's funeral?' The young female officer's face was ardent. 'I heard it was today, I knew he came from round here.' Her colleague gave her a disapproving look, but Sean seized his chance.

'Yes he did. We were old friends.'

'Oh, Mr Cawson, I'm so sorry for your loss,' she said. 'I read about it when it happened, and how you survived. He sounds such an amazing man.'

'Yes,' said Sean, 'he was. Thank you. And I'm sorry to have caused you concern. I feel much better now, and I'll stop at the next opportunity and get some food and drink.'

'You're lucky you didn't have an accident,' she said. 'I mean, again.'

'Yes. I am.'

They diverted the traffic to let him out, and followed for a mile, where he signalled off to the petrol station. Sean got a Diet Coke and a packet of chocolate peanuts for instant energy, and checked all the electronics. Everything worked. He looked in the boot – the blanket, the hat and gloves, all still in their bag. He wanted it to be a migraine, very badly. But he knew it wasn't. Tom was dead and he had survived. The inquest was moving towards him like a great cargo ship on the horizon, and he was locked in its path. When it hit, he would have to go under the ice again.

Two thousand six hundred and sixty-four miles away, on the top of the world, the blue cursors moved slowly across Danny Long's screen as he looked in on what used to be the ice of the North Pole, now just water. It was getting busier, the cargo ships joined by tankers. He clicked on a few. Cosco was sending a lot over the top from Shanghai to Rotterdam, and Maersk went the other way. Some Russian vessels, minding their Ps and Qs. Nothing to report, just as he liked it. He fired off a quick email to his boss, to confirm it.

At supper this evening Peter told some of his remarkable
Spitzbergen stories – *about his comrade Andreas Bek.* 'Well, you see,
it was up about Dutchman's Island, or Amsterdam Island, that
Andreas Bek and I were on shore and got in among all the graves.
We thought we'd like to see what was in them, so we broke up some
of the coffins, and there they lay. Some of them still had flesh on
their jaws and noses, and some of them still had their caps on their
heads. Andreas was a devil of a fellow, you see, and he broke up the
coffins and got hold of the skulls, and rolled them about here and
there. Some of them he set up for targets and shot at. Then he
wanted to see if there was marrow left in their bones, so he took and
broke a thigh-bone, and sure enough, there was marrow; he took
and picked it out with a wooden pin.'
 'How could he do a thing like that?'
 'Oh, it was only a Dutchman, you know.'

Wednesday, 24 January 1894
Farthest North: The Norwegian Polar Expedition 1893–1896 (1897)
Fridtjof Nansen

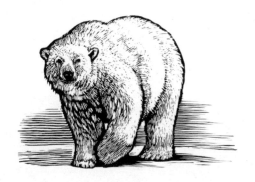

15

The next time Sean saw Parch was a week later, at a summer party on the roof-garden of a bank in the Square Mile. Under a thunderous sky the crowd drank Pimm's and champagne cocktails and ate foie gras and oysters. Parch circled through the crowd until they could spontaneously bump into each other, and Sean remained where he was, to allow it.

'Forgive my ghoulish interest,' Parch said after the first salvo of pleasantries, 'but I've heard that the inquest date for poor Tom Harding has been set. A whole week – is there really that much to say? Yes, I'm a bad person, I saw it on a memo. All right, I peeked. No one likes being disintermediated – I introduced you, but now I'm not supposed to know anything.' He sighed. 'Hashtag bag-carrier.'

'Stowe knows about the inquest?'

'Well, you impressed him, like you do everyone. He takes a friendly interest in your well-being. And before you accuse me of stalking you and throw me over the parapet, here—' He gave Sean a business card, for a Nicholas Sawbridge, King's Counsel. Chambers in Lincoln's Inn, private office in Mayfair.

'Why?'

'Here's what I know about inquests,' Parch said. 'Everyone wants someone to blame. And if my master consults said important lawyer and puts a load of work his way, then he must be pretty good.'

Sean tucked the card away. 'And you're doing this because …?'

'Sharing is caring. No obligation.'
'None taken.'

Rather than his Lincoln's Inn chambers, Nicholas Sawbridge KC chose to meet Sean two days later at his private Mayfair office. After the grandeur of the foyer with its haughty receptionist and mantel-piece dripping marble grapes, it was a surprise when down the stair-case bounded a man much younger than Sean had expected.

In buoyant middle years with a good head of hair just greying at the temples and a lean tennis-player's body, Sawbridge had keen merry eyes behind retro tortoiseshell spectacles. He welcomed Sean into his wood-panelled office that was more of a club room, with its humidor in the corner and dark tartan carpet. After offering Sean a drink and cigar of his choice, both of which Sean declined, and ascertaining he did not mind, Sawbridge re-lit half a Cohiba Siglo VI from the big crystal ashtray on his desk, and they got down to business.

Sean told him how he learned of the reappearance of Tom's body—

'No.' Sawbridge looked over the top of his spectacles. 'You got the traumatic news by phone from Joe Kingston—'

'Kingsmith.'

'Kingsmith, I'm sorry, telling you that *Tom* had been *found*. Talk about his body "*reappearing*" and it might give the erroneous impression that you'd seen it before.' Sawbridge pulled out a transparent file insert, in which Sean recognised his own *Sunday Times* interview from three years ago, part of its Polar Heroes feature.

'Marvellous interview, by the way, hit just the right note. Sorrow, courage, patriotism. And great god, what a feat of survival.' When Sean said nothing, Sawbridge put it down and continued. 'Well, I base my information on your account here, in which your old friend and valued business partner was very much alive the last time you saw him. Correct me if I'm wrong.'

'Tom was alive.' Sean had a strange sense of floating. The smell of the cigar smoke, the fresh shoe polish on Sawbridge's brogues beneath the desk. The muffled traffic sound through the double-glazed mullioned windows onto Brook Street. He reached for his water glass and found it empty. Sawbridge replenished it.

'Jolly good thing you came to me,' he said. 'It's one thing to know on paper what you have to do, it's another to be in the room and feel all those eyes on you. It's not a business presentation, it's not an award ceremony. It's a very intense experience.'

'But it's not a trial.'

'Absolutely separate, purely a fact-finding inquiry. Much as the bereaved frequently want to apportion blame and guilt – which is only human nature, and who can blame them – that's not what the coroner's interested in. So I can promise you there won't be any sentencing or anything like that. We are going to present ourselves in a spirit of respectful cooperation, and assist our good coroner in creating a true account of what happened. Which is to say, it's going to be bloody awful and you need to be ready for that. Are you fit?'

'Fit? Yes.' Sean looked at the wood panelling behind Sawbridge's head. There was a knot, from which the grain swirled out. He looked away.

'Ever seen Tom Harding's dead body?'

'What? No!'

Sawbridge clapped his hands together, as if breaking a spell.

'My dear chap! I'm giving you a taste of what it might be like. A sudden mischievous question out of the blue, like that. Excellent reaction, by the way. We want a clear round, no spooking or refusals – I've got a pony-mad daughter, I've picked up the terms – but to revert: this tragedy occurred three years ago. Now to the conscious mind that can be both a lifetime and, depending on any trauma, five minutes ago. The judge – or coroner, in this case – always says they make allowance for the passage of time, but in fact they tend to press rather hard on areas of uncertainty. Clarity makes their job easier, so we will give it to them. And everyone goes home not exactly happy, but at least with a sense of closure, which is the point of the event.'

Sean understood. He recounted the details of Joe Kingsmith's early morning call, and his own journey up to Svalbard the same day. He heard the change in his voice as he related those details. So did Sawbridge.

'Anything of note, this last time?'

Sean shook his head. The bear stared at him from the edge of the glacier, black light spilling from its knowing eyes, willing him closer.

'Nothing to do with Tom, anyway.'

'But anyway. Just in case.'

'I saw a bear. That's all.' Sean felt an odd sense of betrayal, saying it.

'A polar bear?' Sawbridge's face lit up. 'I really must see them before they're all gone. Reservations just aren't the same, though of course it's the only way to save them now. Was it doing anything?'

'Just standing.' Sean hadn't even told Martine.

'Wasn't there a bear involved in the accident in the first place? I seem to remember hearing something about that.'

'There was an incident with a bear earlier that day. Eclipse tourists. We were delayed in Longyearbyen because of them.'

'That's right! Attacked them, didn't it? Rather gory. But nothing to do with your group?'

'Nothing whatsoever. Except we were delayed overnight because all the helicopters were requisitioned for medevac, including the one we were going to use.'

'So the next day – the day of the accident – you all went up to Midgard Lodge. No bears involved there.'

Sean shook his head. Sawbridge made a tiny pencil note.

'I've been reading up on the Arctic, since knowing you were coming in. Utterly gripping. All those brave fellows. Can it really be peaceful there, like they say? Sounds rather terrifying.'

'It's both. It's sublime.'

'Now there's a word you don't hear very much. I really must go, while it's still there.' Sawbridge studied Sean. 'I do hope you'll trust me. The more you can tell me, the better I can steer our ship. That's how you must think of it: it's a voyage through this inquest, and there will certainly be some weather. And in my experience with my clients, when there's been a close relationship with the deceased, the worst weather comes from within. It's going to hit you again, make no mistake.' He laid down his cigar. 'Let's not pretend that this is not about death. And forgive me for bringing up something else that is painful but pertinent: your divorce.'

'What's that got to do with this? And how do you know?'

'I always research my clients, part of the job. The reason it matters is that, not only did you have the traumatic experience of the accident and the loss of your friend and business partner – one of them, anyway – but that was then followed by your divorce, in the following year.'

He paused, reading Sean's silence as permission to go on. 'For the purposes of context, was there overlap with your current relationship? You would be amazed what opposing counsel might think is relevant to mention, even in the supposedly non-adversarial environs of an inquest. Miss Delaroche?'

Sean looked at the carved nymphs either side of the fireplace, and their small nubile oak breasts.

'Yes, we were having an affair while I was still married. But by the time of the Midgard trip, the divorce proceedings were almost concluded. I'm now divorced and Martine is my partner in both business and life.'

Sawbridge's pleasant expression did not change as he made another tiny pencil note.

'So, whilst business has thrived, on a personal level it's been fairly turbulent. Following the accident, as documented in that marvellous article, you went straight on with business. Barely a week's recuperation.'

'There was a lot to do.'

'And entrepreneurs drive themselves ten times harder than everyone else. How's the sleeping?' Sawbridge peered at Sean. 'Sleep's vital.'

Sean shrugged. 'Could be better.'

'Been bad how long?'

'I suppose … since the accident.'

Sawbridge steepled his fingers and tapped them on his lips.

'I have an idea, if you'll consider it, that might be very useful for us as we approach this process. I'd like you to consider the *possibility* that you *might* be suffering from PTSD. Post-traumatic—'

'I'm not.' Sean said it so fast they both laughed. 'Seriously.'

'No then, that's splendid. However, and I'm not speaking out of turn and she'd never name names, but there is a very fine therapist in London who helps top-level military clients. Going to see her could be an excellent investment before we enter the inquest.'

'PTSD is for people with no legs. Not businessmen who had a shock.'

'You'd be surprised. Jenny Flanders sees some extraordinary people in public life as well as the military. My job is to take all possible measures to prepare you for what is to come. Bereaved families need to complete their grieving process; that is not the aim but a very important by-product of an inquest. They have a hunger for all the details, and to identify the person or organisation responsible for the death of their loved one. This is natural. Going to see Jenny Flanders, a pre-eminent therapist in the treatment of PTSD, shows that you too have suffered, though you survived. It is a signal to the coroner, and it is a signal to the press, should they be there.'

'It's Tom. Of course they will.'

'Right. So expect mud to be thrown. Expect pain and raw grief in that room – and expect some of it to be yours. My job is to help you survive it. To that end, in all good conscience, I urge you to see Jenny Flanders.'

Sean thought of the blizzard on the M20.

'I'll see if I can fit it in.'

I sat in my kayak day after day waiting for the seals. The water was, as the natives say, 'merely oil'. The air was calm as an empty room and the sun like liquid fire on the glass of the sea. The hunter must not move, for the slightest shift of his body will disturb the small craft and frighten the seals away.

It is then that the mind begins to wander crazily. I dreamt without sleeping, resurrected forgotten episodes from my childhood. Suddenly great mysteries became for the moment plain to me. I realised I was in an abnormal, or supernormal, state and revelled in it. I cannot explain the feeling exactly, but it seemed that my soul, or spirit, or what you will, was released from my body, my life and obligations, and it soared impersonally, viewing everything as a whole.

I have often wondered if this was a touch of brain fever, or 'kayak disease' – or merely a state which everyone experiences at one time or another. I have never known, and no one seems willing to talk about it.

Arctic Adventure: My Life in the Frozen North (1936)
Peter Freuchen

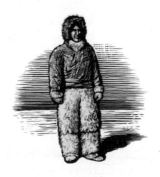

16

Jenny Flanders worked from her home, a gracious house on the far side of Thurloe Square, facing the Victoria and Albert Museum. Her consultation room was on the first floor, in what would once have been the grand reception room. Now the space was piled with boxes and tottering piles of books, as if she were in the process of moving in or out.

Sean took in the good furniture and worn silk rugs as much as Jenny Flanders herself. She was a middle-aged woman with kind blue eyes, a blonde bob, and an all-beige attire that evoked a robustly sprung roll of cashmere. In an armchair against the tall bright window, she waited for him to reply.

Why *was* he embarrassed? Sean shrugged. He felt unbearably scrutinised.

'Well, to be here, in the first place. Complaining about anything, when I've got all my limbs and faculties. I'm a very fortunate man, I know that. I live the life people dream of.' He adjusted to a more at-ease position on the sofa. 'Racing drivers don't look at the barriers, they look at the track.'

Jenny Flanders considered. 'Is that how you feel? Like a racing driver?'

He had told her about the drive back from the funeral, but briefly.

'I mean you don't focus on all the things that could go wrong, or have gone wrong. You look ahead at where you want to go.'

She didn't answer for a while. The room was silent, except for the second hand of a small clock he now became aware of. The ticks alternated in tone.

'What happened on the motorway sounded rather serious.'

'It could have been. But some survival instinct kicked in because I managed to park and put the hazards on. I thought it was a real snowstorm, but when I googled it, it was like a migraine checklist. Snowstorm effect, disorientation, strange noise in my ears like a howling wind. Triggered by stress. And what could be more stressful than Tom's funeral with my ex-wife there who hates me and my daughter who won't speak to me and Tom's ex-girlfriend – that's probably her permanent role in life now, as well as chief mourner – who wants to make trouble. It's not surprising that I had some sort of reaction.'

'Trouble?'

'She said some cruel things to me at the funeral.' He looked at his hands. 'She doesn't accept it was an accident. If something doesn't fit with her world view, she just denies it. It's why she lost her job – she was a field biologist up there – and she'd probably blame me for that as well, if she could. Sorry, but that clock is really distracting, could you move it out of the room? It's like you're trying to hypnotise me.'

'Clock?' Jenny Flanders looked around in concern.

'I can hear it – listen.' Sean looked around but could not see it. They both listened, as a motorcycle went past in the street. When that sound had faded away, so had the ticking clock. Anxiety moved around his body, settling in his hands. He folded them to keep them still. He felt the vibration under his fingers, faint and rhythmic. It was the second hand inside his watch. It couldn't have been that. That would be crazy. 'It's gone now.'

Jenny Flanders did not smile.

'Is there a particular aspect of the inquest that you're focused on?'

Sean let out a slow breath.

'It's all online in the *Sunday Times* interview I did. About how I survived.'

'I didn't read it.'

'Why not? And as I'm going to have to relive it at the inquest, I'm not going to do it now.' He stared at a bowl of tulips on a table by the window, almost prostrate with the weight of their striped ragged heads. The petals were white, splashed with red streaks.

'Everything's online,' he said. 'Everyone's bloody life and death laid out. My divorce, my work, pictures of me with women, skiing – pictures of me and Tom – a ton of pictures. It's like whatever's there becomes the truth.' He sat forward. 'Why didn't you prepare better to meet me?'

She didn't answer. To Sean's surprise, instead of jumping to his feet and walking out, he found himself extremely tired all of a sudden. He yawned, not caring if it were rude. Still Jenny Flanders did not respond.

'You're giving me the silent treatment too, are you? You hope I'll burst, and spill my guts all over your old rug? It's a very nice rug. You must have had it a long time.' A small part of Sean's brain was fascinated by his own attitude. His entire career had been based on networking, on relating well to everyone. His eye went back to the bloody tulips, lolling all over the table. Messy, insolent flowers. He had an urge to knock them aside. 'And people come to you for this once a week? They must be in a bad way.'

'You could come more often.' Jenny Flanders startled him. 'Twice weekly can be useful, at the start of a collaboration.'

'Collaboration? Sounds like Vichy France.'

'That's an interesting association.'

'No, it's not. Sometimes a cigar is just a cigar.'

They sat in silence, Sean determined to wait it out.

'I'm struck,' Jenny Flanders said after a while, 'by how you talk about Ruth Mott. As if she might have been the most difficult part of the funeral.'

So she had paid attention. And it was true.

'She's a very angry woman.'

'You've known her a long time?'

'From the time we were students. Me, Tom, her. And Gail.' He shrugged. The air stilled in the room. Jenny Flanders had somehow tricked him; he'd been about to walk out before. He saw her eyes move, and realised he was fiddling with his empty ring finger. He stopped.

'Sorry, but I thought I was here so you could give me some practical tools to manage the stress of the inquest. I'm not interested in trawling ancient history.'

Jenny Flanders continued to look at him with the same inscrutable expression, that still somehow held kindness. But not enough, Sean felt. Not actually on his side.

'You know I'll have to live through the whole thing again.' He was about to tell her about his fingers, the frostbite, how they were tingling again, when she looked at her watch.

'I'm afraid our time's up. Would you like to make another appointment?'

Yes, he thought, absolutely right. Fake kind, fake concerned.

'No I bloody wouldn't. And I'll see myself out.'

I had a visit from a man named Uvdloriasugsuk, who had come a day's journey to the north-west. He was a big, broad-shouldered fellow with a long black beard; a steady and reliable man, greatly esteemed by all who knew him. Nevertheless, he had shot his own brother the winter before. And it was in connection with this killing that he wished to see me. The brother, it appeared, was a man of unruly temper, who went berserk at times, and had killed one man and wounded others in his fits. His fellow villagers therefore decided that he must be killed, and Uvdloriasugsuk, as head of his village, was deputed to act as executioner. Much against his will, for he was fond of his brother, Uvdloriasugsuk nevertheless consented, regarding it as his duty. He therefore went in to his brother and having explained the position, asked him to choose his own manner of death; by steel, thong or bullet. Without protest or sign of fear, he chose the last, and Uvdloriasugsuk shot him on the spot. He seemed anxious now to hear what I thought about it. I could only assure him that where the safety of all was threatened and all had agreed upon the safety measures to be taken in defence, he could hardly have acted otherwise.

Across Arctic America: Narrative of the Fifth Thule Expedition (1927)
Knud Rasmussen

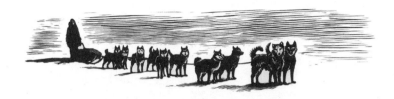

17

October

Sean decided to stay in Canterbury for the duration of the inquest. Early on the Monday of its commencement, he met Sawbridge in the breakfast room of the White Bear Inn, where they had both taken rooms. It was the highest-rated place to stay in the old city, and rather than ominous, Sean felt the name propitious.

His room – the largest – was at the top of some crooked black wood stairs, and from the sloping window he had a view of medieval rooftops and also the car park. A church bell, very loud and close, startled him – he had forgotten what proximity to the cathedral meant – but it was too late to change anything today. He wished Martine had come with him for the whole thing, instead of just arriving on Wednesday for her testimony. But the benefit was on Thursday and she didn't trust anyone but herself to oversee it. It was too important. The Tom Harding Bequest was £100,000, and although there was still an official shortlist, it was going to Imperial College for their newly patented biodegradable Fruit-Fly drones, nano-tiny and with unprecedented manoeuvrability.

In the sitting room of the White Bear, Sawbridge greeted Sean as if they were guests meeting for a wedding, rather than lawyer and client attending an inquest. He reassured him: everyone but Radiance Young had confirmed their attendance – even Joe Kingsmith. Sean's spirits rose at this last item; for his mentor to commit his time was uncharacteristically generous. It was indeed stressful, but it was also a formality that would soon be over, and then all suspicion would be blown away. Sawbridge made it sound as if they were off to see a top-reviewed West End play, and he had managed to get great seats.

Sean followed his lawyer's snugly pinstriped back through a shortcut into the cathedral precincts then out via a private gate in the city wall. As a King's School old boy, Sawbridge knew his way around, and cheerily hailed the flower of wealthy youth as they passed by in their uniform. Sean thought of his own alma mater. One drunken night he had revealed it to Tom, then felt ashamed and denied it as a bad joke. Tom had chivalrously agreed to believe him, and never again referred to it.

The coroner's court was a red-brick building beyond the old city wall, on the far side of six lanes of traffic. The main entrance was on a quiet side-street, with shallow brick steps leading up to the glass box of the reception area. The clerk handed over two copies of the running order for Court No. 1, and directed them to the private meeting room Sawbridge had booked for recesses.

He slapped the pages down on the table.

'I'd say we should be done by Wednesday. Coroner retires to consider for an hour or two if he needs, possibly overnight if he's truly dull – and then first thing Thursday morning delivers his Conclusion, and off we all can go.'

Sean looked through the list of names and time slots. Last night Parch, obviously with Philip Stowe's approval, had left a message of support 'from everyone', but this unexpected solicitude triggered more anxiety than reassurance.

To Sean's relief, Court No. 1 was half-empty. The capacity was maybe a hundred people, and the front three rows of chairs were clearly from some grander environment, high-backed oxblood leather with brass studs. The rest were a mix of serviceable office chairs, with here and there a brightly padded gilt chair commandeered from the Registrar's office down the hall.

It always surprised Sean how little people bothered about their environment, and how simple it was to improve it. As a way of distracting himself from the tension, he considered ways to do this. Clean the filthy sky lantern, for a start; get rid of the vile fluorescent strip lighting, rip out the carpet and put down sound-insulated wood for a sense of quality – find new chairs, all the same – emphasise the formality and get rid of the patched-together air of the room. An older couple in matching jackets sat to one side, and he wondered who they were. They were both tanned with silvery blond hair and the woman had an expensive handbag – and then Sean's attention went to the double doors opening, and his heart started pounding.

Tom's mother Angela Harding came in, his grandmother Ruby leaning on her arm. It struck at his heart to see they were dressed as if going to church, in neat floral dresses with jackets. Granny Ruby had a matching handbag, and they sat down in the second row on the left-hand side. A long trestle table had been set up down that same wall, at right angles to the rows of seats, where sat a very young journalist, tapping away at top speed on her laptop, pausing only to gulp from a paper cup. He stared at her sloppy clothes and flip-flops. He got up and went to her, and she looked up with a smile. Even younger than Rosie.

'Mr Cawson! I looked you up so I'd recognise you – my dad was at—'

'You cannot be here dressed like this.' Sean was appalled. Once he was worthy of a special feature in the *Sunday Times*, but now the only member of the press was this child.

'Do I have to wear something special? I didn't—'

'A man has died. Show some respect.' He saw the alarm in her eyes. He took a deep breath. 'He was my friend.'

'I know, I'm really sorry. I'll change.'

Sean shook his head. 'Sorry. I didn't mean to shout.' Then he steeled himself to talk to Angela and Granny Ruby.

'Sean.' Angela didn't move to embrace him, as she had at the funeral. 'You didn't come to the wake – I suppose you were busy.'

'I don't suppose Ruth invited him.' Granny Ruby's eyes held ancient light as she extended her papery old hand. Automatically, he took it.

She tightened her grip and looked into his eyes. 'Tom admired you so much.' She gripped him harder. 'I'm sure you would have saved him if you could have. Wouldn't you?'

Sean closed his other hand over hers, as much to stop her as comfort her. 'Yes, I would. And I'm glad to be here if I can offer your family support.' He went back to his seat, feeling like the old lady had knifed him. Sawbridge shifted as he sat.

'Best keep this side, for a bit.' He turned as the doors opened behind them. 'Aha. Mob-handed.' An older woman entered, followed by two young men. Each pulled a black document case. Sawbridge rose and bowed politely.

'Mrs Ursula Osman: tremendous to see you.'

The woman paused and blinked at Sawbridge. Everything about her looked slightly battered, from her face to her case to her dusty black suit.

'Nicholas. Good morning.' Even her voice had a rasp.

'Don't tell me you've given up criminal?'

'I give up nothing.'

'So true! Implacable honour your sword and shield. We salute you, madam, and are relieved this inquest is a mere Jamieson.' Sawbridge was as expansive as if he were hosting the entire proceedings.

'No inquest is ever mere,' she said drily.

'Touché!' Sawbridge straightened his creases as he sat. 'Fine KC,' he murmured after she had passed, 'but always looks in need of a good scrub. And my god she's aged. She looks appalling.'

Sean studied the woman who had provoked Sawbridge into such aggressive bonhomie.

She looked in her mid-fifties and was small-framed with the legacy of childhood scoliosis in the hunch of her shoulders. Her sparse hair was dyed an adamant brunette and as she heaved her case over a wrinkle in the carpet, she seemed to Sean to embody the cruelty of the ageing process as well as the vulnerability of the body. Just then a heavy file under her arm slipped and cracked open on the ground. She exclaimed in frustration and Sean went to her aid.

'Leave them.' She crouched on the ground before he could get there, protecting the papers with a crabbed hand. Then she recalled her manners and looked at him. 'But thank you, Mr Cawson.' Her eyes were deep set and black, with an intelligent, knowing expression. With a shock he thought of the bear on the glacier.

Dizzy, he went back to his seat, the tiny buzzing sensation starting up in his right fingertips. The loud distinctive croaks of crows were in the room – their black feet like runes on the dirty glass of the sky lantern. For a moment he saw another window, a cold white lozenge as he lay immobilised in a bed, his arms held in place by straps, an unbearable burning in his fingers. He touched the side of his mouth, then his nose. His fingertips were soft and whole, his skin was warm. He would have to talk about all that, very soon. Sawbridge was saying something to him, nudging him, and Sean realised the courtroom had filled.

'Please be upstanding for His Majesty's Coroner.'

A youthful middle-aged man in a grey suit strode down the aisle, followed by one in his twenties. The coroner took his seat behind the desk on the low platform, and his clerk cleared his throat. 'Please be seated.'

With a scrape of chairs, the inquest into the death of Thomas Walter Harding began.

One of the very remarkable characteristics of the West Greenland 'Husky' is the very varied appearance of different dogs. In the same district one sees animals which look like the old English sheep dog and others which resemble short-legged Alsatians, and neither can be said to be untrue to type. However the majority look more like the Chow than any other European breed. This great difference in appearance suggests that they are a collection of mongrels, like the bastard breed of natives who own them. In point of fact they are probably the purest-bred dogs in the world, being so securely segregated from the rest of the canine world.

Sledge: The British Trans-Greenland Expedition 1934 (1935)
Martin Lindsay

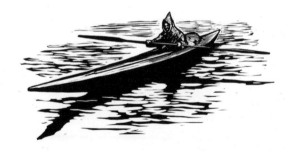

18

'My name is Allan Thornton and I am the King's Coroner for Canterbury and East Kent. I am charged to discover and record, through this inquest, as many facts about Tom Harding's death as is in the public interest.' He surveyed his court with a deliberate gaze and Sean felt a jolt of adrenaline.

'You are all free to come and go at will,' said the coroner, 'but I hope you will respect the process and find the appropriate moment.' Then he indicated the opposite side of his platform, where witnesses would stand to make their statements, and the chair they could use if they needed. There was a television monitor on each side.

'And now, at the request of Tom's family, and for clarity of understanding, I am going to screen footage of the actual moment of discovery of his body, taken in Svalbard in March of this year. I must warn you that at the very end, you will see the body itself. If you do not wish to see this, please leave now.'

When no one moved, officials either side of the room pulled the vertical blinds and put out the lights. The black monitors popped to bright grey readiness. Sawbridge leaned in to whisper to Sean.

'I knew nothing about this – obviously, I would have told you. Terribly bad form – are you sure you want to see?'

Sean nodded, his eyes fixed on the nearer of the two screens. He desperately feared and needed to see Tom's body. The words appeared:

Svalbard Cruise – Property of Mr and Mrs John Burke

The older couple with the silvery blond hair. They held hands, faces rapt.

The footage was slightly jerky and the time code flickered at the bottom. Then the POV lunged to the ship's rail to focus on the face of the left-hand fork of Midgardbreen where the blue ice met the water. The buffeting sound of the wind muffled the excited babble of voices in different languages, then the camera tilted and refocused higher up the glacier. The POV studied the white puffs rising into the air, before rushing down to the front wall of ice at the waterfront as it lifted and bulged before exploding out in the calving. The courtroom heard the deep rumbling sound audible beneath the shouts and exclamations of the passengers.

The camera stared at the great blue floe gliding by, then back to the waterline at the ice-foot. Sean recognised the new cave. It had grown bigger since this footage was taken.

The POV went in closer, tightening on the red shape that had appeared just below the surface of the water. Courtroom No. 1 could clearly hear a woman's voice above the wind and the rustle of clothing.

'John, is that a body?'

The image on the screen was paused. The silhouette of the coroner spoke.

'We are now about to see the recovery of Tom's body.'

No one stirred and the film resumed. The POV on the deck was slightly different, with a new hubbub of voices. The camera focused unsteadily on the blue face of the glacier, then down to the water and a black inflatable boat with four people in orange survival suits. Small pieces of ice fell around them as the boat pilot held its position, whilst the other three pulled the red shape from the water.

It came up long and heavy like a shot seal, but unmistakeably a human body. North Face. Sean remembered Tom's red jacket. The trousers were black. The camera pushed forward over the rail, desperate to see.

The boat then turned around and headed back to the ship and the POV cut out, resuming at a different position on deck. The person filming was leaning over the rail to keep the boat in focus as it returned, the familiar sound of the Zodiac engine cutting through the voices and the wind. The crew on the landing deck below were standing ready, and the camera managed to catch a glimpse of the red shape – and the purplish frozen face Sean can still recognise.

The blinds were opened and also the windows at the top. Pressure popped in Sean's ears and the sound burst loud again. His hands and feet were freezing cold as if all the blood had rushed to his heart. Mr Thornton the coroner consulted a paper before him.

'Tom's family have asked me to explain that they wanted the entire sequence shown to emphasise his concern about the dangerous pace of climate change. That was the biggest ever recorded calving in Svalbard. They feel it's a very powerful way to bring attention to the issue he devoted the last years of his life to bringing to public awareness.'

Angela Harding clapped, others joining in. The sound mixed into something else behind it, a faint plasticky pattering like rain. Sean turned. A couple more journalists – adults at least – had joined the girl in flip-flops. He felt Ursula Osman watching him.

'OK?' Sawbridge leaned in. Sean nodded. Because that twisted horror was not Tom. That was not how he looked.

Tom was handsome in the sleepy-eyed way girls found irresistible and that Sean envied – despite attracting plenty of female attention himself. They had first met thirty years ago, when he was literally waiting on Tom at the Trinity Term dinner held by the elite Lost Explorers' Society. It was the summer term of his first year at Oxford, and the dinner was held in the private upstairs room of the Crown and Sceptre, a fusty conservative pub where he would never have chosen to drink.

He'd specifically asked to work that evening because he'd heard mention of the Lost Explorers' Society, in his obsessive polar reading. The society was several generations old and exclusive, and their focus was on the glory days of polar exploration. It was upper class, extravagant and mounted a serious annual expedition, with sponsorship and risk. He knew he would despise everyone there, but he still wanted to be in the room with them – those fortunate young men of means, whose loud entitled voices he'd heard and hated on the high street, who snapped their fingers at waiters their own age.

It was fascinating. Twelve members were in attendance, they wore black tie – something Sean simultaneously admired and mocked. He was the only waiter and ran up and down the narrow stairs with chilled champagne, then platters of pâté on tiny pieces of toast and yellow wine that smelled like honey, that he discovered were foie gras and Sauternes. When he'd cleared that, he brought up dusty bottles of vintage Pomerol – he had been told to leave them that way – and twelve heavy aromatic plates of Beef Wellington, far too rich for the hot summer evening, but delicious, as he licked his finger of gravy before coming into the room. They wolfed it fast, grenades of laughter exploding around him as he came in to clear their plates. They no longer saw him, but he saw them, how drunk they were, how they shouted over each other, struggling for dominance, and then he heard a magic word: Greenland.

They were talking about their forthcoming expedition in two months' time, in the long vac. This summer! Sean scowled at himself for even thinking of it – he ran back down with their order for another four bottles, and when he came back the leader of the group, whose name, Sean had gathered, was Redmond, stood and grabbed one from him.

He was a thickset young man with a ruddy face and wavy brown hair, and to a roar of general approval, he displayed his father's favourite 1976 Tokay, with the old bastard's compliments – and then Sean was off up and down the stairs again, bringing and clearing plates of apple crumble and cream, port and Stilton, and finally, Armagnac, coffee and truffles.

'You, waiter, stay, will you,' Redmond pointed at him, even more autocratic in his drunkenness. 'Then no one's got to break their neck on the stairs to find you.'

Sean stared back at him for a second, imagining punching him off his chair. But this was the Lost Explorers' Society, formed in the 1930s following the disappearance of Gino Watkins, legendary young polar explorer. He had pored over Gino Watkins' fate, sitting on the curling carpet tiles in his school library. Now he was in the room with the actual people who got to see the real beauty of icebergs. Yes, he would fucking stay. He stepped back into the shadows by the door, and made himself disappear.

Redmond got to his feet and in his booming pompous voice, announced a toast to Gino Watkins – Sean said it in his own mind. When they had downed their brandies – he could not believe how much they'd eaten and drunk – Redmond added that this was also the vetting of the prospective new member of the society: Thomas Walter Harding of Wickton, Kent, who would speak last.

There was a drumming of fists on the table as that young man stood up, tall and handsome, with a disarming smile. He bowed to the assembled company, including, at the end, the waiter by the door. Caught by surprise, Sean reflexively bowed back, and Redmond spotted it.

'Good man.' He turned to his cohorts. 'One anecdote, short and on a polar theme, in order of title which means I go first – yes, still me – new man last.' He looked at Tom Harding. 'Unless you have a title?'

'Mister.' Tom Harding smiled back at Redmond. 'Is that a problem?'

He sat back down too fast and Sean saw him grab the table for balance.

'We move with the times,' Redmond said magnanimously, then launched into his anecdote about his hero, Commander Peary. He was clapped – dutifully, Sean thought – and then the others took their turns, announcing themselves and emptying the bottles as they went. Most of them had some kind of title. Standing in the shadows, Sean forgot he was the waiter and revelled in hearing their stories. It was hard not to jump in and correct their frequent inaccuracies.

And then at last it was the new man's turn. Sean watched Thomas Walter Harding stand up, how he gripped the table. He saw him staring at the picture on the opposite wall, a stag brought to bay. He was clearly very drunk and for a moment it looked as if he would fall sideways, but then he started:

'And now – I shall tell you – an extraordinary story – about – the Arctic.'

Sean could see he was in a bad way. The slow-handclapping started.

'A very – unusual – story,' he gasped. 'Shit, I've drunk a bit too much.'

Before he could collapse, Sean stepped forward and pressed him back down in his seat, keeping one hand on his shoulder until he felt him steady.

'I'll speak for him. I have a story.' He was astonished at himself.

'What are you, his fag or something?'

Sean looked at Redmond sitting in his chair, fat and florid in a few years' time.

'Want to step outside for the answer?' he said. 'Or shut up and listen? Because I've got an Arctic story better than anything I've heard tonight.'

At the challenge to the leader, a frisson of delight ran around the table. Redmond grimaced a smile.

'Love your pluck, waiter. Go on then, tell it.'

Sean stepped into the light and looked around them all. Now he was going to do it, he felt different. They might be dressed up, but they were soft. He could take each and every one of them, if it came to it. They would listen.

'This is the story of Jens Lund and Aksel Søren of the 1902 Kristianborg Expedition to the Greenland ice cap,' he said, and as he did he stood straighter and taller, because whatever happened after this, for this one night he was part of the Lost Explorers' Society. 'And in 1902 there wasn't any reliable data from the ice cap in the winter, but these two men had volunteered to gather it. They knew each other a little, but there was no psychometric testing or anything like that. In October their ship anchored at Daneborg, and the supply team accompanied them to their base, where they had ample provision until the return of the sun in February, when they'd be collected with their data. Then the two men were left alone.'

He saw Thomas Harding drinking water, looking at him gratefully, admiringly. He could feel it, like they were already a team.

'The winter intensifies everything. Both men were diligent in their duties and went out in any conditions to read their instruments, but inside the hut at their evening meal, Søren liked to talk, and read, and exchange ideas. Lund was quiet, and became more taciturn every day, and Søren's cough before he spoke began to annoy him more and more. One day the cough and the questions and the talk became too much for Lund and he decided to go out with a tent alone for three days, and record from further into the ice cap. He completed his work and returned, looking forward to the hot meal he was sure Søren would be preparing.

'At first he thought the hut had vanished, because there was no light on. When he found it, there was no vapour from the ventilation pipe and no friendly smell of cooking when he came in. He got angry because he thought Søren had copied him and gone out on his own research observation, but when he lit the lamp he saw him right there, sitting at the table.'

Sean saw they were all transfixed, even Redmond. No one moved, or drank.

'So Lund decided it must be his turn to make dinner, and made up some seal soup, with some of the dried herbs Søren used. While he was cooking it, he thought of the questions that Søren had asked him, and decided he would answer them over dinner, so he did. He ate his soup, and as Søren wasn't very hungry, he ate his too. All his fears about what Søren would say or think of him were quite unfounded, and he enjoyed talking to him. Usually they took it in turns to cook or clear, but Lund was in such a good mood he said he'd do both, and Søren didn't object.

'In fact, Søren was enjoying himself so much he didn't want to go to sleep, but Lund insisted and helped him to his bunk. Søren wasn't well the next day, so Lund did both their work, but helped him up in time for the evening meal, when they carried on their conversation from the night before. Søren was such a good listener that Lund found himself remembering all sorts of things from his past, even telling jokes, and some personal things that had happened to him, but Søren never judged him. It was a shame he still didn't feel very well, but Lund had energy for two. He told Søren when he felt better, he could get back to it all.

'But after a week Søren was still not better, and Lund had noticed that at their evening meal, he was starting to look quite unwell, and letting his personal hygiene slip. Maybe it was too hot in the hut, and so he took Søren outside and made him a comfortable bunk in a snowdrift, quite near the hut. Søren was much more comfortable because when Lund brought him in for dinner the following evening, he sat up straight at the table, and their conversation continued. They went on like this all winter, and Lund grew extremely fond of his expedition partner, even though he was a bit lazy these days. But he brought out the best in him, like no one else ever had.

'One day he noticed something upsetting. A paling of the darkness. When he checked the calendar, Lund saw to his shock that it was early February, and the ship would be coming back. He told Søren about it that night when he brought him in, but Søren refused to discuss it. Lund didn't want other people invading their happy society and felt his old fearful nature coming back. When Søren refused to help with the dishes or even answer a civil question, he snapped and hit him. Søren's frozen body fell to the ground with a strange sound.

'Only then did Lund truly know what had happened, and that he could not go on bringing Søren in every night, because he was quite dead. He wept then, for the first time in his adult life – we know this because he said it later at his trial in Copenhagen. So he buried Søren outside – which was hard work, digging a grave in the frozen soil, but he did it. When it was ready, he did the thing he hated to do, that caused him all the trouble later. He took the axe and beheaded his friend, so that he could never come to dinner again. Then he buried the head and the body, piled the grave with stones, made a cross, said a prayer, and waited until the ship came.'

Sean found himself at the head of the table: they had moved their chairs back, the better to see him tell the story. He saw Tom Harding gave him a thumbs up, eyes bright with triumph.

'The ship returned with the sun and the supply team came to help pack up the cabin and support the two men. And of course when only Lund was there, they wanted to know what had happened. He explained Søren had died of his cough while he was away, and so he had buried him. That was the truth and he showed them the grave, but when they exhumed Søren to bring him back to his family in Denmark, they found his head had been cut off, and they didn't believe Lund's story. Søren was the popular one and Lund wasn't, so they put him in irons and took him to court back in Copenhagen. Only then, in fear of hanging, did he tell them the whole story, which was written down and can be read by anyone with sufficient interest to find it, and check these facts.' Sean looked around the table. 'And that is the story of the Frozen Friend, and I tell it on behalf of that man there.'

It took a few seconds for the Lost Explorers' Society to realise the tale was told. They stamped and roared and called for more, and more drink to go with it, but the proprietor came up to turn on the lights and kick them out, frowning at his waiter as he did so. Sean's tiredness was gone, he was electrified by his performance, by the story, and he was trembling with his daring. He collected plates and glasses, glad to disappear from view, retreating back into himself, collecting his wages, going back to his room where he lay in bed, smiling in the dark. The world had changed.

The following day he found a note in his pigeonhole at Hertford College. It was on headed Christ Church College notepaper and from Tom Harding, who had traced him. He wanted to thank him in person at the earliest opportunity, and would be in the King's Head pub around the corner, that night. PS He had something to ask him, involving Greenland.

The next depot is – nowhere. Gone, vanished – used for dog-feed. We have already marched as far as we thought to go today, but when we fixed the length of our day's journey we were still in paradise, and never dreamed of any serpent. But now all is changed, the empty tins grin devilishly at us out of wide gashes cut by the axe – we must get in at once, for, in our certainty of finding food here, we have made deep inroads on our stock. It was but a pound a day in all – but it was yet too much; the depot here laid waste speaks ill for what may await us at the next.

It is stern work now: a feverish race with death – the grim death of hunger, and we wonder often as we toil along which is to win in the end.

Lost in the Arctic: Being the story of the 'Alabama' Expedition, 1909–12
(1913)
Captain Ejnar Mikkelsen

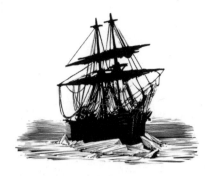

19

Angela Harding was next to take the stand. She asked, on behalf of the family, for as much information as possible.

'If we know,' she said, and her voice was small but strong, 'we can stop imagining. I don't enjoy that, I'm better with facts. Don't think you're sparing us by not saying.' She went back down to her seat, and then the coroner called Inspector Pal Brovang of the Sysselmann's Office, Svalbard, in the Kingdom of Norway.

Sean twisted round as Inspector Brovang came in, a quiet-looking man in his fifties with close-cropped grey hair, the lean compact frame of a much younger man, and a light tread. He and the coroner nodded to each other as equals. Mr Thornton thanked him for making the time to attend this inquest, then Brovang took the oath in fluent English, a skill in Sean's experience shared by 100 per cent of Norwegians.

Though he had been in contact with Brovang before, in every sense, Sean had never been conscious and in the same room. This was the first time. The thought of his own hands, cold and frozen, in that man's warm armpits, was embarrassingly intimate.

'Inspector Brovang,' commenced Mr Thornton, 'you attended both the aftermath of the accident on the Midgardbreen glacier, during which Tom Harding is believed to have lost his life, and also the subsequent discovery of his body in June of this year, by the cruise ship *Vanir*.'

Brovang nodded. 'A sad coincidence, but it meant I was well placed to help.'

'If you would please summarise the events of the accident to us?'

'Certainly.' Brovang looked out across the court. 'But first may I offer my condolences, and that of my whole team, to all Tom's family. We greatly regret we were unable to recover his body for you at the time.'

'Thank you.' Sean knew the small clear voice of Granny Ruby.

'So then. Late on the twentieth March 2015, the day of the solar eclipse, the coastguard received emergency calls made from the buildings now known as Midgard Lodge, by Miss Martine Delaroche and Mr Danny Long.' Brovang's eyes searched the court before he continued. 'She reported there had been an accident at the Midgardbreen ice-caves and said that two people – Sean Cawson and Tom Harding – were still inside, and there had been an internal collapse. Three people had managed to get out because they did not want to go so deep and had stayed near the entrance. These were Miss Delaroche, Miss Young, and Mr Kingsmith. Mr Cawson and Mr Harding wanted to go in to see the feature that was known as the Great Hall.'

'Was?' asked the coroner.

'Since this accident we put warnings against exploring ice-caves everywhere on the archipelago. The stability of the permafrost is compromised in many places; houses and mines are also collapsing. In Greenland too, and in Russia.' Inspector Brovang looked out at the silent courtroom. 'In the Arctic the weather can change very fast, and this is what happened that day, all over Svalbard. We had many incidents of people in difficulty.'

'Is Miss Delaroche testifying today?' The coroner consulted notes. 'I see, Wednesday. Very well. Please go on.'

'Also at the location of the cave – not inside it, but at a vantage point higher up the glacier – Mr Long and Mr Bjornsen had been standing bear watch. But because of the rapid change in the weather they were already heading down to the cave when the three got out. Then because of the fast-approaching storm, they made the decision to get the three visitors back safely rather than further risk all their lives. Our phone records show that the storm had stopped their phones working. The best satellite technology is no match for Nature.'

Brovang poured some water from the jug on the stand and drank. Sean realised he was holding his breath. He knew this story like a fable: the solar storm that knocked out all the satellite phones, the collapsed cave, the blizzard. Then they all went back to Midgard Lodge and left him and Tom under the ice.

Brovang's eyes found his. 'You know they had to do it: they could not clear a collapsed ice-cave with their bare hands, and a storm coming in. They acted with sense, but they were very distressed when they got through on the telephone.'

Sean nodded, to show *Yes, of course. They had to abandon us.*

'We had many emergencies on Svalbard over this period, and because of the storm and the fog it was impossible to travel to Midgardbreen for four hours after we received the distress calls. Fog is the most dangerous condition if you want to render aid, because you risk also having an accident and … compounding? – compounding, the first crisis with a new one. We had to wait until it was safer to fly, then locate the entrance to the ice-cave. It was difficult because of all the new snow.'

He turned to the coroner. 'Whenever there are high numbers of visitors to Svalbard, we see a corresponding increase in the need for the emergency services. This was the case on the day of the solar eclipse. It is sadly ironic that my department had already called upon the search and rescue facilities offered to us by Midgard Lodge, for use in other incidents. It is possible that without the arrangement Mr Cawson had with the Sysselmann's office, aid would have come sooner. But it is my opinion that, because of the storm, the outcome of the situation would have been the same.'

Brovang's eyes now found Tom's family. 'It is normal for the family to want to know everything. I would be the same. So I will tell you that, by our records, from the time of the phone call from Miss Delaroche, to the time we arrived, it was nearly seven hours since the cave system collapsed. The fact that the other three members of the party survived is because Mr Long and Mr Bjornsen got them back to Midgard Lodge. Then it was night and we could not continue searching. We sent the three survivors back to Longyearbyen for medical support; we stayed on at Midgard Lodge, and in the morning by first light we resumed the search for Tom and Sean.'

Sean felt a peculiar pang at how Brovang had changed to his first name. He had a fleeting fantasy of Brovang as his older brother. He had that quality; someone you could lean on and trust, who would make the thugs think twice before taking him on.

'We called reinforcements from Longyearbyen,' Brovang continued. 'Some of the search and rescue staff from Midgard Lodge had also returned to help. But it was impossible to open up the cave without further risk of life. We had to accept the strong chance that both men were lost. Then we had news of another storm coming in, so we had a maximum thirty to forty minutes more to search. It was during this time that I discovered Sean in an old polar bear den. In the Arctic, we say you are not dead until you are warm and dead, and so I did that: I warmed him.'

Brovang stopped. In the silence everyone heard Angela Harding sobbing quietly. Another mother's son found, and hers lost. Sean didn't know it was a den. He thought he had burrowed that hole himself. Explorers did that, he knew. That was what he'd said in the interview, that was what he remembered. A polar bear den was a much better story, and it was even true.

Suddenly he didn't know what was his own experience, and what were things he'd unconsciously gathered from other sources, and wanted to believe. Like the stories he'd told about his supposed father, the lost polar explorer. Inside him he had felt that it was true. He was taking deep breaths of air, and he felt the deliberate pressure of Sawbridge's arm against his.

'Steady now,' murmured his lawyer. 'Steady.'

'It is important, I think, to say that Svalbard is an unrestricted environment,' Brovang addressed the courtroom. 'We are there on Nature's own terms, and at our own risk. Sean and Tom knew this, they were experienced travellers. Also, I believe the cave was checked by Danny Long and Terry Bjornsen two days prior to this visit, and they found no unusual risk factors – beyond of course that going into a glacier has an inherent risk.'

Brovang paused, and looked directly at Angela Harding. 'In my opinion, this is a tragic example of a true accident. The weight of the collapsed ice and the lack of oxygen would be similar to being caught in an avalanche, which is what I said in my report. When I interviewed Mr Cawson in hospital, he told me about Tom's fall to the deeper level, and it was only at that time I gave instructions to stop the search. We could not go down any further, and the time had passed to expect to find him alive.

'And now, three years later, we have more than one hundred pieces of evidence of how his body was found, from all the passengers on the *Vanir*, who were in the fjord because of a bear sighting. Otherwise no one would have known, because his body would have sunk within minutes.' Brovang looked back to Sean. 'This time Mr Cawson's men were on hand, to offer assistance, but the Coastguard was already there so we did not need them.'

The coroner sat forward with a frown. 'Mr Cawson's men? I don't understand. And how did they know?'

The courtroom became quiet.

'Mr Cawson's business, Midgard Lodge, is further down inside the fjord, almost at the boundary of the National Park. They would have picked it up on the radio, when the *Vanir* called us with the emergency.'

'Why would they do that?' asked the coroner.

'In remote places like Svalbard, your life might depend on a good neighbour. If you are a little nosy, well, OK. An emergency on the doorstep would be important to know about. I am guessing that is why they were there so soon.'

The coroner made a note on his pad.

'I'll be coming to Mr Cawson's business later, so I'll save further questions about that for him.'

Sean felt the room shift in awareness. People moved to take a better look at him. So he had a business there did he, he was nosy, was he? He heard the tiny plastic rattling of keyboards, but he did not look. He could feel Sawbridge tapping his foot.

'There is one more thing,' said Brovang. 'At the time of the accident, I asked for photographs of both Tom and Sean, to show my team. I also took samples from their clothing, for DNA, which has been held at the Folkehelseinstituttet in Oslo. So when Tom's body was found, I could still recognise him, and his family kindly provided a DNA match also.'

Sean kept his eyes forward. All these things going on, and he hadn't even known Tom had been found.

'A question,' said the coroner. 'When you identified him, I believe you first notified Dr Ruth Mott, the tourist lecturer. Why her?'

'Ah.' Brovang took off his glasses. 'Because her name and number were in the back of Tom's passport. I had the details from before.'

The coroner looked out. 'Mrs Osman, Mr Sawbridge, any questions?'

They both nodded, but Sawbridge waved her forward.

'Ladies first.'

Mrs Osman stood crookedly, and spoke in her rasping voice.

'On behalf of Tom's family I would like to thank you, Inspector Brovang, for your diligence in all matters concerning the search for Tom, your care in assistance with his repatriation home, and your time in attending this inquest. First, I'd like to ask you a bit more about your choice to call Dr Ruth Mott, rather than Mr Cawson, whose details you also held. And who, after all, had been in the accident with him.'

'Yes.' Brovang spoke quietly. 'But he had not written Sean's details in the back of his passport.'

'Is that the only reason?'

Sawbridge half rose. 'Terribly sorry,' he called out, 'but the relevance of the question is … what, exactly?'

Mrs Osman addressed the coroner, not Sawbridge.

'I believe Tom Harding's relationship with Ruth Mott will prove to be significant in illuminating the circumstances of his death. My other question concerns the exact nature of these "search and rescue" staff at Midgard Lodge?'

'I don't know.' Brovang said it simply. 'But they are good neighbours.'

'Where is this going, please?' Sawbridge leaned forward.

'Agreed,' said the coroner. 'We have a lot to get through. Mr Sawbridge?'

'Thank you.' Sawbridge pushed his spectacles up his nose and smiled respectfully at Inspector Brovang. 'You said people visit Svalbard "on Nature's terms". Could you explain that a little more?'

'The simplest way to put it is to say, be humble. Every single time you step outside, respect her power.'

'No matter how experienced you think you are?'

'Especially then.'

'Thank you, Inspector Brovang, no further questions.'

*

Sean stood on the side-street with Sawbridge, his mouth and eyes burning dry. People from the courtroom ducked their eyes as they passed. Sawbridge aimed his match hard and accurate into a drain, then puffed on his cigar for a while.

'Exploitative and unfair, showing that footage. What's Osman playing at, going in so hard right at the start? That's the worst, though: seeing it. How're you doing?'

Sean felt the warm brick wall against his back. The gritty air near the ring road was refreshing after the stillness of the courtroom.

'I needed to see it.' His voice did not sound his own.

'Sean?' Brovang had followed them. He nodded to Sawbridge then shook hands with Sean, his grip warm and vigorous. 'I heard you were fully recovered,' he said. 'But it is still good to see with my own eyes. And also to say thank you for the generous donations,' he went on. 'Midgard Lodge helps Longyearbyen stay Norway's Most Generous Town every year. But you know it was our duty to help. You don't need to keep paying for it.'

'You're sure,' Sean said, 'that it was a polar bear den? Perhaps if they'd known that, people wouldn't have thought so badly of me. A polar bear sells anything.'

Brovang smiled.

'Oh yes, we are quite sure. Higher up the glacier, and we think long unused. I did tell you, afterwards when we spoke in the Sickehaus. You were very pleased – you said you were lucky, because it might have been occupied!'

'I don't remember that at all. But it would be a pleasure to see you at Midgard Lodge, I'll be there much more often now. I just couldn't face it for a while.' He felt like he was apologising to Brovang.

Brovang nodded. 'That is very easy to understand. I think many people will be glad to know you are in charge.'

'I've always been in charge. What do you mean?'

'Ah.' Brovang looked at his watch. 'I must make sure I catch that train. Good luck, Sean.' He hurried away and Sean watched him go, thinking.

When a human being dies, the soul leaves the earth and goes to one or the other of two distinct regions. Some souls go up into heaven and become Uvdlormuit, the People of Day. Their country lies over toward the dawn. Others again go down under the sea, where there is a narrow belt of land with water on either side. These are called Qimiujarmuit, the People of the Narrow Land. But in either place they are happy and at ease, and there is always plenty to eat.

Those who pass to the Land of Day are people who have been drowned, or murdered. It is said that the Land of Day is the land of glad and happy souls. It is a great country, with many caribou, and the people there live only for pleasure. They play ball most of the time, playing at football with the skull of a walrus, and laughing and singing as they play. It is this game of souls playing at ball that we can see in the sky as the northern lights.

The greater among the angakoqs, or wizards, often go up on a visit to the People of Day, just for pleasure. Such are called Pavungnartut, which means, those who rise up to heaven. The wizard preparing to set out on such a journey is placed at the back of the bench in his hut, with a curtain of skin to hide him from view. His hands must be tied behind his back and his head lashed fast to his knees; he wears breeches, but nothing more, the upper part of his body being bare. When he is thus tied up, the men who have tied him take fire from the lamp on the point of a knife and pass it over his head, drawing rings in the air, and saying at the same time; 'Niorruarniartoq aifale' (Let him who is going on a visit now be carried away).

Across Arctic America: Narrative of the Fifth Thule Expedition (1927)
Knud Rasmussen

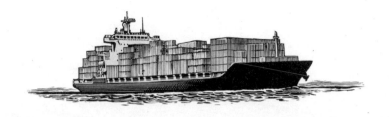

20

Flip-flops, as he had mentally named her, rushed up to Sean before he sat down with Sawbridge for the second session. At first he didn't recognise her – she had changed into 'the most boring clothes I could find', she told him breathlessly. 'I am so sorry to dress disrespectfully, I didn't know.' She looked down at her black shoes and skin-coloured tights. 'Sorry.'

'You weren't to know.' Sean thought of the strange outfits Rosie wore. This girl was about the same age. He looked over to the long trestle, where a couple more journalists, a man and a woman, had taken up positions a couple of seats apart. 'Who are you with?'

'With?' The girl followed his eyes. 'Oh. I'm freelance.' She gave him a card, her name handwritten in block capitals. BETH BURNHAM, ENVIRONMENTAL CORRESPONDENT. He tried not to smile.

'That's right.' She looked at him earnestly. 'You have to imagine yourself where you want to be, then it can happen. You said that in your *Sunday Times* interview.'

'Shouldn't you be in school?'

'This is more important.'

'Than your education? No, it's not.'

'It is! The Arctic is melt—'

'The Arctic, the Arctic: do you have any idea what you're talking about? It's not a theme park with indigenous dolls, you know, or some kind of fantasy game with polar bears against the oil demons. You

can't save it. You can only manage it. Understand that, first of all.'
Sean saw the alarm in her eyes, but she didn't back down.

'I know it's complicated and I know I don't understand it all. That's
why I'm here, because you are, you're really involved so I thought—'

'Here's what I think' – Sawbridge peered at the handwritten business card – 'Miss Burnham. You're doing media studies and thought
this was a good project.'

'How'd you know that?' Her indignation made Sean fond of her.

Sawbridge smiled. 'I'm also guessing you're local, you heard about
the inquest and you saw the words "interested party" and thought to
yourself, ooh yes, *I'm* interested, why don't *I* go along, and observe
other people's grief, and other people's business, and I'll put it down
to environmental awareness. Or did you not consider that part?'

The girl frowned. 'It's a public hearing. I'm allowed to be here.'

'Mm. Thing is, you're not.' Sawbridge dropped his voice so only
they could hear him. 'Unless you have a demonstrable vested interest,
or are with a recognised official press organisation, you need to leave.'

'Official press organisations,' she retorted, 'are stale, male and pale.'
She stood up straight. 'I've changed my shoes, which was a fair
comment from Mr Cawson, but in case you didn't know, things have
changed. I *am* a global citizen journalist and what happens in the
Arctic affects us all. So I would call that a very strong vested interest,
thank you.' She was breathing hard at her own defiance. 'And if people
like me don't take a stand—'

'Or a seat by the socket,' said Mrs Osman, a gleam of amusement
in her hooded eyes. 'Oh dear, too late.' They all turned to see a new
male journalist, large and slobby and vaguely familiar to Sean, sweeping her things down the table and taking her place. He ignored Beth
Burnham's glower as they were all upstanding again for the second
part of the morning. Sean recognised him, he was the coiner of the
'Dirty Davos' nickname, and was constantly trying to join one of
Sean's clubs, under false names. Sean knew he bore him nothing but
ill will, but he still felt for him. The man craved status.

*

The American cruise tourists, John and Trudie Burke were next on, Mrs Burke speaking for both of them. Sean listened as she described how the passengers yearned for a bear and how passenger power had got that drone up, and found that bear, that led them, like some kind of animal guide, wasn't it? to where they needed to be. Even if the captain hadn't wanted to go there and there was some sort of to-do about it. But it was the right thing, because then they found that poor man's body. She was ready to give forth their views on the warming Arctic, but the coroner glanced at the clock and thanked her.

'A moment?'

The coroner nodded to Mrs Osman.

'Do you mean, there was a disagreement about following the bear?'

'Something about going up that fjord,' Mrs Burke said. 'One fjord, another fjord – we wanted to see the thing they'd sold us on: a polar bear! Nine days of glaucous gulls and fulmars – then some walrus we weren't allowed close enough to see properly in case we upset them. Let me tell you, there were people on board who have died natural deaths, God bless them, since that voyage, and seeing a polar bear was on their bucket list! So first they announced over the PA system they'd seen it and we all rushed out and some people even got a glimpse, then all of a sudden they changed their mind and we couldn't sail down that fjord where it was headed. Kingdom of the Ice Bear or Lord of the High North or whatever, and there he was but we couldn't take a look?'

She smiled. 'You can trust a bunch of oldsters to make trouble. The attorneys got up a memo for the tour operator who took it to the captain, and that's how come we went down that fjord, and then – well. The calving and all.' Her bright tone fell away as she looked at Tom's mother for a second, and bobbed her head in deference or condolence. 'I just hope it was a good thing, in the end, that we followed that bear. We're going to light a candle in the cathedral for him.'

'Thank you, Mrs Burke.' Mrs Osman sat down.

Sean felt his heart beating harder and composed his face to show nothing but calmness. Osman must know something of the activities of Midgard Lodge, she must be curious or she wouldn't have asked about the passage of the ship into the fjord – but this process was simply about the circumstances of Tom's tragic death. Not the favour

Sean was doing, for both the governments of Norway and Great Britain.

Parch was coming to the benefit on Thursday night; he would collar him then and tell him they could stick their knighthood. He wasn't going to dance on a chain for anyone any more – he was a very successful British businessman willing to put his entrepreneurial talent in harness to the greater good of the nation and they could show a bit of respect, or fuck off. But even as he thought these things, Sean knew he still wanted Philip Stowe to keep his word. He wanted to believe.

Sean declined Sawbridge's offer of the guilty pleasure of a cheap bacon sandwich, in favour of clearing his head with a walk. He bought some peanuts then ducked through the concealed gateway to the cathedral precincts, lifting his hand casually to the porter as his lawyer had done. With some time to spare, he decided to take a quick look in the cathedral.

He stepped out of the wind and into the vaulting stone space, where jewelled light fell down between the pillars onto the paving of ancient tombs. Traders in the temple, in the form of two gift stands, were overhung by the tattered regimental banners once held by living boys and men.

Sean moved deeper, drawn by the sound of a choir somewhere in the cool stone depths. The nose-less alabaster effigies and curlicued marble scrolls recording noble young death after death, reminded him of the legless soldier, on his new career path of medical re-enactment. He hoped his Equity card had arrived.

He went up scooped stone steps, shaped by centuries of footfall, heading towards the music. Two black-robed clerics talked intently at the top – comparing budget flights to Rome these days. The choir kept pausing and returning to one musical phrase, like a many-throated bird – and then Sean saw them, their young faces angelic in the light falling from hundreds of feet above. Their music master set them off again, and to stay and listen for longer, Sean wandered across to a small chapel within their chapel, where a large book was set on a low stand. A pen dangled from a string.

It was a prayer book, and visitors to the cathedral were invited to write their requests. Many people had already done so, and Sean looked closer as the music washed over him.

For my mother's operation, said one.

For my lost family, said another.

And then further down, in writing so hard the page was almost torn, someone had dug the words into the paper: SHOW YOURSELF GOD.

He looked around. The force of the words and the writing itself was like a challenge to anyone reading it. Whoever had written it might even be in the cathedral now, might be watching him read it. All he saw was the choir, distant tourists, a few clerics walking quietly. He picked up the pen and – a respectful distance under the great spiritual demand, added two words: *forgive me*.

He stared at what he had written. Then he put a ten-pound note into the donation box and went to light a candle, not because he was religious but because he liked the act of doing so. To his horror, John and Trudie Burke, the cruise passengers, were heading towards him. He looked back across at the book – if they read it and had seen him write it, they would get completely the wrong idea.

They were coming closer, it was definitely them, he could hear her distinctive voice. Sean lowered his head as if deep in prayer and walked in the opposite direction. It turned out to be a one-way aisle with arrowed signs pointing ahead, which led to a small landing above a flight of candlelit stone stairs, and another sign To The Crypt and Way Out. The second part was what he wanted.

Naturally there were frequent storms and intense cold, and in regard to the storms of the Arctic regions of North Greenland and Grant Land, the only word I can use to describe them is 'Terrible', in the fullest meaning it conveys. The effect of such storms of wind and snow, or rain, is abject physical terror, due to the realization of perfect helplessness. I have seen rocks a hundred and a hundred and fifty pounds in weight picked up by the storm and blown for distances of ninety or a hundred feet to the edge of a precipice, and there of their own momentum go hurtling through space to fall in crashing fragments at the base. I have been there and I have seen one of my Esquimo companions felled by a blow from a rock of eighty-four pounds in weight, which struck him fairly between the shoulder-blades, literally knocking the life out of him. I have been there, and believe me, I have been afraid.

A Negro Explorer at the North Pole: The Autobiography of Matthew
    Henson (1912)
Matthew Henson

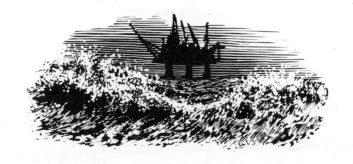

21

Even after the Svalbard accident, Sean had been fine on the London Underground, but then a few months ago there had been that thing at Knightsbridge station – or more accurately, his experience in the tunnel just before. Heading down towards the crypt made him think of it, but he pushed fear away. Becoming phobic about being underground meant too many places where he would no longer be able to go.

The Piccadilly line train had just stopped for a few minutes between stations, nothing massively unusual in that. But it was the morning rush hour and, without a seat, Sean faced out into the blackness as without warning the engines and lights went off. In the crowded silence he felt the press of flesh and backpack around him, he heard people breathing. The feeling oscillated through them all: they were trapped in the dark earth in a metal tube.

Sean was already physically tensed with his effort to keep maximum headspace, and the collective body heat rose around his face. He shifted against the interconnecting doors to the next carriage and squeezed the two metal latches to drop the heavy glass window, letting in more air. The only light was from the hundreds of oblongs of phones, underlighting people's faces in a horrifying way.

The same was happening in the next carriage. He listened to the silence of the tunnel, which smelled alien and industrial and ancient all at the same time. He had the idea that they were all dead, that some

disaster had taken place but his consciousness lingered in anaesthe-
tised death-lag. Soon he would feel the pain of the explosion or atroc-
ity or whatever had befallen his train. His body might already be
indistinguishable from the red shreds of others, they were carbon,
atomised back to stardust, the tunnel blocked for months—

—he was in the ice again – he was blinded with terror, he had to
plunge and kick and force—

Commuters shouted angrily at him as with a great cry the tall man
by the connecting door went crazy, shoving them all back, his eyes
wild – and then the lights went on and the train resumed its motion.
The driver's distorted voice apologised through loudspeakers for the
delay, and Sean stared at the shocked faces of the people around him.
He was on a train.

When the doors opened onto the platform of Knightsbridge station,
he burst out and ran through the tunnels, up the sliding metal teeth of
the escalator, he slammed his plastic card against the ticket barrier and
did not stop until he was out on the roaring street.

The crypt was completely manageable, however, nothing like the
closed-in darkness of the tube tunnel. There were only a few steps
down to it, and it smelled of stone and incense, not soot and sweat.
He walked on to where the passageway opened into a little chamber,
a large pillar candle flickering in the middle of flagstones. A guide with
a small respectful group told them of the murder of Thomas Becket in
this spot on 29 December 1170.

Who will rid me of this turbulent priest? Thomas the
troublemaker.

Sean's Thomas had a gift for it, even in death: appearing in such a
dramatic way to the Burkes.

He looked back – they had not followed him, and he had been
stupid to be spooked. His private prayer – if that was what it was –
was none of their business. He was spooking at everything and it was
ludicrous. He ran up the exit steps and out into the bright day. A small
group of grey-robed monks were gathered together, and Sean stared
at their high-tech hiking boots, and cross-country walking poles. They
were youthful and fit, more like young explorers than monks. He

longed for another expedition. When this was all over, he would find one to join.

Sawbridge was waiting in the lobby when Sean arrived, and hurried him in. Straight-backed, tall and in good clear voice, Sean took the stand and the oath. Going to the cathedral had worked – those banners, that vaulting spiritual environment, his ability to face the crypt – let them all look at him.

'You kindly submitted a prepared statement of the events of February fifteenth,' said the coroner, 'but I will trouble you, if you can, to tell the court in your own words, what happened.'

'Of course.' Sean had worked on this statement precisely to avoid what Sawbridge had predicted could turn into a lengthy testimony.

'I appreciate that it's three years ago now,' said Mr Thornton, 'so I don't expect your memory—'

'Oh no,' said Sean. 'It's pin sharp.'

'Then if you would take us from your arrival with Mr Harding, in Svalbard, and why you were there.'

'Yes. Of course.' Sean could see Ursula Osman poised and still, like a cat in the bushes. He needed Martine here, she was the antidote to whatever charge Osman put out into the atmosphere.

'The party I took up to Midgard Lodge consisted of the five members of the consortium that bought the property – myself, Tom, my long-term backer Joe Kingsmith, another investor called Radiance Young, and my partner in business and now also in my personal life, Martine Delaroche.' Sean felt the catch of tension before the keyboards rattled again.

'I'm the director and CEO of Midgard Lodge, but everyone on that trip had a financial stake. Tom didn't contribute equity but he received a large signing-on fee, plus he would have been entitled to a salary and dividends for his directorship, and for his ongoing work: helping tailor best environmental policy for the business leaders we hosted on retreat.'

Sean felt the reins now. 'The Arctic is melting, whether we like it or not. The summer sea ice has gone and while some people are wringing their hands, treaties fall wildly out of date and business capitalises. So choose denial, or choose – like I did, like my partners and I have actively and responsibly done – to be at the vanguard of those changes and make sure they happen in the most positive way. If the opportunity is there, someone will seize it. Better it be us. Tom wanted to speak truth to power, and he knew he needed to be in the room to do that. And you have to have a stake in the Arctic to have a voice there – or you're just a bleeding heart southern liberal.'

'Mr Cawson—' The coroner held up his hand, but Sean went on.

'I knew that if Tom believed in Midgard Lodge, then what I was trying to do was truly worthwhile. Not just for the money.' He stopped. The fat journalist stared at him, then started typing fast.

'I've done a bit of research myself,' said Mr Thornton, 'and I'm surprised you got permission to develop at Midgardfjorden. Isn't it a national park?'

'Just outside the boundary,' Sean said. 'We've done it very sympathetically. If we weren't so discreet, the architect would have surely won awards. That was part of the reason for our trip – no one but myself had seen the completed work. Nor had we all been able to meet in person before, so it was a double celebration. Plus the solar eclipse happening, which was best viewed in Svalbard ...' He paused. 'We said the stars were in alignment.'

When a mature male appears on the scene, all the other bears pay attention. The general rule is, the more mature, heavier, and stronger the bear, the more dominant it is in any interaction. However, there is another rule that says a bear that approaches confidently and without hesitation is accepted as a potential threat by the bear that is being approached. Even a mature male may be frightened by a young bear under certain circumstances. Polar bears are powerful animals; they are also intelligent. They realize they can hurt one another, and they avoid situations in which their power might be put to the test. They also know that the outcome in any particular situation depends on a bear's personality, current motivation, and individual circumstances. Where possible, they err on the side of caution.

Polar Bears: Living with the White Bear (1996)
Nikita Ovsyanikov

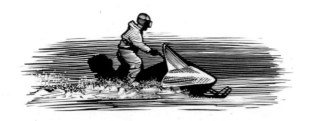

22

Three years earlier

A private Boeing 747 cruised at 36,000 feet over the Greenland Sea heading in a north-easterly direction for Longyearbyen airport, Svalbard. Inside it, Joe Kingsmith napped in the larger of his two bedrooms, while out in the salon his steward attended the needs of the four other passengers, variously relaxing.

Having flown with Kingsmith before, Sean was familiar with the luxurious environment, but it was the first time for Martine, Tom, and for Radiance Young. She was currently engaged in a game of online chess with someone from her cosmonaut training programme – which she was doing privately in Moscow, 'for fun'. This joined a list of activities that included polar exploration, motor racing and collecting important estate jewellery. She frowned as she considered her next move. Sitting nearby, Tom ignored her bare red-nailed toes wiggling towards him, and her occasional glances.

Behind them, Sean and Martine observed with discreet amusement. He was browsing an online portfolio of interior designers for the new building in Cochin and she had laid her iPad aside and was looking over his shoulder. In the white heat of early lust, Sean had welcomed her involvement in the interior of Midgard Lodge – with spectacular results – but the process had revealed Martine's dominant personality, and he had declined to involve her in the design of his other businesses.

'Checkmate!' Radiance lifted her own iPad in triumph. 'He is senior and thinks he beats me, but he never does!' Her accent was an odd mix of English private school and native Mandarin. She turned to Tom. 'Now you.'

Tom put his book down. 'I'm hopeless. Ask Martine, she's a good strategist.'

'Martin likes to play with men better, like me. Right, Martin?'

'I'm very happy to play with you, if you'd like.' Martine forced a smile.

'No, it's OK. I see Sean eye-boss you to say yes.'

'He didn't.'

'Oh yes he did!' Radiance had evidently been to British panto-mimes. She returned to her first target. 'Tom, why are you single? No children, no ex-wife?'

Sean looked up with interest. Tom shrugged.

'There was someone, once. It didn't work out.'

'Why not? It's OK I'm asking?'

'Radiance, stop torturing him. He doesn't know how to fob you off with a lie.' Sean caught Tom's grateful look, but she was not so easily dissuaded.

'What happened?'

'We fucked it up. And then it was too late. OK?'

'Huh. Doesn't sound OK!' Radiance held up her left hand with its empty ring finger. 'Look at me: sad face: no kids. Still time though if I hurry, before I'm old and dry. Husband too. Maybe I adopt one, like Martin!' She laughed for a second. 'Martin, you want kids too? How old are you, little bit more than me? Thirty-nine? Forty? We should get busy!'

When Martine didn't answer, Radiance winked at her. 'We talk more later. You can tell me how you make Sean leave his wife. I need to learn that trick!'

'Considerably younger and it was no trick.' Martine pointedly returned to her own iPad, but Tom looked round at Sean.

'You've done it?'

'It's in progress,' Martine said immediately. 'We need to be honest.'

Radiance pointed at Sean. 'Oh! Angry smiles are dangerous! Don't be angry, Sean. Martin's right.'

'Mar*tine*.'

'That's what I said: Martin.'

'Radiance, lovely special, talented Radiance,' said Sean. 'Shut up.'

'Sure.' Radiance was impossible to offend.

Down the cabin, Kingsmith emerged from the bedroom, freshly showered and changed. The PA system chimed and the captain announced they were starting the descent to Longyearbyen. He took his seat.

'Everything OK? It's gone very quiet.'

'Joe, you want a baby?' Radiance leaned forward. 'Let's do this thing!'

Kingsmith patted her hand. 'I'll take that in a friendly spirit, thank you. But can we discuss it a bit later, over a drink?'

'Sure!'

Kingsmith shot the others a look of panic. Sean winked.

'Take one for the team,' he mouthed to him. Then they began the descent into Adventfjorden and conversation ceased. Sean looked out as they entered the narrow channel of the mountains, the sharp black peaks tipping the snowline. Ahead was the small runway of Longyearbyen which terminated in a headland on the south shore of Isfjord, against which the Barents Sea burst against the rocks. The approach was notorious since 1996, when a Russian Tupolev transit plane, arriving to rotate coal workers in and out of the settlement at Pyramiden, crashed with the cost of every life on board. Sean thought of it compulsively, every time he came in.

The Arctic year is made of four very long days: the midnight sun of the summer months, from late April until mid-August, when it does not set at all, then the brief season of dusk at the change of the year in autumn, when the polar night is coming and the light shrinks faster every day. By late October there are only a few hours of twilight in the middle of the day, and by mid-November total darkness has fallen, with no day at all. For three months, or about two thousand hours, there is no natural light. For some people, this is a relief compared to the high-crime season of the summer months, when the bars manufacture night inside, while on the other side of the door, the sun bleaches all sense of time. There is endless liberty to work, travel, or make any kind of mischief – there are no restrictions, except on peaceful sleep. For some, it becomes a time of madness. For others, that is the polar night. For a few, the madness can strike at any time; it quivers in the Arctic silence that can be spiritual, or demonic as it claws reason off balance. When survival is the ultimate value, many inhibitions are released.

For Sean's party, touching down on the ice-swirled tarmac of Longyearbyen in the smoky blue February twilight, it was a time of great excitement. They readied themselves to transfer to the helicopter that would be waiting to take them straight up to Midgard Lodge – but as they disembarked, Sean couldn't see it. The captain hurried up to Kingsmith with the message that it wasn't there, they had to go in. Sean shouted through the wind for everyone to get inside, and they hurried over to the small terminal building, mini-snow cyclones rushing along the ground and bursting against their ankles.

It was nothing serious, the captain told Sean and Kingsmith, at least not for them. There had been an incident with a bear and a big bunch of tourists up at Dronningsbukta, and all the helicopters on the islands had been scrambled to help. Danny Long, as an experienced Arctic pilot, had been commandeered for search and rescue by the Sysselmann's office, along with the Midgard helicopter.

The captain apologised for not having more information. He looked at his watch and asked Kingsmith what he wanted him to do.

'Passports and on your way,' Kingsmith told him. 'While you still can.'

Sean could tell by the set of his shoulders and the particular smile, that Kingsmith was displeased. They waited by the motionless luggage carousel, presided over by a medium-sized stuffed polar bear, every tourist's first picture. The captain returned with the passports.

'Mr Long has left another message, sir: he'll pick you up in the morning and he's very sorry, but you can't get to the Lodge tonight, all men are required by the Sysselmann.'

'In the *morning*?' Martine and Radiance said it together.

Sean took the message from the captain and read it.

'Nothing to worry about. We're aiding search and rescue – remember, Joe?'

Kingsmith frowned. 'Danny had his instructions.'

'Tell the Sysselmann that,' Tom said pleasantly. 'I'm sure it would make a big difference. What men, by the way?'

'Lodge staff,' Sean said, truthfully. They were. 'Fortunately, we've got rooms booked in town too. Always have a contingency plan.'

Kingsmith patted Tom's shoulder. 'You're right to rag me. I'm getting old and inflexible. Of course we should be helping out.' He turned back to his waiting crew. 'Happy returns to Benoit. Tell him to have fun.' The captain confirmed he would pass it on. The crew hurried back to the plane.

'Who's Benoit?' asked Martine.

'A pal, a mere kid turning fifty. Lending it to him for his celebrations. But they've got to stop in Riga to pick up the other guests.'

'Where's the party?' Tom said it in the casual way Sean knew meant trouble. Kingsmith too, by his smile.

'Central African Republic. Though I'm guessing they'll probably bar hop.'

'Where the beautiful pink wood comes from,' said Radiance. 'So popular now in Asia.'

'Pink mahogany? I hope you're not importing that—'

'Of course not, silly. But I've got eyes in my head, it's everywhere. Hey, Tom, come visit with me, while you're still single. I show you all the sights of outrage.' She grinned at him.

He ignored her. 'I hope those guests from Riga are of legal age.'

'Thomas! As if I'd compromise my crew like that. Everyone's a fully consenting grown-up.'

Tom didn't smile back. 'So you've started up in the CAR again?'

'Sure. Last time I looked, mining was legal, as was helping the local economy, setting up health centres after the epidemic, and bringing prosperity to a lot of people. Tom, you'll give yourself a hernia trying to police the whole world.'

'I don't want to police it, I just want—'

'Things done your way – I remember. The good way, the green way, the right way. I know, and please god, don't change – it's why we want you here. But let me tell you, you go looking under stones and you know what you'll find? Good clean dirt and the creatures that live there. It's called a financial ecosystem, and I'm just as keen on protecting that one as you are with any of yours. That's how the world works and it's prudish to deny it, any more than your own bodily functions. Come out of denial and join the party!'

'What am I denying, Joe?'

'That the ice is going going gone, and there's nothing we—'

'There absolutely is: all of us together—'

'Time's passed, there's no political will. Look at the US! Much easier to make all you bleeding hearts feel guilty for flying on vacation than change a trade deal. Governments would rather invest in space and leave the mess behind. Few centuries later, and it all turns to holy relics anyway. Your beautiful idea of everyone pulling together only happens in the movies, war, and sport. Real life, it's everyone for themselves and their families – and there is nothing more selfish than a new family.'

'Joe, you're wrong.'

'I'm not.'

'But it's my job at Midgard to convince people exactly like you.'

'There's no one remotely like me—'

'—that it's better to think collectively than selfishly, and you'll make more money when you do.'

'You're fighting human nature.'

'People are better than you think.'

Joe Kingsmith turned to Sean. 'I love this boy.'

'Man.' Tom didn't smile. 'And we both know you don't.'

'OK. But I give you respect.' Kingsmith stopped the joking. 'So seriously, Tom, let's get you down to the CAR, the DRC, even South Sudan, if you want.'

'Are you crazy? You're in there?'

'Aha, you see – right there, that's what I'm up against. South Sudan has a lot of talented, hard-working people developing the infrastructure – come see for yourself what I'm up to, I'll set your mind at rest.' Kingsmith paused to admire his plane rolling past towards the runway.

When it had gone, a small figure was revealed in the arc lights, crossing the snow-swirled tarmac towards the terminal building. She entered in a blast of cold air and the glass slid shut behind her. She wore a long brown parka with a fur-trimmed hood and rummaged in its pockets for her ringing phone. They all watched as she unzipped the parka, trying to get to it in time – revealing it was in the pocket of a bloodstained white lab coat. She cursed as she missed the call, then realised people were watching her. Her look turned to shock as she saw Tom.

'I look that bad?' He went up to her. She was speechless. They kissed so clumsily, their past as lovers was blatant. Martine and Radiance exchanged a look.

Sean took a deep breath and went forward.

'Ruth!' he called out. 'Fancy seeing you here!'

They greeted each other like the old friends they once were.

'Everyone,' Sean took control, 'this is Dr Ruth Mott, eminent biologist specialising in …'

'Ice-obligate marine mammals,' said Tom. '*Ursus maritimus* in particular.'

'No longer in the field,' she said, 'but covered in the blood of the one I've very sadly just prepared for autopsy.' She looked round them all. 'Hello. Sorry about the gore, I've just removed the head. And, um, more small talk like that.'

She looked at Martine and Radiance, then Tom. 'Well, I better …'

'No. Don't go.' Tom looked at Sean. 'We're here for the night, aren't we? So we have to eat.'

Sean knew what was coming. Get out in front.

'We are. Ruth, if you're free, would you like to join us for supper?'

'Thank you, but I wouldn't want to gatecrash your party.'

Radiance pointed to Kingsmith. 'That one's mine tonight.' She pointed to Martine, and Sean spared them all.

'Martine is with me.'

'Martine?' Something went through Ruth Mott's eyes. 'Hello.'

'Yes, the Terrible Homewrecker herself.' Martine smiled. 'Please don't hate me until you know me first-hand.'

Despite herself, Ruth smiled. 'I can't promise, but I'll try.'

'Good enough.' Martine focused her charm. 'And please do join us.'

'You must.' Tom was completely focused on Ruth, Kingsmith forgotten.

'You can tell us about the bear!' Radiance was as eager as a child for an ice-cream. 'Or maybe we could even see it now? I'm fine with blood. What happened?'

'Tourist stupidity. I'm sorry, right now I'm really upset about it all.'

'Were there many casualties?'

Ruth Mott looked at Kingsmith.

'Upset about the bear.' She turned to Tom. 'What are you doing here?'

'Going up to Midgardfjorden.'

'That's – *you*? But that's amazing! The whole world was after that.' She turned to Sean. 'Wow. You are never to be underestimated.'

'That's the truth.' Tom looked as proud as if she'd meant it for him. Sean felt a mixture of shame and gratitude, and a lot warmer towards Ruth. She'd only ever been a loyal friend to Gail. And until Rosie had involved her, she hadn't interfered.

'Guilty as charged, this is the purchasing consortium. Ruth, if you are free, please do join us tonight. It's been ages.'

Ruth smiled, and Sean noticed how Tom smiled too. 'I'm supposed to be talking to drunken eclipse tourists after dinner,' she said. 'Let me see if I can find a stand-in.'

Auks pickled in oil. This is done by killing a seal and skinning it through its mouth without splitting the skin. Not every hunter can do this, but when it is accomplished satisfactorily it makes a magnificent poke, because most of the blubber still clings to the skin.

The person intending to fill the hide takes it along with him to a spot where the birds are thicker than fish in any aquarium and, with a net attached to a long stick, he catches the auks as they fly past, often bagging enough in one day to fill his sealskin, which is then latched and covered with stones. The sun must not reach it or the oil will turn rancid. During the summer the blubber turns to oil and soaks the birds, which decompose slowly without interference from the air.

This makes a dish which tastes like nothing else in the world, and one loved by young and old alike. The white feathers turn pink, and may be easily plucked out. The birds are often eaten frozen, but some connoisseurs say they are better warmed up. In fact, frozen meat never tastes as strong as it does when it is thawed out. When frozen the diner must chop the birds out of the poke with an axe, but after they become soft, they may be eaten with grace and elegant manners. The gastronomist takes them by the legs and bites off the feet. Then with a deft twist of his hand he removes the feathers – or most of them. After that he skins them, from the bill backwards, and, having turned the skin inside out, sucks the most delicious fat from it. Finally he swallows the skin at one gulp, and then begins on the meat.

Arctic Adventure: My Life in the Frozen North (1936)
Peter Freuchen

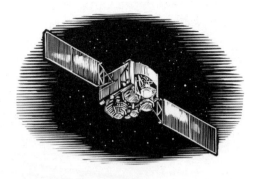

23

Across the courtroom and without directly looking at her, Sean felt the force of Ruth Mott's steady stare. He wanted to be kind, but in case she did not – and the way she'd spoken to him at the funeral suggested she wouldn't – he had briefed Sawbridge about her. It had to be done.

'We all checked into our hotel,' he said, 'the Polar Dream – then we went for supper at a restaurant called Amaruq, where Dr Mott joined us. We had supper, then we came back to the hotel.'

'All of you?' asked the coroner.

'Ruth was staying somewhere else. In the morning, we met in the lobby and took a car back to the airport, where Danny Long flew us up to Midgard as planned.'

'When you say *we*—'

'Myself, Tom, Joe Kingsmith, Martine Delaroche and Radiance Young. Just the consortium partners.'

Amaruq, which the menu explained meant Wolf in the Inuktitut language, was the new restaurant just outside the town limits. Already famed for its bold interpretation of traditional gourmet Inuit dishes alongside its regular Nordic menu, its proprietors were a Danish couple who had lived in Greenland, and supported one of the last remaining traditional communities through exporting their food. They offered a literal taste of a lost world, and it was impossible to get a reservation for the whole of the summer season. Sean felt gratified that one phone call to Skadi Larssen's secretary in Oslo had sorted that out.

They'd had one round of cocktails before Ruth Mott arrived, flushed from her skidoo ride. The men all rose to greet her, and Sean enjoyed the eyes of the other diners on their glamorous table. Both Radiance and Martine, au fait with wilderness chic, were understated but had each put on a serious cocktail ring as a token to their status at this business dinner, even if was happening in the Arctic. Ruth wore jeans and a black silk shirt, which gleamed – Sean could not help noticing – where her breasts pushed against it. Her eyes had changed too. She was wearing makeup.

'Something wrong?' She smiled at him.

'You haven't changed a bit.' He thought the opposite; she was much less strident, and seemed to have softened with the years. More drinks came. Sean ordered one Inuit tasting menu to share, and the six-course Nordic set menu for each. Both Tom and Ruth asked for substitutions for the 'whale beef', which could be served either as carpaccio or seared as a steak. Sean looked forward to his, which tasted like nothing else and he ate on every ethically sourced and defensible occasion, which was the great USP of the restaurant.

Kingsmith ordered vintage champagne from the extensive wine list, and they toasted the success of Midgard Lodge. Ruth Mott was preoccupied by the bear, she said. They should not mind her. The animal was pregnant but with strange complications. And in the wrong season.

'Don't say any more.' Martine shuddered.

'I wasn't planning to.'

Radiance studied Ruth, unabashed.

'You and Tom. Exes, right?'

Ruth glanced at him before she answered. 'That's right.'

'If that's your final word.' Tom looked at her.

Radiance grabbed up a menu and fanned herself.

'Something on fire here!' She nudged Kingsmith. 'Hey: sexy old man: when do we have our special talk? Like you said, on the plane?'

Sean burst out laughing at Kingsmith's look of agitation.

'Radiance, you're too good for me. Also, you might kill me.' Then he said something in her ear that made her slap him playfully. Ruth and Tom sat side by side, not speaking, but obviously intensely aware of each other. The waitress passed among them with the bottle.

'Bad idea,' Martine said it so low Sean barely heard it, but they were both thinking the same thing: Tom must not invite Ruth up to Midgard with them.

'So, Ruth,' Sean broke them apart without knowing what he was going to say next. 'How is the world of tourism?'

'Disasters waiting to happen. Oops, they already are. The Arctic's the new Mediterranean, and Svalbard its Ibiza. Watch this space.'

The waitress brought the first course of the Inuit tasting menu. She set down a board of small blocks of terrine, fine strands of a dark meat, threaded with translucent lines of fat.

'This is pickled auk,' she explained. 'The little birds from the cliffs? We serve it just thawed, so it melts in the mouth like foie gras. Enjoy.'

They each took one, Radiance's eyes bulging as she tasted it. She had another. Joe Kingsmith took one, looked like he was going to throw up, and had a big gulp of his wine. Sean did the same, Ruth ate one and declined more, Martine shuddered and passed, so Tom and Radiance ate all the rest.

'You know how they make them?' he said.

'Don't,' said Sean. 'I remember.'

'He's right,' said Ruth. 'Seriously.'

'But what about my knowledge of the minutiae of Greenlandic culture?' Tom said to her. 'And my superior knowledge that I like to parade, even when other people might know better? Or have jobs equally valid?'

'Well, that's not me, not any more,' Ruth said. 'Now it's just you. I hope.'

'What if I've changed? Lost all my bad qualities?'

'I'd be very sorry. I haven't lost mine.'

'Good.'

'We saw them made,' Sean announced loudly. 'In Greenland – remember, Tom?'

'That's right.' Tom smiled but he didn't want to relive it, he wanted to stay connected to Ruth.

Sean continued, trying to catch Ruth's eye. 'We spent some time in an Inuk village, while we were students, living with the people, eating like they did.'

'I didn't know that.' Martine didn't look like it pleased her either.

'What was the girl's name, who made us those mittens?'

'I can't remember any girls.' Tom looked at Ruth. 'Not one.'

Sean turned away from their separate dinner for two, feeling a dull wash of deprivation that he didn't have that kind of communion with Martine. They shared lust and excitement and passion, and thrilled to the deals to be done – here they were, right this very moment, in the middle of one – but where was that ineffable sparkle between a man and a woman? With a stab of pain, he recognised it as love.

'Sean: don't stare.' Tom winked at him.

Sean laughed, despite himself. 'I'm not fucking Roxy.'

'Who's Roxy?' Radiance looked at Martine for a reaction. 'Cute name.'

'Their Greenland rescue dog,' Ruth said. 'Who ruled them.' She looked at Martine. 'You must have heard.'

'Many times.' Martine forced a smile. 'Forgive me,' she said, 'but being an Arctic biologist sounds so fascinating. Why did you stop?'

'I haven't,' Ruth said calmly. 'I am still a scientist or I wouldn't have been asked to carry out the post-mortem of the bear today. That's not a job for a cruise-line speaker. Hasn't Sean filled you in on why I left fieldwork?'

'He hasn't,' Martine lied. 'But please excuse me: I didn't realise it was a painful story for you.'

They were all silent for a moment. Then Radiance tinged her fork against her empty champagne glass. 'Very serious! I have the glass with the hole!'

Kingsmith agreed, and requested more champagne when the waitress returned with the whale steaks and cloudberry sauce. This, she stated with cheery defiance, was a traditional food from sustainably harvested right whale, which was plentiful in the region and whose stocks were restored. There was evidence. She strafed the table with her smile, checking for troublemakers.

'If you really want to know,' Ruth Mott said to Martine, when the waitress had gone, 'I'll tell you. I killed a bear by accident. A sponsored bear, of viable reproductive age. We were due to take new readings and I darted her.'

Ruth Mott paused, and Sean watched Tom take her hand under the table. 'She suffered a reaction to the tranquilliser,' she continued, 'and she died. No reason, correct dosage, it just – happened. But they said that I'd got the dosage wrong, that I was over-tired. I was forced to take a sabbatical. While I was gone, the story got twisted. Now I can't get another research job. But I still love the Arctic, so I've found a way to be here. And, as you saw earlier today, I can still be trusted with dead ones. If there's no one better around.'

'There never has been, there never will be.' Tom said it so directly, she looked at him in shock. To cover her feelings, Ruth took out her phone and scrolled for a picture, hiding her shining face as she searched.

'But today, look what I found.' She showed Tom her phone. 'A lip tattoo like we did in Qarrtsiluni. Imagine if she'd come all the way from there.' She put it away, her face glowing. 'Sorry. No one needs to see that. I don't need to talk about this any more.'

'Everyone makes mistakes,' Martine said. 'It's healthy you've moved on.'

'It was not a *mistake*.' Ruth looked at her fiercely. 'I know it wasn't.'

Kingsmith replenished her glass.

'Qarrtsiluni?' he pronounced it effortlessly. 'You know that place?'

'Do you?' Ruth gratefully disengaged from Martine.

'Sure. We were considering a couple projects with the government – when I say *government*, I mean everything was clear from the Danish side, but the natives – the Greenlanders—'

'Inuit,' Ruth said. 'That's what they call themselves.'

'Sure,' Kingsmith agreed, 'the Inuit – so tricky to work with. Charming, extraordinarily talented people, but no idea of timekeeping, non-existent administrative system – long story short, things just didn't pan out.'

'Pan out,' Ruth Mott repeated. 'Things, meaning mining? In Qarrtsiluni?'

*

When he thought back to this moment, Sean knew that what was about to happen was completely his fault. He could have headed this off at the airport, he might have prevented all that followed. Instead he had succumbed to that old competitive urge with Tom where women were concerned, and got in first to invite Ruth to join them. Now here she was, facing off with Kingsmith. Two elements that should never have been mixed.

'Prism Mining.' She stared at Kingsmith. 'That was you.'

'Proud to say so.' Kingsmith could not have been more relaxed. 'Back in the day, what a great company! Sadly, long gone. Too many delays, too much bureaucracy. Leave them on the table too long, and some deals spoil like meat. Prism Greenland was one. We wanted to bring prosperity to those poor people – if you've worked there you know how desperate their lives are. My god, the poverty, and the problems it brings. All very well being nostalgic for Arctic Past, like these two boys here – but you and I know that old romance is a complete crock. Arctic Future is what they want: TVs, iPads, foreign travel, all the rest of it. You can't keep kids in the last century.' He went back to his food. 'Losing battle, but we gave it a good go.'

Ruth spoke too carefully.

'Some people there, some young people, still wanted to choose. They did not want to be resettled. They didn't want Prism's money, or to be bullied when they refused. I know that for a fact.'

'Delicious, this beef.' Kingsmith looked at her over his whale-loaded fork. 'How's that then?'

'My research guide was one of the local leaders. He told me that, before he disappeared. Tom, I'm so sorry – for all that. He wasn't—'

'I know.'

Radiance held out her glass. 'You've got a lot of stories, Bear Lady.'

'No story, Mad Lady,' Ruth said to her. 'But not everyone wanted mining.'

'Here's the thing,' Kingsmith said, and Sean heard the edge cutting through the charm. 'If you take the money, it's a done deal. Right, Sean?'

'Your company tore up denning sites that were used for generations.'

'Oh, Ruth, please.' Tom put his head in his hand.

'No, she's got a point,' Kingsmith said. 'Life's constant change, and survival's the prerogative of those who adapt quick enough.' He smiled at her. 'People and animals migrate. Old ways change.' Now all the other diners were listening. 'They serve whale here because the whale stocks have restored, so once again they're a food source. Like cows. Neither of them want to die and be eaten, but we've all got canine teeth in our heads, whether we use them or not. I do, because I'm not just an animal, I'm a natural predator. So be sentimental and angry about how business is developing the Arctic, or get on board to make it a positive thing.'

'You destroyed a human and an animal community, for profit! You call that a positive thing?'

'Sunny side up, please,' Radiance interrupted. 'Tell the shipping story! So much less fuel in transit across the North Pole, so much less pollution – you know how many days you save?'

'You know how many whales are hit by ships?'

'No, and you don't know either,' retorted Radiance, 'because no one does, no one can, because there aren't any statistics. You say that to make me feel bad? Go on then, open the Suez Canal again, go make the terrorists be nice – oh no, you can't. So we better send all those things another way, right? I better send them over the North Pole! Where there's no more summer sea ice and climate change has made it quicker and cheaper for everyone! It's not bad, Bear Lady, it's progress. But new shoes hurt, right?'

Ruth turned to Tom. '*These* are your partners?' She pulled a handful of notes from her pocket and put them on the table. 'Wow.'

'Ruth! Don't be so silly!' Sean called after her, but she didn't stop. Tom grabbed the money and ran out behind her. The whole restaurant remained paused, listening to their raised voices beyond the entrance curtain. Then there was the sound of a skidoo engine. Tom returned, holding the money.

'May I?' It was Osman. The coroner nodded permission. 'Thank you.' She cleared her throat with the small rasp Sean was growing to hate. He noticed a long scar just above her clavicle – surgery probably. Or an attack.

'Mr Cawson, thank you for your very brief account. You alluded to Dr Mott leaving the restaurant first – do you know why?'

'Dr Mott took offence at something my partner Joe Kingsmith said, about the future of the Arctic. They were coming to it from pretty much opposing points of view, and she stormed out before the meal was over.'

'Was Tom involved? In this ... disagreement?'

'No. But he went after Dr Mott, to try to talk sense to her.'

'She seems eminently sensible to me.'

'She very rudely threw down some money, even though it was my invitation. He wanted to give it back to her. He was embarrassed at her behaviour, she was very ungracious.' Sean left a pause. 'Some people hold their drink better than others.'

Mrs Osman shifted slightly, her crabbed shape now blocking his sight line to Ruth Mott. 'Yet I believe she is godmother to your daughter, Rosie?'

'She is.' Sean was wary. 'She's always loved her, even if she led her astray.'

Ruth Mott jumped to her feet. 'I've done no such thing! I know exactly what you're referring to and that was completely her own idea – just because you lied to her did not mean I had to.' At Mrs Osman's look, she sat down again.

'Thank you,' said the coroner. 'If you do not observe the protocol of the court, Dr Mott, you will not be permitted to remain. And let me remind you, Mrs Osman, Mr Sawbridge, that this is a Jamieson inquest, in which all we are seeking to do is understand by what means the deceased met his death. It is not an Article Two inquest, in search of all the circumstances surrounding that fact. And it is emphatically not a criminal trial, much as you would both like to show off your rhetorical abilities on such a stage. Is that clear?'

Mr Thornton waited until both Mrs Osman and Mr Sawbridge had respectfully nodded. 'Then Court is recessed for fifteen minutes, after which, if you are able, Mr Cawson, we will hear of the events of the following day and the accident.'

*

The event to which Ruth Mott referred was bitter to Sean to this day. At the age of fourteen, during a half-term at home, Rosie had heard a savage row. Gail knew about Martine, and pleaded with Sean to either stay or go. Not yet ready to do either, and in miserable desperation to buy time to think, Sean lied. He swore to Gail that she was wrong, she had misheard, he had been foolish in the past with silly girls, but now she was paranoid.

Gail had wanted to believe him more than the truth. She had comforted Rosie, who came down in tears and stood between them, and told her she had made a mistake. Rosie had wept in relief, and for two or three days Sean felt like a good man and loved his wife and daughter with a fierce protective passion. Then Rosie heard him answer his phone in a different tone, and speak to Martine, who had been calling repeatedly.

Rosie hid, and heard her father apologising, and promising. She noted the time, and when her father left his phone for a few minutes, she noted the number that had called. A friend hacked it to an office location, and as Sean found out later, Rosie did not go to London to meet friends, as she'd told her parents, but to Martine's work – where, dressed as a bicycle courier, she delivered an envelope to her hand. She said she needed to wait for a reply and watched as, at her desk, Martine pulled out photographs of Sean and Gail's wedding, of Sean and Gail and Rosie on their most recent holiday, and of Sean and Gail watching television, Harold the cat sprawled between them.

'Leave my family alone!' Rosie shouted in her face, before snatching back the photographs and running faster than the security guards coming to get her. Distraught, she'd gone to Ruth Mott's. Ruth had applauded her courage, let her cry it out, and kept her for two days. It was the beginning of the end for Sean and Gail, and because he could not blame his own child for his own lies, he blamed Ruth Mott. So had Gail, for a few years, until the truth of Sean's infidelity had become impossible to ignore any longer.

It was my boy O-tah who disclosed to me that Peary was to leave me behind in the final few miles to the Pole, and with E-tig-wah he witnesses the disappointment of Commander Peary when a few miles from his camp, his observation told the lieutenant that he had overstepped and gone past the Pole, which we had reached the night before. Our camp itself was practically situated on 'the top of the earth'. For the crime of being present when the Pole was reached Commander Peary has ignored me ever since.

After twenty-two years of close companionship he refused even to say good-by when we separated in New York. And at Fort Conger, nearly ten years before, we had carried Peary nearly 200 miles with his feet frozen, traveling days and hunting nights for food to keep him and ourselves alive!

A Negro Explorer at the North Pole: The Autobiography of Matthew
    Henson (1912)
Matthew Henson

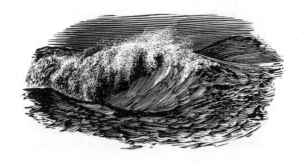

24

The press bench had filled up some more. Flip-flops was pushed further towards the end by reporters who checked emails and sent texts until the last possible moment before being upstanding. Sean saw they all had a photocopied sheet – and so did the front two rows of lawyers and family. He had one too, on the stand: a large-scale map of Midgardfjorden with an inset showing its location on a map of the whole of Svalbard. At Mr Thornton's request, he resumed his account of the eclipse trip.

'Danny Long picked us up at the Polar Dream after breakfast and then we flew to Midgard. The mood was very upbeat, everyone was excited. The Lodge was looking great and it was an extraordinary experience to watch the eclipse from there …'

Danny Long was all contrition. Sean reassured him: always better to be owed than owing, and this was the first time the Sysselmann's office had required them, and must surely have been impressed? Danny Long admitted they'd done Midgard proud. Their twelve-man Dauphin had clocked nearly 500 kilometres ferrying the hapless British stag party out from the accident scene and back to Longyearbyen. He assured them no one else had flown it, nor noticed its many capacities. He added that they'd all been pleased to have the chance to serve.

They put on their headphones and strapped themselves in, Kingsmith insisting, despite Radiance's protest, that he ride shotgun with Danny Long. Radiance had also trained as a helicopter pilot, but everyone – even Tom – instantly protested against the suggestion of her showing them her skills.

Airborne, no one spoke much. Tom was lost in thought, gazing out at the pale blue mountains. They flew north-east from Longyearbyen over Isfjord, banking to the right as they passed the Russian settlement of Pyramiden, so that Sean and Kingsmith could look down on the new constructions. The speed and scale of the expansion was impressive. Or, if you were Mrs Larssen, disturbing.

They continued north over the great glacier of Mittag Letterbreen and then its delta into the steely water of Wijdefjorden. Martine and Radiance photographed the rippled strata of the mountainside, its layers of colour piled up and swirled like ancient stone marble cake.

'It's the only place on earth where you can see this much geological time.' Tom's voice came over the headphones again. 'Each of those stripes represents about two thousand million years.'

'Nice numbers,' came back Kingsmith. 'Keep talking.'

Sean relaxed as Tom, now with permission, released the brake on his geological passion and talked them through what they were seeing: the clasts and the tillites, the glaciofluvial moraines, the time banks of plant and dinosaur fossils where armoured fish forever swam through seas of rock, the Devonian age, the Silurian, the Ordovician, the Cambrian …

'We've got to record him, so we can have this on every flight,' shouted Kingsmith, as Danny Long banked to show them the green glittering ribbon of rock as Tom pointed it out. 'It's like poetry – I don't understand but I love to hear.' He twisted round to see Tom. 'You and Dr Mott, you two could be a lecturing duo. She talks whales, you talk rocks—'

'Like a light entertainment double act? Joe, if that's all you wanted me for—'

'It wasn't.' Sean stepped in quickly. 'He meant, you're fascinating.'

'That's exactly right. And I have huge respect for your knowledge.'

Tom didn't answer, and Radiance put her hand on his arm.

'Tom,' she said, 'I could listen to you for strata.'

212

'Your English is brilliant, Radiance,' he said. 'Where did you learn?'
'Roedean,' she said. 'While English girls still went.'

Sean recognised the volcanic chimneys on the edge of the ice cap
where the glacier pressed down towards the sea. It gave him an
immense satisfaction to begin to recognise parts of the terrain; it
connected him to his explorer gene. Then they clattered out over the
middle of Wijdefjorden for the central approach between the high
walls of Midgardfjord, the Dauphin a noisy mechanical insect lowering itself down onto the gravel beach.

As the rotor chop slowed, Sean listened to them exclaim as first
they saw the silvered wood of the old whaling station, and how subtly
the scale of the building and its artful materials revealed themselves.
The blackened wood was not a pile of driftwood, it was the upper
part of the wall, made of a huge shelf of granite rock-fall.

The whole edifice was an angular flow, an aesthetic paradox in
Svalbard, where colossal geological actions formed cubist patterns on
a massive scale, and the lack of man-made anything – buildings, signs,
roads – was disorientating. Midgard Lodge met the eye as a restored
old whaling station on the beach – and grew backward into the mountain from which it became indivisible.

'Ye gods.' Tom was beside him. 'What a brilliant job!'

After the bear all-clear had been radioed down to Danny, they ran up
the beach to the steps, where Terry Bjornsen's wife Anne was
waiting.

'Welcome to Midgard Lodge, even if you own it,' she said in her
soft South African accent. 'It's thirty minutes to the eclipse, so please
make yourself at home and let us look after you.'

Midgard Lodge looked as fine as Sean could wish. The reception
area smelled of fresh coffee and cinnamon pastries, and was paved in
under-heated stone strewn with worn sealskin rugs. The space was
half-timbered with the same silvery wood used to restore the exterior:
specially treated driftwood from the Russian taiga forest, washed up

(actually shipped) across the Kara and Barents seas. A wide turning staircase led up to the rooms, each (a diplomatic essential) as good as the next.

Silver nitrate photographs of the early Pedersen family, heroes of polar exploration, and photographs of the whaling station at work adorned the walls, and a silver samovar stood ready with Russian tea glasses on a colourful enamelled tray. The mezzanine seating area was walled with polished, fossil-embedded stone, before wide shallow steps rose to the main salon. Here, the central freestanding fire-pit with bench-height stone surround, gave the feeling of a chieftain's hall, and the great triangular window wall looking down the fjord gave the aspect of a chapel to the primeval view. Today the water was mercury-coloured, but Sean had seen it gold.

Anne Bjornsen brought out cloudberry cocktails, crystal tubes of dill vodka, and water from icebergs thousands of years old. Then ruby-red reindeer carpaccio and soft pearly wafers of halibut sashimi, to eat with moist black bread and sweet Norwegian butter.

And then, Sean showed his guests the wardrobe full of furs from Sami or Greenlandic Inuit collectives. If they were going to watch the eclipse from the deck, it would be cold. Or of course, they could wear what they had brought.

But the furs were irresistible. The weight of them, the sensual illicit touch ... Even Tom succumbed to the childish pleasure of dressing up in the romance of the north. Kingsmith chose a polar bear parka, and Martine let Radiance grab the long blue fox coat with dramatic hood. She then debated between a wolverine jacket with a black-tipped sable pelt, or a narrow dark sealskin parka with a hood. She chose the wolverine, and was pleased to catch Tom staring. Her triumph was spoiled by Sean excitedly calling him over to show him the two old jackets he had at the back: ragged and worn sealing anoraqs, handmade, exactly like Gino Watkins wore on the British Arctic Air Expedition—

—No, like Knud Rasmussen had, Tom said, equally happy. Like Peter Freuchen had when they were in Greenland, and Sean had forgotten that, yes more like that, and they marvelled over them. The wolverine stood impotent in her beauty, then followed the blue fox out to join the polar bear on the deck, and Anne Bjornsen made sure they all had sunglasses. Two telescopes were positioned ready. Tom and Sean came out in glacier glasses with the leather eye guards and their old sealing anoraqs and their arms around each other's shoulders, posing and grinning.

'Beards,' said Tom, 'we should have thought.'

'With frost,' Sean agreed.

'Photoshop you.' Radiance shot them on her phone. 'With ice eyelash too, looks so hot – you're welcome.'

There was no need to time the eclipse: the birds told them it was near. At 10.40 they shrieked and wheeled across the long V of fjord sky, then disappeared. The grey mountains filled with black ink. The rippling water turned to sheet metal and the clouds stopped. All that moved was the colour of the sky. Changing faster than any dawn or dusk, from pink to violet to blue, a fast dark shadow pulled night over the mountain as Earth moved behind its moon.

One telescope was shared by the polar bear, standing between the blue fox and the wolverine. The two sealskinned explorers shared the other. Or rather, Sean did, but when he pulled back from the telescope to offer it to Tom, he saw his friend standing in the dark of day, lost in thought.

'You're missing it,' he said.

'I've got this feeling I am.' Tom looked at him in the darkness. 'But what?'

'The eclipse—' Sean stepped aside and Tom put his eye to the scope.

'We decided not to go round the headland in a boat,' Sean's underarms prickled with stress, 'but to go by skidoo – snowmobile – up to the ice-caves on the other side of the glacier tongue. It was a better use of the time we had.'

'We've found an image of the topography,' said the coroner, as behind Sean the screen glowed to rectangular life. Projected on it was a line drawing of Midgardfjorden, which changed at a click to a satellite photograph.

'Where did you get that?'

'Google Earth, I think,' said the coroner's clerk. 'Whole world's there.'

Sean stared. There was the beach and the grey oblongs of the whaling buildings. But, as they had always planned, the rest of it disappeared into the contours of the mountains and the moraine. He repressed the urge to point out the architectural brilliance.

He felt the force of eyes pushing at him like a tide. His hearing, always good, had become acute. The rattle of keyboards. The sound of clothing rustling. Someone eating – he could smell the mints.

'Mr Cawson.' The coroner leaned forward. 'Please go on.'

'Do you think you could ask the press bench not to type as I talk? It's very distracting.'

'Press bench,' said the coroner, 'please be aware of the witness's preference, at your discretion. Go on, Mr Cawson.'

'After the eclipse we went to the ice-cave on skidoos. It was on the other side of the ridge – you can see it behind me. It had been checked the day before, and passed as safe. People have gone there every season.'

'I believe that's not now possible, though, is it?' said the coroner. 'Because the demesne of your property goes to the water's edge, blocking access – if you choose?'

'It's remote and it's always been private property,' said Sean. 'But the Pedersen family pretty much abandoned it, and so there were no regulations enforced.

'Two of my experienced and trusted staff visited it the day before and went all the way down to the chamber known as the Great Hall ...' He waited for the typing at the press bench to keep up. 'And these very experienced men found it safe.'

There was silence, and he knew he'd given them that already, but he was mindful of Sawbridge's advice: *The heart of your testimony is due diligence, personal responsibility of each party, and your blamelessness.*

'So we had checked it the day before. We went in good light with a good weather report. We posted bear watch overlooking access to the cave and the snowmobiles parked near the mouth. We were half a kilometre from the Lodge. We had planned to be in the cave for a maximum of thirty minutes. We could not have been more careful. No one' – and now Sean did look at the press bench, and out at the courtroom, at Angela Harding, at Ruth Mott, at Ursula Osman and her black hooded gaze – '*no one* could have predicted the collapse.'

Directly after the eclipse, Tom disappeared. He was not in his room nor any of the public areas. Then Sean saw him, rifle on his back – he had helped himself from the gun safe, he must have seen Terry Bjornsen key it open – walking across the beach. He should have asked Sean, he was behaving like he owned the place as well. And now – Sean and Kingsmith watched from the chapel window – he was heading to the boat hangar.

Sean ran down to the beach, calling to Danny Long – currently sitting in the Dauphin with a coffee, on bear watch – then he went down after Tom.

'Hey!' he followed him into the cavern of the boat hangar. 'You should have said – I could have showed you round.'

'No time like the present.' Tom emerged between the two stacks of Zodiacs. He wasn't smiling. 'Lot of boat here. How many people are we planning to host?'

'Varies.' Sean kicked himself for not mentally rehearsing this. 'We had the space. And search and rescue – we just proved our community credentials.'

'Right. Search and rescue for the Sysselmann.' Tom looked around the hangar. 'Where's the manpower, right now?' Without asking Sean, he went up the three steps and opened the door at the top.

'That's the dorm,' Sean said, as casually as he could. He could see the room Tom was looking into: an insulated and ventilated space with stacked bunks. Tom climbed up a ladder beside one set of bunks, and received the view down the fjord. He looked back at Sean.

'A barrack lookout. Where are they right now?'

'On leave, after yesterday.' Sean followed him out.

'I thought the retreats would bring in their own people. That's what it said in the proposal.'

'We're trialling a new idea, I'll tell you about it later, or we'll miss the light—'

'What's that?' Tom pointed his powerful pencil-torch beam at the keypad on another door in the rock.

'That's the strong room.' Kingsmith stood silhouetted in the doorway.

'Strong room?'

Sean walked past Tom and tapped in the code. 'I want to tell him.'

Kingsmith shrugged. Sean pulled the big steel door open, activating the light inside a smaller cave. Tom looked at the stacked arsenal.

'Just how big have the bears got up here? Are we expecting trolls or an aquatic assault from a sea monster?' He picked up a shoulder holster. 'These are for RPGs. This is an armoury for guerrilla warfare.' He took out his phone, but before he could photograph it Sean pushed his arm down.

'Tom, don't. I'll explain it all.'

Tom shook him off. He stood in front of Kingsmith.

'What exactly are you doing here?'

They were equal height; Tom was younger, but Kingsmith far bigger. They held each other's stare. Then Kingsmith smiled.

'So serious! Tom, I'm bankrolling your conservation campaign, I'm investing in the Arctic, and I'm helping Sean boy get his boy scout badge for being neighbourly. My immediate concern? Let's not miss the window of opportunity – I want to see this Great Hall.' He turned to go. 'And, boys, do not leave me alone with Radiance: I'm not sure I can keep up the good daddy routine much longer.' Kingsmith went back out onto the beach and they heard him exchange pleasantries with Danny Long. They stood in silence as his footsteps receded towards the Lodge. Sean closed the door to the armoury. The locks whirred.

'Four RIBs,' Tom said very quietly. 'Body armour and harnesses for RPGs. Quite a lot of kit for an ethical retreat. So talk. Because my name is on this.'

'Tom, please trust me. I was asked to do this.'

'By him?'

'By Philip Stowe. You know, our Defence Secretary.'

'*Stowe?* That crook? You know he's bloodstained, don't you – he sells British arms to the highest bidder, he cares fuck-all about human rights – you're telling me you're doing something for *him*, and *I'm* involved?'

'Sean!' Martine called in to them. 'Danny says we need to go now or we'll miss it. Are you guys ready?'

218

'Just coming!' Sean turned back to Tom. 'Long story short, as well as everything that you do know about, we're also protecting radomes for the Norwegians. Now NATO's gone, they're really scared – Tom, think about what could happen if a hostile power knocked out friendly satellites controlled from Svalbard—'

'Wake up! You're protecting the means of warfare for Philip fucking Stowe and his business cronies! This isn't about patriotism, it's about money—'

'And you're so up your own holy arse now you can't even see that Midgard is helping with the stability of the whole region—'

'What I see is that Midgard is being used, and so am I. By you.'

Sean couldn't bear the look in his eyes. 'I want to explain everything to you, so that you understand. I'm sure, *I'm sure*, Tom, that you'll be OK when you do. Everything you want to achieve here – you still can. Everything I said about the business and the retreats is still true. Private security isn't a crime: you of all people know how it works. How do NGOs do their work? Peace-keeping means having a big stick.'

'What about that little thing called the Svalbard Treaty? The one that specifically prohibits any warlike purposes—'

'Everyone ignores it! It's out of date!'

'Like our agreement. It's void. And I'm blowing the whistle on you.'

Before Tom could go, furious with fear, Sean grabbed him by the arm and pulled him back. They stared at each other in the gloom of the strong room. Sean took his hand away. They heard the skidoos starting up, and Radiance cheerfully calling them.

'Please,' said Sean. 'Please, let's just go to the cave. And then I'll tell you everything you want to know.'

'I don't want that. I want the truth.'

'I promise.' Sean said it to Tom's back. He followed him out.

'I need to pee,' Tom yelled, heading for the Lodge. 'Wait for me.'

The bad news was brought this afternoon that 'Job' is dead, torn in pieces by the other dogs. He was found a good way from the ship, 'Old Suggen' lying watching the corpse, so that no other dog could get to it. They are wretches, these dogs; no day passes without a fight. In the day-time one of us is generally on hand to stop it, but at night they seldom fail to tear and bite one of their comrades. Poor 'Barabbas' is frightened out of his wits. He stays on board now, and dares not venture on the ice, because he knows the other monsters would set on him. There is not a trace of chivalry about these curs. When there is a fight, the whole pack rush like wild beasts on the loser. But is it not, perhaps, the law of nature that the strong, and not the weak, should be protected? Have not we human beings, perhaps, been trying to turn nature topsy-turvy by protecting and doing our best to keep life in all the weak?

Wednesday, 11 October 1893
Farthest North: The Norwegian Polar Expedition 1893–1896 (1897)
Fridtjof Nansen

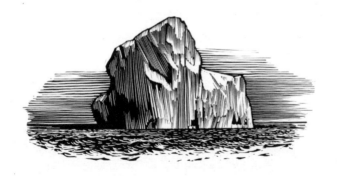

25

Five skidoos went up the glacier, the roar of their engines muffled by the deep snow. Up ahead, Tom kept pace with Terry Bjornsen who led the way, then came Sean with Martine pillion, and close behind, Radiance with Kingsmith on the back. Danny Long brought up the rear. The snowmobile trails glittered pale pink and the sky glowed all shades of rose above the sharp violet peaks. Sean had never seen Svalbard so beautiful, but he focused on the immediate problem of Tom's anger.

He guided his skidoo in Tom's tracks. Now was not the time to lose his own cool – he must stay focused on the super-objective of Midgard: an inspiring venue in which to promote the reconciliation of business and environmental ethics. And here they were, the two of them, actually living out that conflict, at this very second. He wanted to laugh – of course Tom would see it too. And the solution was to keep talking, arguing if necessary, but always in pursuit of that shared goal. Sean's heart lifted. As long as Tom did not act rashly, they could get through it. As long as Tom and Kingsmith were not left alone – that would be a recipe for disaster. He knew he and Tom could argue above their solid bedrock of friendship – but Tom and Kingsmith had never clicked.

They came to the first saddle in the ridge between the two tongues of the Midgard glacier and crossed over, leaving the Lodge behind and out of sight. They dipped down onto the other side where the snow shadow was pale blue, Terry Bjornsen leading them around a darker blue track to an easy further ascent. Two small fluorescent orange pennants fluttered ahead like candle flames, marking the entrance to the ice-cave.

They parked the skidoos in a line angled for the descent. The pennant flags were mounted on whippy plastic masts weighted deep in the snow, from which emerged a length of orange nylon rope. One end was hooked halfway up a mast, and the other attached to the cave cover, revealed when Terry Bjornsen kicked away the snow to show them a scarred white plastic slab. Sean knew Tom was avoiding his eye, but that was better than conflict, for now. They were still together.

Radiance, ever the expert traveller, was checking all her equipment, tucking in her own loose straps and then fussing over Kingsmith. He allowed her, rolling his eyes at Sean. Martine called Sean to help with hers. When their heads were touching, she whispered, 'What's going on?'

'Nothing to worry about.'

She nodded, but her eyes went to Tom, standing alone, still as a stone cairn. Sean had a terrible fear that at any second he was going to turn and denounce him. But Tom remained looking back towards Midgard Lodge. Then Danny Long, who had already climbed to a lookout ridge, radioed the first all-clear and Sean put the unpleasant thought of their impending conversation aside. He watched Terry Bjornsen take up his pre-planned spot on the opposite side to Danny. The cave was well positioned for surveillance: this side of the glacier narrowed between the rocks and a bear would easily be spotted. The spotters had flares as well as bullets and would be in constant contact by iridium satellite phone. Sean had two, and had intended to give one to Tom. He changed his mind.

To reach the Great Hall and return would take thirty minutes, max – most likely they'd do it in fifteen. Beneath the plastic slab the entrance to the cave system was a neatly edged circular hole in the ice, a metre wide. A few centimetres below, a wooden ladder had been secured to the ice wall with large and reassuringly new steel clamps and screws. This fed down three metres to the first landing, where weak daylight illuminated the area called the Lobby. Black plastic grids were half-sunk into the hard ground to aid progress and along the wall, new rope fed through steel rings where the tunnel sloped away into darkness.

Sean climbed halfway up the ladder to phone Terry Bjornsen – everything looked good. His crackly laugh came back, saying it bloody should, they'd killed themselves making it pretty. Then they all switched on their head torches and Sean led the way in, followed by Tom, Radiance and Martine, with Kingsmith bringing up the rear.

The sound quality was very different inside the ice. When Sean spoke to make sure they all wanted to go on, he had to project loudly because the frozen density sucked his words away. But they all called out to show they were keen, even Tom, who the others ushered into second place in the line. Radiance went behind him, then Martine, Kingsmith last. They followed Sean down the slope away from the Lobby, along the ice corridor where their torch beams bounced and shone on white curves.

Sean called reassurance as he led the way down rough steps cut with an ice axe, and was relieved to see Tom slipping naturally into an authoritative role, helping Martine, who was grateful. Radiance didn't need him, and turned to help Kingsmith down. They all waited for him, passing through a smaller landing, then out into a wide passageway where even Tom could stand upright in the centre.

'Everyone's fine.' Tom's tone was still curt.

'Thanks.' Sean was grateful he was helping. He tried not to feel too happy that they were doing their favourite thing together, even if all was not well. Surely Tom was glad he hadn't sulked and missed it?

They went on.

The rope holds continued, the floor had been graded and black grip-tiles filled gaps or places where the walls were glassy either side. As the passageway continued its descent, they paused to marvel at the changing colours of the ice, from white to a fairytale pale blue. In one place a streak of sulphurous gold matter ran diagonally across the wall and into the ice, and a few metres further on, down another set of ice-axed steps, the passageway became a domed room with a natural porthole in one ice wall.

They crowded around it to look. Their torch beams showed a deep narrow chamber filled with ice stalagmites and stalactites, stretching up and down towards each other and sometimes forming delicate ice columns. Their breath came in clouds, drifting into the cavern and trailing between the frozen forms.

'Where's that air coming from?' Tom had moved closer to Sean, his voice low.

They watched the pale vapour from their lungs move around the stalagmites, then disappear.

'The air vent from the hatch.' Sean said it automatically. He watched the five halogen beams from their head torches shifting the shadows and making the ice strobe and gleam with light, as if stirred to life by their observation. Radiance exclaimed in frustration that her micro camera, guaranteed for polar conditions, did not work.

'So expensive,' she said. 'Complete rip-up.'

'It's too cold for the battery,' Tom said. 'But you don't need a camera. Use your eyes. This is truly awesome.'

Standing beside him, Sean smiled at the excitement in his voice. Everything was going to be all right.

'OK, team?' Sean avoided Tom's face, but let his beam rest for a moment on Martine, who smiled, Radiance, who gave him a thumbs up, and then Kingsmith, who was looking up at the roof. He looked back at Sean and nodded.

'Tom,' Sean said, 'go first?'

'Sure.' There was no need for explanation; Tom understood Sean's concern for the others, and immediately moved a few paces into the darkness ahead, waiting.

'Don't you worry about me,' Kingsmith called. 'I'm doing just fine.'

Sean fell into second place, and was glad to feel Martine squeeze his shoulder. They went on, Tom's beam showing the way. The passageway continued to descend, its shape changing as they went – sometimes wider around the head area, sometimes narrowing, sometimes with a ledge protruding at waist height that they had to pass by, taking the ice by their mittened hands and feeling it glide as the friction melted it.

They came into a broader section, and again Sean checked their faces. They were all smiling, but he could hear their breathing was faster.

'Still OK?'

The three of them nodded, then Tom called out softly that the ice was good.

'I can make out a big arch ahead – that's got to be the Great Hall. There's this narrow bit, then a couple of big shelving steps down, it's right here.'

Sean could hear the excitement in his voice.

'We're coming!'

'No, I don't think so.' Kingsmith's voice came from further back in the tunnel. 'I'll see you guys back up top.'

'Hold up, Tom,' Sean called ahead. 'Joe's not OK.'

'I'm fine,' Kingsmith called back irritably, but Radiance and Martine were already with him, and he did not look at all OK to Sean. He was leaning against the ice wall and smiling, but it was more of a grimace. He deflected Sean's torch beam from his face and started back along the passageway.

'You take care of things down here, I'll see you up top.'

'Hey, old man,' Radiance said. 'You need me. Admit it.'

Kingsmith laughed weakly. 'Radiance, you kill me.'

'What are you talking about? I save you! I make your life so fun!' She grinned back at Sean and Martine, her teeth white in the darkness. 'Martin, come on. I save you too, no fee.'

Martine did not reply, but Sean saw her tense expression.

'Go,' he said. 'Tom and I will just have a quick look.'

'Or we can take them back.' Tom had returned to Sean's side.

'We'll be fine!' Radiance winked at them. 'I'm their leader now.'

Martine rolled her eyes at Sean. 'Don't be too long.'

'Ten minutes,' Sean said.

'Fifteen, realistically,' said Tom.

'I'm the leader,' Radiance called back. 'Fifteen is OK.' She herded Martine and Kingsmith back up the passageway. Sean grinned at the thought of what Martine would say later.

'Might as well take a quick look,' Tom said. 'We've come all this way.'

'We have.' Sean looked at him, and this time Tom met his gaze for a second. They went down the passage together, towards the ice-cave known as the Great Hall.

*

'We went inside,' Sean told the court. He felt like the ice was taking his breath again, he almost expected it to come out in clouds. 'Tom went in first.' His lungs worked fast and shallow at the thought of it all.

They were so excited neither could speak, but they turned to each other to confirm they really were seeing this marvel. They were in a huge cavern, like some ice giant's baronial hall. At first they looked around separately, then, by unspoken instinct, they moved their two torch beams together, like a single pair of eyes.

Parts of the structure glowed to life under their double gaze. Slowly, amazed, grinning at each other, they went a few steps deeper, nudging each other to point out the blue ribs and rafters of ice above them, a cathedral crossed with the inside of a whale. They gazed on a massive slab resting on smaller blocks, like a chieftain's table. Below it, softer-shaped extrusions formed huge sleeping dogs. Here and there were stalactites spreading like candelabra, and other strange forms twisted into ropes hung with ice tassels.

Sean saw gargoyles and effigies, and then one eye of the double beam shifted, and Tom was looking at him.

'Tell me now,' Tom said. 'While the cat's away.'

It took a few seconds for Sean to remember what he meant. Kingsmith. That whole mess above the ice. Tom had broken the spell and now they stood looking at one another in the Great Hall, each face pinned by the other's beam.

'Fine,' Sean said. 'You have to understand though, no one's doing anything wrong.' But as he said it, he didn't sound convincing even to himself. 'We're just protecting the place we both love.'

'With a private military.'

'Tom, I told you – it's standing security for guests.'

'You let Kingsmith do this, didn't you? Of course you did.'

'Yes, I left that side of it to him, but, Tom, if your own government asks you to do something ...'

'You're delusional.' Tom's breath came in bigger clouds.

'You know something, Tom?' Sean's breath billowed out as well, they were like dragons facing each other. 'There are lots of ways to protect the Arctic, but you think you've got the only answer, you want a vital new trade route just taken off the table – you think the world really will put ice and whales and—'

'Climate change first? Yes! I'm hoping—'

Tom stopped suddenly. He turned away, his beam flashing over the blue-and-white ice walls. Then back to one spot, where the blue ice gleamed more vividly.

'Shit. Look—'

Sean's torch beam picked it out too. A narrow thread of water trickling from high above, following the curve of the vaulted wall, down into the cavern floor, through the crack they both saw, running beyond the range of their light.

They stopped arguing, hearing the tearing sound. Only a second, then it stopped. Then came another sound – the high-pitched moan of ice squeezing ice.

Sean held on to the lectern. The eyes of the courtroom were on him and felt like ants, he wanted to scrape them from his skin. The carpet tiles smelled dirty, someone was wearing too much hairspray. He was close to it. He wanted to push his fingers under his jacket, into his shirt and the warmth of his sticky armpit – they were burning like they had when he was recovering. He put his fingers into the glass of water on the stand, and heard the tapping of keyboards, no doubt recording this strange gesture. Sawbridge was looking at him with an urgent expression.

'Your Honour,' he called out, 'a break for my client, I think?'

'Do you need that, Mr Cawson?'

Sean heard the metallic scrape of the louvre windows being opened. He felt a trail of air move through the room and over his face.

'No. I'll go on.' His voice felt deadened, as if still in the ice. 'A massive blow hit us under our feet then we were – we lifted up as the ice shifted and I fell sideways, there was nothing to hold on to, there was this rumbling noise and even as I was slipping I knew the cave was collapsing.'

He put his hands back on the lectern. 'I tried to push my feet against something so I could get upright – I was still on my side – but I couldn't find any purchase because everything was slippery and my torch had got knocked sideways so I couldn't see. Then the rumbling stopped.'

Sean closed his eyes. No one moved in the courtroom, not a finger on a keyboard or a hand in a pocket. He could hear his breath, loud and shallow, and he didn't know if he was at the lectern or in the ice.

'I called for Tom. I called out – and then I heard him, his voice was coming from somewhere below me. He was alive but he'd fallen. I called to him to hold on – I got my boot against something and I pushed up so I could secure my torch – and all I could see was a jumble of huge ice fragments. I called out again and when he answered I saw the hole it came from.'

The sound of Angela and Ruby Harding's weeping brought Sean back to the courtroom for a moment. He spoke directly to them.

'I said to hold on. I said the others would be out by now, they'd raise the alarm. I kept saying, "I won't leave you, just hold on, Tom, hold on."'

Sean braced himself against the ice, his belly against a freezing slab of it, the hard edge of his boot soles scraped in behind him to get a hold. With one hand he felt for his torch and secured it, then shone it down into the black chasm.

'Tom!' He waited. '*TOM!*'

There was no reply. All he could hear was the great bloody gulp of his own heart. He was completely alone in the ice, deep below the surface. Tom was gone.

Sean stared into blackness for a moment. Then the court came back into focus. The staring faces. The sound of the traffic.

'I don't remember much after that.' He did not wait for the coroner to release him, he left the stand and walked back down to his seat. Sawbridge stared at him with grave concern and patted him on the arm. No one spoke. The coroner cleared his throat.

'We'll adjourn for today. Mr Cawson, thank you, but I'm afraid I'll need to ask you back to the stand tomorrow morning for questions.'

Sean nodded, then did not move until all the motion in the room was over, the scraping chairs, the stares, the chiming of phones released from silence. When he finally looked up, Sawbridge was waiting at the end of the row.

The traffic of Canterbury's ring road looked like a film, as unreal and alien as the jerky Inuit of Nanuq of the North.

'A drink, that's what we need.' Sawbridge steered him in the other direction, around the corner into the back streets where kebab shops jostled medieval walls and an old pub stood waiting.

They went into its gloomy womb of beery carpet and ugly dark-wood furniture, the only people except for the barman, his belly prominent under a sports shirt. He looked at them disapprovingly as he sloshed a pint of water down in front of Sean – the only thing he wanted – and a tomato juice for Sawbridge. Somewhere in the background a fruit machine whirred and pinged. Sean stared through the darkness that still clotted his vision.

'You did splendidly.'

'I failed.'

'Rubbish! If it were water off a duck's back, if you just sang your song all well-rehearsed, it would be a disaster. You went through hell to survive.'

'I failed Tom!'

Sawbridge held up his hands appeasingly, as if to show he understood. He opened the peanuts and ate them in meditative silence for a while, then hailed the barman. 'Don't suppose there's anywhere I might fire up a very small cigar?'

'The street.' The barman was unimpressed. 'You from the inquest?'

'Ah, you know about it.' Sawbridge pepped up his charm, just in case.

'Know the family. I knew Tom.'

Sean looked up. 'A friend?'

'Village cricket, when he was around.'

Sean stared at him.

'You were one of the pall-bearers.'

'That's right.' The barman looked at him. 'I remember you, too.'

Sean held out his hand. 'Sean Cawson.'

'Yeah. I know.' The barman hesitated fractionally then shook. 'John Burnham.'

Sawbridge stood: 'A great tragedy.' Sean ignored the signal.

'I couldn't save him.'

'I'm not asking. Mate, you look in a bad way.'

'He's doing extremely well and we are almost at the finish line.' Sawbridge tapped Sean on the arm and went to the door. 'Very best to you,' he called to the barman. 'I'm sure we'll stop by again.' Out on the street a safe distance away, he stopped. 'Important you hear this: discretion is most certainly the better part of valour. Quite serious now. Absolutely no vino veritas-ing with anyone, please, and I include myself in that.'

'I wasn't planning to.'

'Who ever does?'

They walked back to the White Bear in silence. Sean changed his clothes, did not check his phone or email, went down to the restaurant and ate before Sawbridge arrived. They were both relieved to miss each other for dinner and, back in his room, Sean stared at whatever was on the television and drank vodka, until he was able to pass out.

Now we are in the very midst of what the prophets would have had us dread so much. The ice is pressing and packing round us with a noise like thunder. It is piling itself up into long walls, and heaps high enough to reach a good way up the Fram's rigging; in fact, it is trying its very utmost to grind the Fram into powder. But here we sit quite tranquil, not even going up to look at all the hurly-burly, but just chatting and laughing, as usual.

Such an ice conflict is undeniably a stupendous spectacle. One feels one's self to be in the presence of Titanic forces, and it is easy to understand how timid souls may be overawed and feel as if nothing could stand before it. For when the packing begins in earnest, it seems as though there could be no spot on the earth's surface left unshaken. First you hear a sound like the thundering rumble of an earthquake far away on the great waste; then you hear it in several places, always coming nearer and nearer. The silent ice world re-echoes with thunders; nature's giants are awakening to the battle.

Friday, 13 October 1893
Farthest North: The Norwegian Polar Expedition 1893–1896 (1897)
Fridtjof Nansen

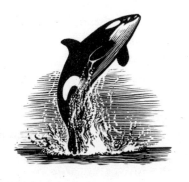

26

Summer, 1988

The first time Sean stood on Arctic ice in Greenland, sponsored by Kingsmith and with Tom Harding by his side, he wanted to shout in triumph. He was here, he had made it. There were no green-tinted icebergs or radiant pink light, as in the painting, but the cold on his face, the sunny glitter of the air, the bluest sky and the sound of excited sled dogs howling at their approach, filled him with real joy.

It didn't matter that Redmond was a tosser, that the whole thing still smacked of elitist privilege – he was here and that was all he cared about. Taking part in the Lost Explorers' Society point-to-point dog-sled race on a section of the route of the 1935 Oxford University West Greenland Expedition.

They would be in six two-man teams, with no backup save each other. They could wear modern base layers, but the aesthetic was strictly 1935, and Redmond looked forward to his photographs being displayed at the Royal Geographical Society. He enjoyed documenting Sean and Tom's fumbling attempts at harnessing their team. They could not help noticing they seemed to have been given the smallest dogs.

'It's like he wants us to die on the ice,' Sean muttered.

'Fuck him,' Tom agreed, as they were the last to set off.

Redmond was pleased to humiliate them but not quite to the point of death, so he sent a couple of teams to escort them safely to the first base camp.

Inside an alarmed perimeter fence, to protect them against bear attacks, and with the thirty-six Greenland sled dogs, they all felt quite safe. The twelve young men fed their dogs, pitched their tents, gathered to share a communal meal of rehydrated chicken curry, followed by rehydrated apple crumble with custard – then they retired to try to sleep. Each pair had a rifle, just in case.

Sean was excited beyond being able to rest, but Tom insisted they try. They lay in their glowing orange tent, talking in low voices.

'Thank you,' Tom said after so long a pause that Sean thought he was asleep.

'What for?'

'Coming with me. Partnering up on this.'

Sean lay silent for a while, absorbing this. 'This is my dream, to do this. If you hadn't asked me ...'

'You'd have found another way. You're resourceful.' Tom wriggled around in his sleeping bag so that they were facing each other. 'I really admire you, Sean. I've had everything given to me, and I know you wish you hadn't told me, but you—'

'Shh—' Sean heard a dog's short whuff outside.

'No let me say it – you've done it all yourself—'

As the dogs began baying they were both on their knees scrabbling for the rifle. Sean was out first with it, loaded and cocked, Tom right behind him – and there, two hundred feet away from their encampment, was a huge female bear with a yearling cub, coming to investigate.

'Flare!' Sean shouted, and Tom grabbed one and released it into the air. It arced towards the animals, almost invisible in the sun. All the dogs were baying now, everyone was scrambling from their tents. The female stood straight ahead, curious and unafraid. Her deep pelt was cream against the blue-hued snow but her cub was pearly fluff. As she stood up on her hind legs, she looked so human, so intrigued, that Sean would not have been surprised if she had called out to know who they were. She was the most beautiful, most thrilling creature he had ever seen.

Tom fired two more flares and at their screech, the cub ran behind its mother. That seemed to decide her, she gave them one last look and turned to leave, but Redmond was taking aim with his rifle.

'Mine!' he called out.

'Don't shoot! she's leaving!' Tom yelled, but Redmond fired. He missed and when the mother and cub began to run, he took aim again. People were shouting to release the dogs, hold the dogs, the dogs were howling and barking—

Before Redmond could fire again, Tom hurled himself at him, knocking his rifle skywards and wrestling it from him. Redmond struggled for it but Tom hurled it away into the snow, before catching a furious punch on the jaw. As Redmond landed it, Sean was on him, slugging him back then kneeling on his chest and holding him down in the snow, one arm across his throat like he'd learned as a kid, putting his face close and telling him to be calm, be calm—

Sean knew how fights went, and this one was his. No one was coming to Redmond's aid. He pressed down a little harder, and Redmond stopped struggling. Sean got off and offered his hand to help him up. Redmond spat at him, murder in his eyes.

'You fucking oik.'

'I think what Redmond is saying,' said Tom, rubbing his chin, 'is that he won't shoot the fucking bears unless he fucking needs to – is that right?'

'We could have died!' Redmond screamed at the rest of them.

'Anyone can panic,' Sean winked at him, 'don't feel bad.'

'You fucking morons! Never touch my gun again!' Everyone stared at him, even the dogs. He turned on Sean and Tom. 'You're off this expedition, do you hear!' He glared at Tom. 'You and your fucking oik servant—'

Tom grabbed him by his jacket. 'Don't talk about my friend like that.' He shoved Redmond back so hard he fell over his feet, and the others laughed.

Sean turned to the rest of them. It was a surreal sight, the bright orange tents glowing in the midnight sun, the dogs, Redmond holding his nose, the red seeping through his fingers, dripping on the snow. 'I've paid my way,' Sean said, with all the confidence he could muster. 'I've got a right to be here. Anyone who disagrees, say now.'

'I do! This is my expedition.' Redmond was staggering to his feet, still murderous. 'Shut those fucking dogs up!' He looked around for support. 'Who's with me?' No one answered.

'*Fram*,' Tom said to Sean.

'Fucking right, *Fram*,' Sean agreed.

They walked back to their tent, not daring to look at each other, half expecting to feel a blow from behind – but all they could hear was Redmond's furious hissing at the others, and the yelp of one of their dogs.

They settled their own team, they checked for bears – they caught each other's eye with a glint of triumph – but only when they were back in the orange glow of their tent, the rifle safely stowed by the flap, did they turn to each other and high five, then lie on their backs and kick their legs in the air, laughing until they cried.

They did sleep, but a couple of hours later they woke to the sound of barking again. Looking out, they were astonished to see the other five teams had packed up and were harnessing their dogs. They were being left behind. They watched in amazement as, led by Redmond's sled, their fellow explorers abandoned them, although they did leave them the tripwire fence.

'Bastards.' Tom scratched the head of Roxy, their lead dog. 'Like we care.'

'We don't need them.' Sean looked at him. 'From now on, we can do our own expeditions. I bet Kingsmith'll fund us.'

'Fine. But let's come back alive from this one first.'

They decided to make a circular route of their own, and as they sledged and switched over, and as Sean ran with the sled and leapt on, and the pure clean wind rushed over his face, and the jingle of the dogs' traces made music, he thanked Joe Kingsmith with all his heart for this chance.

And then finally we were back on our own glacier, and far below lay our own fjord and the dots that were Thule and home – the spot we had been longing for during the endless, tedious months.

We called a halt and waited for Uvdloriark to explore the crevasses between us and home, and while I sat there Knud walked over to me and gave me his hand.

'Many times during the summer,' he said, 'I didn't believe we could go on. But now that we have completed such an expedition together, we ought never to be apart again. Wherever we go in the whole world, we must always stick together.'

I have heard many speeches in my life, most of them stupid libels on friendship and loyalty at banquets or meetings, but there on the glacier Knud dared put into a simple declaration exactly what he felt. I replied in kind. It is seldom men have the courage to do what they want to do and say what they really think, especially to other men. But Knud said these things, and I never forgot those words while he lived, and I shall never forget them so long as I live.

Arctic Adventure: My Life in the Frozen North (1936)
Peter Freuchen

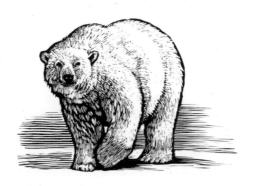

27

On Tuesday morning, like a general achieving the ridge before the opposition mustered below, Sean was the first in court. He'd slipped out of the White Bear early and walked the city walls, then gone to a chain café in the town. Its soothing weekday hustle calmed his racing mind. Tuesday, Wednesday, Thursday: Over.

He felt the brisk heavy tread on the floorboards and caught the aroma of a Cohiba Siglo VI before his lawyer was upon him, ebulliently well-rested and thumping down into his seat with a cheerful grin. Then came Mrs Osman, looking as if she might have slept in her black suit, and today allowing her two young aides to pull the document cases for her. They had the air of monks from some martial sect. She returned her counterpart's greeting pleasantly enough.

'So showy,' Sawbridge murmured after they had passed. 'But makes the family feel cared for. Done it myself.' And then he allowed Sean quiet reflection, before the ordeal to come.

Sean kept his eyes from any one face, and his testimony simple.

They were in the cave. The cave had collapsed. Tom was on one side, he was on the other. Tom tried to get back across but slipped and fell into a crevasse.

'It was completely black, except for my head torch. But I crawled to the edge, and there was nothing. My beam went about twenty feet, and I could see the sides where the ice had broken apart. It was very deep, and then my beam wouldn't reach any further. I couldn't see Tom's head torch. It was just black. I called out, I called to him. But there was nothing. I was frightened. I thought I was going to die too. But I pulled myself back and I felt my way along, trying to get up to where I thought the opening was. I was terrified I would slip into the crevasse as well. I didn't know how long the torch would last. I couldn't hear anything and I didn't know if the others had got out in time. Everything had fallen and crashed, the whole cave had collapsed, there were bars and huge chunks of ice everywhere and I had to crawl. I just kept trying to move up and find the tunnel. I can't remember clearly after that.'

Sean is on his belly, he can hardly breathe but he knows oxygen is vital so he forces himself to control his gasping. The beam of his head torch picks up a jumbled plane of surfaces, matt and shiny, white, grey, blue, transparent. His mind and body are throbbing, he can't tell if he's injured, if he's bleeding and that's the pumping feeling – but he knows he has to move or die.

He hauls himself forward on his elbows, a huge weight of ice dragging on his right leg. He hauls through and keeps going. Too much vapour – overspending – slow the breath or suffocate. Slower … can't call to Tom because no shouting, no disturbing vibration, he remembers that too – burning feeling on his face – takes his forehead off the ice, do not stop! Keep moving up, keep forcing forward – get help – buried alive if he stops, then they're both dead. In training: under an hour to survive before hypothermia or asphyxiation or both set in. The torch beam is still steady, but batteries don't last forever. Find a gap, keep moving, stay calm.

There: a black triangle in the jumbled plane of ice. He might be imagining it or there might be air movement, he closes his eyes to feel it better.

Tom.

He calls it, but in his mind not with his voice and lungs. It's death if he stays and it might be death to try, but he worms forward on his elbows into the black hole until his helmet jars and stops him, so he has to try to take it off, fumble the strap and clip – he uses his teeth to pull off his glove – and push the helmet aside. It drags hard and painful on his ear and scalp, but he pushes on, feeling it scrape deep into his back as he forces forward into that hole where there is different air—

—like an animal, he can taste it, taste air, because his rational brain has gone. In his panic, he forgot his torch was on his helmet and now there is only dark and cold and the pressure of the ice around him, death touching him on all sides, but like a blind worm he does not stop, he uses his bare head as a ram when he has to because pain is a sharp tool and even a parasite has the will to live and this is what he now is, some ancient ice parasite working its way through the ice-giant's gut—

That thought fires him with rage and powers his boots against the great bastard's intestinal wall; he will get himself out through the mouth or the eye or the arse or the skin – he makes himself a great pulsing worm for the rhythm to keep moving, writhing, the friction melting just enough space to give him passage—

Sean's will powers him on, hauling and forcing this length of meat and bone and cartilage through the tight hard spaces, even though the ungainly weight is too much and he only wants to rest – but thought of failure whips him on and gets that sack of meat thrashing its legs and almost vomiting with the effort—

He shoots forward into black air – and a wall of ice slams him from underneath.

TOM – the name does not stir his lungs or tongue but drops down instead into a hole in his mind and vanishes.

In the blackness, Sean's mind moves, then his body. He is not dead. He feels space around him. He fell.

'Tom!' This time the sound comes out. He hears the acoustic bounce. He calls again in different directions. In the blackness, one side is solid, but the sound quality changes to the other. He crawls forward, blind but sensitised—

Tom, Tom, Tom—

In the blackness like a drum beat, reaching forward using Tom's name for echo-location, he feels a drift of air ahead. The ice beneath is starting to dip down. He slips and grabs but there's nothing to hang on to, steeper and faster – then a gasp as something blocks his hurtling force. Impact but not pain. His mouth full of soft snow. He struggles out into a howling black snowstorm.

Sean turned to the coroner.

'I was so lucky. Somehow I got into another part of the cave system and was able to get out. The rest of it is all in the *Sunday Times* interview I did afterwards, that Mr Sawbridge submitted.'

'I know, Mr Cawson, and thank you. But as I am not a *Sunday Times* reader, I missed it three years ago, so what you say is fresh to me. I did see you had included it, but I chose to wait to hear your own account live, rather than an edited version. Though of course we all edit our memories, it is unavoidable.'

Sawbridge did his push-up move on the chair in front. 'Your Honour, it sounds as if you're suggesting—'

'That memories are subjective; indeed I am, Mr Sawbridge. Mr Cawson, can you continue?'

Sean nodded. To his surprise, he saw Martine's face, a pale beacon in the spot beside Sawbridge. He had not registered her arrival.

'I knew we'd gone in at midday, an hour after the eclipse. At that time of year, the light's almost gone by about three, and when I – when I came out into the drift, it was dark. So it could have been three, or ten – I had no idea. I couldn't see any lights, I couldn't hear anything over the wind. The weather had totally changed. All I could think was that I couldn't be on the ice cap because I'd fallen, but I couldn't see the mountains. I didn't know what to do except get back into the tunnel, because at least that would provide shelter, but I couldn't find it.'

The wind is a devil screaming in his ears, trying to kill him with the sound. With numb hands, Sean struggles to tighten all his toggles: jacket hem, sleeves, hood, trousers. No Tom. No skidoo, no survival suit. He is going to freeze to death on the Midgard glacier, or a bear will get him – that thought sparks his vision fractionally keener, searching for a different movement in the snow. The pumping fist of muscle in his chest goads him on. Shelter or death.

A wind of a thousand fists screams him off his feet and he's face down again, pummelled and kicked every time he tries to stand. A tiny part of his brain understands he's facing down the slope – the blows spin him but most seem to come from behind – it's coming down the mountain. His brain clings to that information, it's important – yes! Because katabatic wind comes off the land towards the sea. The wind will drive him down to the fjord, to take his chances with the bears.

The wind has another idea. It lifts him up and hurls him about like a ragdoll thrown in a tantrum. Sean stumbles and falls until he can't get up any more. The wind shrieks in triumph and he knows exactly what is happening, but it's really not so bad at all. Because he's stopped struggling, his mind unclenches and he lets it wander. He feels as safe and comfortable as if he were in an igloo, like the Inuit made so cleverly.

Knud Rasmussen and Peter Freuchen learned the skill. The best of friends, like him and Tom. Rasmussen and Freuchen, Cawson and Harding, the four of them in sealskin anoraqs, they would build one in no time.

We don't need to make it big, not everything has to be big to be good, Sean, we'll just do what we can – get up, you lazy bugger.

Sean turns his face to Tom's voice, the effort coming from a thousand miles away. Tom is right there beside him in the snow, showing off how he can dig with his bare hands. He grins as Sean copies him, but much, much slower. They keep going, they're getting there, they've made a hole in the snow – or rather uncovered one, and Sean gets into its smooth curved sides and curls into the foetal position, out of the howling wind and punching fists. And somewhere on the slopes of Midgardbreen, beneath the ice cap of Midgardfonna in the archipelago of Svalbard, two men lie lost beneath the ice, one deep, one shallow.

'It was a miracle I survived. I don't remember being found, just waking in the Sickehaus the next day. I only know I gave statements because I was told. But I don't remember.' Sean clamped his right hand under his armpit and felt it moisten. He became aware of his shirt sticking to his back, and the adrenal sweat smell that rose from him.

'All I know is that cave fell in on us and Tom slipped down. Somehow I got out. Inspector Brovang found me.'

'Thank you, Mr Cawson.' Mrs Osman adjusted her ill-fitting jacket. 'Thank you for revisiting that ... ordeal ... for us. My questions are less to do with the fact of your survival, and more to do with how Tom was not so ... lucky.'

Sean nodded respectfully. Here it came.

'We will later be hearing from an expert witness ... a glaciologist ... that the structures of ice-caves, wherever they are found, can never be relied upon for stability. But that you had every reason to think that this one ... on Midgardbreen ... was safe enough to venture with your partners.'

'I did. Yes. And so did Danny Long and Terry Bjornsen, both of whom have masses of polar experience and live there year-round.'

'Yes. I did note that. So a gap opened up in the ... floor? Of the cave known as the Great Hall. Is that correct? How wide was it? Could you describe it? I am trying to get a sense of the danger.'

Sean stared at her a moment.

'It was very hard to see. Everything under our feet had shifted. There was water, it made everything slippery, or Tom could have jumped it.'

'It sounds very frightening.' Mrs Osman frowned down at her open file. She shook her head and used both hands to lift the mass of papers, bristling with Post-it notes. 'I'm sorry, a moment ...'

Sawbridge's deep audible sigh signalled his opinion of her competence. The coroner tapped his pencil.

'Yes. I'm sorry, here we are ...' Mrs Osman looked up again. 'How would you characterise your relationship with Mr Harding?'

'We were friends from college. From 1988 to Tom's death. Three decades.'

Mrs Osman inclined her head encouragingly.

'Would you say it was a stable and constant friendship?'

'Very much so.' Sean felt a tremor as he said it.

'Though it was not without its ... gaps. Was it?' She looked down and turned a page. 'Because when I looked at your written statement delivered to my chambers, and also to the coroner ... apart from finding it very helpful – for which I thank you and Mr Sawbridge for the foresight – I did wonder ... If there was a time when you might not have been ... so close. A gap of maybe seven or eight years, during which time you had no contact with Mr Harding.' She studied her file again. 'Until you resumed contact, and shortly afterwards, Mr Harding came on board with your consortium, the – Fairlight Group. That you used to make your purchase bid, for Midgard Lodge. Registered in Jersey.'

'Might I ask my learned colleague where exactly she's going with this?' Sawbridge tipped his head to the side and smiled. Mrs Osman ignored him.

'I ask because it looked to me as if a ... gap ... might indeed have opened up between you. And I wondered why.'

Sean interlaced his fingers and took a deep breath, the way he had read could work as a stress management technique. He wanted to yell at Osman to say what she wanted, not lay traps – but that would alienate the room.

'You're right,' he said. 'We didn't exactly fall out, but there was a serious difference of opinion. Political not personal, but there was fallout.'

It was a Sunday in February. Tom had come for lunch and to discuss his latest breakup with Ruth Mott. Sean was of the opinion he was better off without her, but Gail thought he should propose and be done with it, then they would both know where they stood, and commitment could carry them through the difficult bits.

Somehow the conversation had strayed into the minefield of what shape that could take, between a man and a woman, and having recently strenuously denied his latest philandering, Sean felt increasingly under attack. Thinking to save him, and simultaneously drawing a picture with Rosie, Tom had changed the subject to next Saturday's march in London, to protest the imminent invasion of Iraq.

'I can't,' was Sean's immediate reaction. 'I've got a meeting.'

'On a Saturday?'

'Sean's a workaholic now.'

Sean heard the sadness in his wife's voice, and the guilt made him angry.

'Yes, on a Saturday. It's the only day everyone can do it.'

Tom added a shark to Rosie's picture, and she nodded seriously, approving it.

'Sean, you've got a profile. People would take notice if you joined in. There is absolutely no evidence of weapons of mass destruction, this will be an illegal invasion.'

'But if there are—'

'IF! But so far, there aren't! Tell me one good reason we should go ahead.'

'I'll tell you a reason it *will* happen,' Sean said. 'I'm not saying it's a good one, but it's the truth. This invasion is going to happen whether you march or not, because it is in the interest of the global economy to end the uncertainty.'

Tom and Gail stared at him. Then Tom laughed. 'I'm sorry; for a moment there I thought you said—'

'Yeah I did.' Sean felt suddenly quite drunk. 'It's very simple. The banks want war. So that's what's going to happen.' He looked at Rosie's picture. 'That's brilliant.'

'It's completely immoral!' Gail cried.

'It's a *shark*.' Rosie was upset by the atmosphere.

'I didn't say it was *right*, I said it was what was going to happen.' Sean felt the cat rubbing his ankle, as it did when it detected stress in the family. He took the picture from Rosie. 'A very scary shark! But listen to me, marching will not make a blind bit of difference. The money's decided. That's how it goes.' He gave the picture back to Rosie, hating how Tom was looking at him.

'I cannot believe I'm hearing you talk like this.'

'It's economic realpolitik.'

'Sean it's disgusting, it can't be true—' Gail looked like she was going to cry, and Rosie actually started.

'For god's sake I'm not saying *I* want war' – Sean took a huge slug of wine to control his own anxiety – 'but the banks hate uncertainty, everything is on slow, people's livelihoods are going to suffer it if goes on much longer.'

'More people are going to die very soon if it doesn't! You're going to sit back and do nothing?' Tom covered his glass against a refill, and Sean thumped the bottle down.

'Tom, don't talk to me like I'm responsible for all this and you're trying to save everyone – you know you've been a bit too sanctimonious for a bit too long.'

Tom got up. He folded his napkin, kissed Gail, and turned to Sean.

'Thank you for your hospitality.' He bent down and kissed Rosie. 'Oh please don't tear it up, it's such a good drawing.'

'You see how you've upset everyone?' Sean stood up. 'You can't go, you can't bloody well drive! I'm just telling it like it is!'

'Mr Coroner!' Sawbridge did his half push-up on the seat in front. 'Long friendship has its ups and downs, and I believe Mrs Osman is diverting our attention away from our common interest.'

'Agreed, Mr Sawbridge. Mrs Osman, in view of the limited time and availability of all parties, please confine your questions to our remit: how and in what manner, did Tom Harding meet his death. We do not seek existential causes that may extend back several years to wars illegal or otherwise, nor to plumb the psyches of our witnesses.'

'Hear hear!' called Sawbridge, and clapped his hands slowly.

'Your Honour, with respect.' Mrs Osman turned to him. 'Is it not also the function of any inquest to fearlessly investigate all causes and seek out and record as many of those facts concerning the death as the public interest requires—'

'Yes, thank you, Mrs Osman. I am quite up to date with Lord Lane's pronouncements, and the requirements of my own office.' Mr Thornton laced his fingers and bumped his hands down on the table with each word. 'Can we go on?'

'Certainly. No further questions, thank you, Mr Cawson.' Mrs Osman sat.

Sean had sweated throughout his testimony and wanted a shower at the White Bear, but there was no time. Concerned for him, Martine had come down earlier than he expected, and had researched a small bistro a short walk from the court. They repaired with Sawbridge, who primed her for her own testimony.

'Smile, but not too much. I say that because if beautiful women don't smile, they're perceived as aloof and threatening. But if they smile too much—'

'Everyone gets the wrong idea,' Martine finished. 'Believe me, I know.'

'Try not to finish anyone's sentence either.' Sawbridge tucked into his veal. 'So clever of you to find this place.'

'Maybe you should give me some performance notes.'

'I hoped I might.' Sawbridge grinned, refusing to take offence. '*You* are the brilliant, soignée, femme-fatale who is responsible for the breakup of this poor chap's marriage – best you get over it now, because that's what they'll say about you.'

'It could be worse.'

'Ha. It might well be. But regardless, you did everything you could to save Tom, and Sean here has been distraught ever since.'

'I have.' Sean had barely spoken since they got there. He felt hyper-sensitised – he saw a trace of makeup on Martine's face, and then he saw it everywhere. All over her skin, on her eyelashes – even some clever paint that gave her hand a pale shimmer. He took her hand and looked at it. Tiny little flecks of mica, suspended in lotion. Misinterpreting the gesture, she smiled and squeezed his.

'Darling. It'll be OK.'

'Of course it will,' said Sawbridge. 'Tell him to eat or he'll keel over.'

'He can't, when he's agitated. I'm the same.' Martine took a mouthful of food. 'Tonight he'll be hungry.'

'I do hope so. He needs his strength.' Sawbridge winked at him. 'Join in whenever you feel like it, or not. Anyway, this afternoon should be OK. We've got a video postcard, I believe they call them, from Miss Radiance Young. Then it's Martine. And the glaciologist, Professor Roger Kelly. Ocean Physics at Cambridge. Controversial with the oil lot, adored by the green lot, so we'll have to watch out for him.'

Martine leaned forward, her hand on Sean's thigh.

'You're the hero of this story, don't you worry.'

Sawbridge grimaced.

'What?' she asked.

'The survivor is rarely the hero,' Sawbridge said. 'We must go carefully.'

Gangrene, as it develops in a frozen limb, is not so painful as it is odorous. It stinks fearfully and one cannot get away from it. The nurse had a special cure. She captured small lemmings – the Arctic mice that multiply faster than guinea-pigs – killed them beside me and laid the warm skins on the open wounds, bloody side down. After some hours, during which she caught more, she peeled off the skins, the decayed flesh adhering to them, and replaced them with new ones. She also muttered magic formulas over the foot and sang pain-killing songs.

Nevertheless, the flesh fell away until the bones protruded. I could endure no blankets touching them, and the sight of them sent my nerves jangling. If the room was warm the stench was unendurable; if it was cold, I froze. I went through a living hell, and each night felt that the old man with the scythe was close after me.

When a man is sick and cold and lonely he gets strange ideas, and one day I told the nurse that I wanted to have those toes off. She thought that might be the best thing to do, and she knew just how to do it – bite them off at the joints and prevent the ghosts from occupying my body – her mouth would close the wounds immediately. I thanked her very much, but took no stock in her method; instead, I fitted a nail puller over each toe and banged it off with a hammer.

I cannot attempt to describe the physical pain – but there was a spiritual pain, too – in discarding a portion of my own body, even a part that would never be of any use to me again.

Arctic Adventure: My Life in the Frozen North (1936)
Peter Freuchen

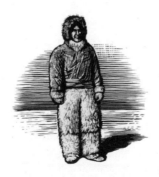

28

The courtroom absorbed Martine's business glamour as she took the oath in her unlocatable accent of cosmopolitan privilege. The coroner's clerk stared at her slightly too long. Mr Thornton, unsmitten, asked for her account of the events at the ice-cave.

Martine channelled demure respect. She told Mr Thornton how thrilled she had been to work on such an important venture. How delighted to bring such exciting value to her green-minded investors, all hungry for rare ethical vehicles such as Midgard Lodge. She was excited herself to go to Svalbard for the first time and believed in the power of spending real time with one's partners, as people, not just financial co-investors. She expressed her deepest condolences to Tom's family, and told them how Tom believed Midgard Lodge would be a place where great things might be accomplished, to the benefit of the whole world.

'Confine yourself to the facts and avoid speculation, Miss Delaroche.'

'Yes, sir.'

Sean knew Mr Thornton's neutrality would have offended Martine on other occasions, but she understood her role. He had seen her protean ability before, matching herself to the taste of the dominant force, before gradually moulding it to her agenda.

She described how they prepared with every precaution to go to the cave, how Sean could not have done more for their safety. Everyone travelled at their own risk, she was herself intrepid when it came to skiing and diving and driving – she'd been allowed to drive her father's collection of sports cars from a young age – so it was a great surprise to her when she did not like the cave experience. When Joe and Radiance decided to go back, she did too. Only when all three were in the last part of the tunnel with the ladder in sight did they hear the sound of the collapse behind.

When they got out, Mr Long and Mr Bjornsen – Danny and Terry – were already on their way down because they'd seen the sudden change in the weather. As soon as they realised they couldn't break through what had fallen, they hurried back to the Lodge to raise the alarm. Despite insisting that she must stay to try to save Sean and Tom, she'd had to submit to being taken back to the Lodge.

And then the most terrible sleepless night of the storm, not knowing if they were alive or dead but fearing the worst, and in the morning came the Sysselmann's team and then thank god – and here Martine shamelessly crossed herself like the good Catholic she was not – they found Sean, out in the snow. Miraculously alive. Martine looked out at Sean, tears in her eyes. Then to the coroner, lest he miss the full benefit of her emotion. That was all she had to say.

'Not quite all, Miss Delaroche, I believe both counsel have questions. Mr Sawbridge, please go first this time.'

Sawbridge would rather have mopped up any damage Mrs Osman might have tried to inflict, but could only agree. He spoke gently, to signal Martine's fragility.

'Miss Delaroche, what do you think this project represented to Mr Harding?'

'The chance to influence the environmental conscience of the business community, from a position of soft power.'

'Soft power?'

She allowed herself a small smile.

'When people are sharing important experiences, when the stress of the deal is put to one side and they are enjoying themselves, it is so much easier to come to agreement. That is one of the most important things about the Lodge; how the environment itself speaks every language. The spiritual quality is stronger there, it touches people inside. It's truly humbling.'

'Quite.' Sawbridge looked genuinely impressed. 'How would you characterise the mood of the participants on this expedition, to see the eclipse at Midgard Lodge? We have heard about the unavoidable delay, and you were all very busy people. What was the mood like, on the day of travel?'

'Very upbeat. Like an amusing, wonderful, school trip.' Her smile faded. 'But with a tragic outcome. At least we have resolution now.'

No, don't say that, shouted Sean in his head. Resolution of what? Osman will go there – you were doing so well. Come on, Nicholas, bring it back.

'I understand.' Sawbridge was aware of the danger. 'The pain of not knowing where Tom was lost.'

'That's right.' Martine wiped her eyes again. Sawbridge held a look of deep compassion for several seconds. 'No more questions. Many thanks, Miss Delaroche.'

'May I?' Osman was up before Sawbridge was back beside Sean. 'Miss Delaroche, you work in a so-called "clean-tech" equity firm, is that correct? Raising capital for environmentally friendly businesses?'

'I'm very proud of that,' Martine was considerably less charming to women than men. 'It's something I strongly believe in.'

'I notice your company stresses its business ethics, and the ethics of all its partners, of which you are one. Is that also correct?'

'Why would anyone trust us otherwise?'

Mrs Osman considered this.

'Do you think personal ethics have anything to do with business? Or, to put it another way, do you think a moral code is important?'

'Of course.' Her eyes went to Sean for the briefest moment. Mrs Osman turned to follow Martine's look. Other heads did the same.

'Yes. I would have thought it was,' Osman went on smoothly. 'So, for instance, someone with a ... flexible attitude ... to morality in their personal life, might also carry that over ... into business dealings.'

'Are you accusing me of something?' Martine became poised and still.

'Is it not a fact,' pursued Mrs Osman, 'that you were accused of stealing jewellery – a necklace, I think? – from the wife of a man with whom you were having an affair? While you were living in Geneva? I do have the dates, somewhere.'

'That was a vile accusation, and withdrawn!' Martine flushed, the first time Sean had ever seen her do it. 'It was a gift, I had no idea it belonged to her. I returned it.'

'But only after being threatened with court proceedings.'

Martine made a sound of contempt and exasperation. 'She was old and jealous and she wanted revenge.'

'Not very sisterly of you, Mrs Osman,' called out Sawbridge. 'Aren't you supposed to be a feminist?'

'Justice is my interest,' Mrs Osman continued in the same calm tone. 'And my professional experience shows that people in the habit of having affairs, are also in the habit of frequent ... economies ... with the truth. And because, Miss Delaroche, I have reason to doubt the trip to Svalbard was as harmonious as you present it. I believe that, despite your shared endeavour, there was no love lost between yourself and Tom Harding, because he was a friend of Mr Cawson's ex-wife and, rightly or wrongly, held you responsible for their divorce. I believe you disliked Mr Harding, Miss Delaroche.'

'I'm still sorry about the accident! And you blame the woman because the man falls in love with her?' Martine dropped her eyes. 'Sean pursued me and I couldn't resist. I didn't know he was married at first. I'm not proud of that.'

Sean sat forward in shock. Martine in the sauna of the Kempinski hotel in Berlin, asking him if he liked her tan lines. He was trying to keep his word to Gail, no more dalliances. Martine naked, tanned dark and pale, telling him she knew he was married, it suited her better. Getting up to stand above him, his weakness plain to see.

'I wanted Tom to like me,' she told Osman. 'I knew how much his friendship meant to the man I love. And yes, I wanted him to respect what I had brought to the deal, not to behave as if he was the single thing that made it happen, and I was just one more corrupt piece of the business.'

Mrs Osman spun the silence before she spoke, very quietly. 'There was corruption?'

'I didn't say that! I meant his attitude was that we were all corrupt capitalists and he was the holy one coming in to set us all straight. So no, I didn't like his attitude. And no, he didn't like me. But that had nothing to do with the accident or how hard we tried to find them both, or how sorry I am that he died! I don't know what you're trying to say to me, or make of me, or why you're questioning my integrity. It's insulting!'

Sean removed his hand from his mouth. Unmasked by Osman, Martine could not have projected a worse image. Sophisticated, defiant, aloof. He heard Sawbridge's low intake of breath beside him and knew he felt the same. Mrs Osman nodded gently.

'I'm simply searching for the truth about—'

'I'll *tell* you the truth,' Martine broke in. 'The ice-cave collapsed, Tom fell and died. It was a terrible accident and I had *nothing* to do with it. I would never have come here if I'd known it was going to be so' – she looked directly at Osman – '*ugly*.'

'As the truth so often is. Thank you, Miss Delaroche.' Mrs Osman sat down. Sean looked at his hands as Martine stalked back to them, furious. A PR disaster. How on earth could Osman possibly have known about Tom blaming Martine? Then he understood. From that reliable troublemaker, Ruth Mott.

Stunned by Martine's misrepresentation of the start of their affair, Sean did not trust himself to speak to her until they were in private. She had twisted it completely. When the break was called, he made an excuse and went to the lavatory, leaving Sawbridge to cajole her out onto the fire escape to keep him company while he had a quick puff – and, Sean knew, deliver a cautionary briefing. He returned to his seat and busied himself with his email until they came back. Without a word, she knew he was angry, and he knew she did not care.

The next testimony was 'a video postcard', the coroner announced, from Miss Radiance Young, a partner in Midgard Lodge. He had requested a testimony by Skype if she could not attend in person, but believed she was literally in space as they spoke. She had however, sent the answers to his questions.

The screen behind him brightened and Radiance's face smiled out at them. She was wearing a white zip-up sports top with stripes down the arms, and sat against a blue tessellated background with a Cyrillic logo. Her hair was pulled back in a ponytail revealing small but sparkly diamond earrings.

'Hi, Sean,' she said to the camera. 'Hi, all court officials. Hi, Joe, you naughty man, if you're there too. Hi, Ruth Mott – Bear Lady.' She dropped the smile. 'Hi, Martin.' Then she leaned forward.

'First I want to say please tell Tom's family sorry we couldn't find him. Very sorry. Thank you for passing on this message.' She looked down at something in her lap. 'I'm going to answer all the questions one time, right? OK. We all had a good time together, no argy-bargy except stressy Bear Lady and Joe at the restaurant. But everyone loved Tom, no arguments, everything was great! Joe's plane was very nice, Midgard Lodge is very beautiful, so well done Martin for that. Good taste bad person – no joke!'

The coroner paused it. 'When Ms Young says "Martin", I take it she refers to Miss Delaroche – is that correct, Mr Cawson?'

'I believe so,' said Sean. He felt Martine tense beside him. Sawbridge had clearly failed to pour oil on troubled water.

'Joe rode with me to the cave,' Radiance said from the back wall. 'Very strong man but an old man too, right? No good in tight spot, I said to him, when we got out. Breathing like this' – Radiance closed her eyes in a grimace and demonstrated rapid, panicky breathing. 'I thought he was dying of heart attack. But it got worse! The bad sound inside – then Martin starts shouting all weak and screamy, and the bad weather comes from nowhere. Nowhere, like it happens there.' Radiance shook her head sagely.

'We got back to the first place under the ladder, but you can feel the shaking in the walls – like this' – Radiance shuddered her whole face and body, raising a few titters. Granny Ruby looked around indignantly. On the film, Radiance seemed to remember the camera.

'Storm cut out phones, right? Solar blasts. So interesting but bad news here. Long and Bjornsen treat us like kids, made us go back to the Lodge to call for help. Martin useless, Joe no good. Even me. We thought: Sean dead, Tom dead. For sure.' She shook her head. 'So sorry, to Tom's family. Very beautiful man. I liked him a lot.' She looked down, then back up with a big smile. 'OK – and by the way, Martin, if you're there: "I must tell you friendly in your ear, sell when you can, you are not for all markets."' She blinked innocently. '*As You Like It*. Just popped into my mind when I thought of you.'

The screen went black, and the clerks opened the blinds. People whispered, and Sean could hear a few muffled laughs, then the room quieted for the coroner.

'Perhaps some of you are familiar with the physics of glaciers, with their caves and calvings. I'm not, so I'm pleased to have the benefit of an expert witness in Professor Roger Kelly, chair of Ocean Physics at the University of Cambridge, who has kindly made time for us.'

Sean watched him take the stand, and the secular oath. He was a kindly-looking donnish type who gave the impression he'd be more at home in a country pub than roaming the oceans of the world, as was his preferred habit when not teaching. Professor Kelly looked out.

'Go ahead,' he said. 'I know the Midgardbreen glacier, I've been in that cave system. What can I tell you?'

'How it might have collapsed,' said the coroner. 'How Mr Harding's body might have emerged. And how, out of interest, Mr Cawson managed to get out.'

'Isn't that last part interesting?' said Professor Kelly. 'Suggests a hidden structure of tunnels, made accessible by the shifting of the glacier. That's probably what caused the collapse of the caves. They've been on record since the end of the nineteenth century, then the Oxford Air Arctic Expedition mentioned them in 1929. At least, the Great Hall was mentioned, named after college hall, I believe. Sounds to me like that chamber collapsed unevenly, part of it dropping into a chasm and part of its structure falling to block that drop.

'Looking at the footage, I think it's possible that after the initial collapse the whole inner structure of the chamber called the Great Hall slipped down a very long way within the interior of the glacier – and was eventually forced out as an underwater shooter during that calving event witnessed by the cruise ship. Fascinating, but diabolic in meaning.'

He looked over at the press bench.

'The most likely cause of this cave collapsing is climate change. We know for a fact that the warming seas are increasing rain over the Arctic, creating lakes of meltwater all over the ice caps. They look very beautiful as you fly over, but it's one of the worst sights in the world, because now it's not snow collecting and compressing any more, it's just water. So it seeps through into the glacier, weakening its structure. Caves collapse. Calvings increase in magnitude and frequency. The summer sea ice has gone twenty years ahead of predictions. People who want to get at the minerals unlocked by the thaw, or to exploit new sea routes, want us to believe this is a good thing. Accelerated warming, rising sea levels, increased disruptions of global weather patterns – how is this a good thing?'

'Professor Kelly, if you could confine yourself to the singular matter of this particular cave system.'

'Sorry, but I absolutely cannot, any more than we would sit here feeling safe if there was a fire raging in the next room. I have shifted everything to be here this afternoon – and the press bench need to report my testimony, not least so that Mr Harding's very valuable life's work might also be supported by his death.'

'Professor Kelly, this is not a political forum—'

'I'm sorry, Your Honour, but we're in a burning building together! Tom Harding died in a caving accident, which can itself be attributed, I believe, to the reckless endangering of our planet by every industry that ignores the environmental recommendations for how to operate, and to every government that fails to abide by the Paris Agreement and reduce the emissions of greenhouse gases to 1.5 degrees – 2 degrees is not enough! The world is going crazy, the president of the United States calls climate change a hoax invented by the Chinese – the world is governed by lunatics and we just sit quiet?'

'Professor Kelly, you will please vacate the stand—'

'I will. But only when I have told you it is my expert and considered opinion that the destabilisation of the ice-caves was a direct consequence of climate change.' He looked to the press bench: 'Those exact words please – and if you have space, also that the seeping of the meltwater down from the Midgard ice cap probably fatally compromised the structural integrity of the caves. I believe this is why they collapsed, and also that Mr Cawson escaped with his life because in the collapse a hitherto unknown section of these same caves was opened up, with a shallower lateral exit. Tom Harding's body probably emerged through that same action, the water taking him out into the fjord. We're seeing this in Greenland at an unprecedented rate and at glaciers all over the polar ice cap.'

Professor Kelly noticed the stewards at the doors and came off the platform before he could be ejected. 'Wake up!' he called out. '*Wake – up!*'

They broke for the day, Professor Kelly at the centre of Tom's family group, Ruth Mott part of it. The journalists vanished. Sensitive to their tension, Sawbridge left Sean and Martine to walk back together.

The late afternoon was balmy for October, the cathedral bells were ringing. Martine had lied in court, and Sean did not know what to say to her. She talked brightly about the benefit – and again he had to force himself to acknowledge that it was still going ahead, and he was an integral part. A grand black-tie dinner, in forty-eight hours' time, at the Carrington. He had to make a speech; Martine assumed he had it all ready and it was easier to lie. The main thing was to get through the inquest.

The restaurant was full when they arrived and she was pleased at her acumen in finding out about it and booking it, despite how busy she was. Sean listened to her talking about stress, and agreed with her advice of what to order, and what wine. He listened until the wine made the lights seem softer and beautiful Martine sat there with him, her skin gleaming gold over her bones. It was relaxing just to listen, after the intensity of the courtroom. He didn't argue when she told him he was exhausted, and they should both go away after this was over, maybe on Kingsmith's yacht, as he had suggested.

Brisingamen, the nearest thing Kingsmith had to home, was an exquisitely converted Canadian frigate whose muscular capacities lay hidden beneath the best taste in ocean-going luxury. Sean had been on her a long time ago during his stint as Kingsmith's assistant – but things were different now. There would be no admin to keep at the forefront of his mind, Kingsmith liable to ask him about anything at any time. With Midgard under his belt and Martine in a bikini, he would feel distinctly equal to his mentor. Life was going to improve, unlike the steak, which was overdone – he'd ordered rare. He raised his hand for the waiter, who turned from a nearby table and came over.

'How can I help you?' Tom asked through his crushed and purpled face.

Sean leapt up, overturning his chair and wineglass. He looked at Tom in horror.

'Sean!' Martine scanned around. 'What is it?'

'I know.' Tom winked gruesomely at him. 'I look all washed out.' He offered the menu.

'Get away from me.' Sean backed into another table.

'Sean!' Martine grabbed him. 'Look at me.'

He saw her. Then he saw the waiter standing there in confusion, a young man in a black apron, a frightened stranger. Sean looked around the restaurant. Diners stared in astonishment. He bent to pick up the bottle of wine that had spilled all over the pale boards and took a napkin to blot it with. He enjoyed how the red soaked into the white. In the distance he could hear Martine's voice, paying, apologising, lying.

They walked back, her arm through his like a mother shepherding a child after a tantrum. He was not at all OK, she told him, he needed a break, the coroner must adjourn, Sawbridge would want that too – and he must share with her what just happened in there and not treat her like a stranger.

They reached the White Bear. Martine's voice was percussion against his head. Sean still could not speak and to stop her talking he turned her to him and kissed her. He needed air, he would be up soon. When she left him, he sat on the flint wall in great relief. For the first time since morning, he was alone. He stared into the darkness. He had seen Tom and although the sight was shocking, there had also been something perversely cheering about the encounter. Sean remembered the feeling of true friendship, a feeling he had missed for so long.

In Svalbard, in Midgard Lodge where the October wind slammed and screamed at the windows, Danny Long sipped his coffee and checked his screens. He went wide, checking on the number of vessels in line, slowly making their way over the North Pole. He clicked on them for their vital statistics, port of origin, flag of registration – and found the one he was looking for. The *Zheng He*, coming from Dalian. Making steady progress, in very sporty conditions. He wondered what sort of bonus the captain would be getting when he exchanged cargoes in West Africa. Then he put it from his mind, and rang down to Anna Bjornsen to see what she was cooking.

The Great Bear

A woman whose child had died left her home and walked away. Then she came to an igloo and went inside. She found the skins of bears, left like coats. The people who lived there were bears in human form, and she stayed with them.

The big bear would put on its skin and go out to hunt. It might stay away a long time but it always came back with food.

The woman had stayed away from her people a long time and felt homesick. She wanted to see them again. So the bear spoke to her:

'Do not speak of us when you return to men,' it said. It was afraid lest its two cubs should be killed by the men.

The woman returned to visit her people, and the need to tell burst inside her. One day she said to her husband,

'I have seen bears.'

And now many sledges drove out, and when the bear saw them coming towards its house, it felt so sorry for its cubs that it bit them to death, to spare them falling into the hands of men.

Then the bear hunted down the woman who had betrayed it, and broke into her house and killed her. But when it tried to return home the dogs closed round it and fell upon it. The bear struck out at them then all at once they rose up in brightness to the sky, and became the stars called Qilugtussat, which look like a bear beset by dogs.

Since then, men speak carefully of bears, for bears hear what men say.

Inuit legend, as told to Knud Rasmussen, 1921
Across Arctic America: Narrative of the Fifth Thule Expedition (1927)
Knud Rasmussen

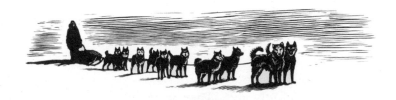

29

Dr Ruth Frances Mott took the secular oath, the picture of academic respectability in her black linen suit and white blouse, her thick hair neat in a ponytail. Sean reflexively studied her the way he did all women, for sex appeal. Still those bright eyes and air of focus he'd found so alarming when they were all young, still that don't-care style, a provocation to this day. That beautiful girl in the pub with Tom had the same quality, but at a lower strength.

Martine glanced at him, then back at Ruth Mott, now answering the coroner's questions.

'I am a marine biologist specialising in ice-obligate mammals of the Arctic. Over twenty-five years I've gone from being a generalist on different species of whales, to studying the walrus, the population dynamics of different seals – bladdernose, ringed, harp – then specifically, the polar bear, focused on the reproductive cycle of the female. My most recent peer-reviewed work is on the denning behaviour of the East Greenland population, the least studied of the twenty-two known population groups.' She looked out at the court. 'At least, that's what I was doing until the area I was studying was destroyed by mining activity.' She cleared her throat. 'Now I work in the tourist sector, in my capacity as a biologist. Lecturing. That was the reason I was in Svalbard for the weekend of the eclipse, and met Tom again.'

'Thank you, Dr Mott.' The coroner made a note. 'Would you please describe your relationship with Mr Harding?'

'We were mates.'

'As in, friends?'

'As in, the primal bond.'

Mr Thornton paused.

'I'm not sure I know what that is. Would you give me a context in time?'

When Ruth smiled, Sean saw that, unconsciously, people mirrored it. Except Sawbridge, still and watchful.

'First at college,' Ruth said. 'Then we lived together in London, before our careers started pushing us apart. Tom finished law school and went straight into activism and journalism, so he was off the whole time. I was getting positions on different field studies in the Arctic, but we'd find different places to meet. We were together in Alaska when the Parrish oil pipeline failed, which was when he joined Greenpeace full-time. I was taking part in a field study in Nunavut for the season.'

She paused. 'That was the beginning of our end. It was too painful to go on trying. We kept hurting each other. So we let it go.'

Sean counted the brass studs on the chair-back in front of him. He could smell the mints someone was eating, and the tired air in the room. He wanted to be outside.

'Except,' he heard the coroner say, 'when you met in Svalbard, the day before the eclipse. But that was not planned.'

'Not unless that bear planned it.' Ruth Mott's smile faded. 'I followed up on the autopsy results, and it came from East Greenland, from the very population I'd been studying when my project was cancelled.' She looked out across the court. 'Is Joe Kingsmith here?'

'He's coming later, Dr Mott. Please confine yourself to answering my questions, not asking them.' The coroner held her eyes. 'But why do you ask?'

'I think Tom found something out he didn't like. I think something happened at Midgard that led to his death. I don't think it was an accident.'

It was not her words so much as the complete silence that followed them.

'You know, Dr Mott, that there is no doubt the ice-cave on Midgardbreen collapsed, trapping Mr Cawson and Mr Harding.' The coroner leaned forward and spoke clearly. 'You are making a serious allegation, so please explain it.'

She nodded. 'You know how we met at the airport because I was performing the autopsy on the bear that was shot in the tourist incident. Tom invited me to join them for dinner at Amaruq, and I did. They all invited me, or I wouldn't have gone. I should say that Sean and I had sort of fallen out sometime before, so I was pleased he did that.' She looked at him. 'I really was.'

Everyone in the courtroom turned to look at Sean.

'Is that falling out with Mr Cawson significant, Dr Mott?'

'I interfered in a marriage. I was wrong. I'm sorry, Sean.'

He shook his head – it no longer mattered.

Sawbridge leaned closer to Sean.

'No more of that please.'

The coroner observed the silent exchange with a raised eyebrow.

'Dr Mott. Regarding your opinion that Mr Harding's death was not an accident: I would like to know more about that.'

'I was really shocked Tom was involved in Midgard Lodge. Like a lot of people, all I knew was that some British group had bought the property and developed it, and it was all top secret. The rumour was that it had nothing to do with environmental concerns and everything to do with protecting the satellite company over the ridge, or something like that. Why else would they be allowed to fly in and out with helicopters? No one else on Svalbard had those privileges. It seemed crazy that Tom was involved – even after he explained about the retreats.'

'When did he do that?'

'At dinner. They all gave me sound bites about what a great thing it was and how global rapers and pillagers of the environment would come on Arctic jollies and do deals and some of the fee would go to Tom to fund climate change education, or something like that. I told Tom he was a lackey – and then there was another row.'

'Another one?'

Ruth nodded and pushed her hair back in the way Sean remembered, her tell before steaming into some ethical brawl and ruining a nice evening. Tom was the only person who could ever rein her in.

'If I'd known that Joe was Joe Kingsmith, I'm not sure I'd have gone. Because he was the owner of the mining company that closed down my survey in East Greenland.'

'Objection, Your Honour, this really can't be allowed.' Sawbridge stood up, smiling. 'My client does *not* recall the events as Dr Mott relates them. Additionally Dr Mott has no evidence for her irrelevant accusations against Mr Kingsmith. After she left the restaurant she took part in no further conversation.'

'I did,' she called to Sawbridge. 'Tom spent the night with me after leaving the restaurant.' Sawbridge looked quickly to Sean, and she almost smiled at their shock. 'You didn't know?'

Sean did not. His mind raced. Ruth nodded slowly.

'At the airport, I thought whatever god there was that I didn't believe in, had brought Tom back to me. Then at the restaurant, I thought he'd sold out, and I was so upset I had to get back to my shitty broom cupboard of a room where I could cry.' She paused, and when she spoke again, everything about her was softer. 'But he followed me. He tracked me and found me.'

'And ... you talked?' The coroner sounded almost embarrassed.

'Talk? Oh yes ... we talked ... all night. And we planned that when he came back from Midgard Lodge we would be together. We'd both been long enough in the wilderness but we'd found each other again. Suddenly it was easy.'

'But you said you thought his death was not an accident.'

'That's right. We talked about what Sean was really doing up there. About Kingsmith. I don't know about the other two. Radiance was into shipping and hotels. Tell me how that's a good thing for the Arctic. The other one, Sean's current whatever, she's just into the money, as far as I could make out.'

Sean felt Martine glitter in anger beside him. Part of him wanted to high-five Ruth Mott for being as combative and difficult as he had ever thought her.

'In the morning, Tom left me and went to the hotel very early to meet them and go on to Midgard Lodge. We thought it was better to be discreet, for him not to say anything. That was the last time I saw him. We joked about bailing on everything and staying in bed – but he wanted to see Midgard. He completely believed in Sean again. Even though he'd apparently already told him not to bring me – "for confidentiality", but I knew it was because I'd upset his billionaire friend Kingsmith.' She looked at Sean. 'I did, didn't I?'

The press bench turned its hydra head to observe Sean for reaction.

'Dr Mott.' Mr Thornton was impatient. 'This is not a platform for debating matters that do not concern my inquiries. Did you discuss the matter of Midgard Lodge and its affairs with Tom?'

Ruth hesitated. 'No. He'd signed a confidentiality clause. And he was honourable.'

Mr Thornton had no more questions for Dr Mott, and he allowed Sawbridge the first opportunity to question her. Sawbridge gave her his eyebrow-flash smile as he rose.

'Thank you, Dr Mott. Given your relationship with Tom, this must be an extremely sensitive process for you.'

'I want the truth. I'm fine.'

'Very good.' Sawbridge narrowed his eyes. 'We're talking here about the tragedy of Tom's death, and your belief that it was "no accident". This raises very serious questions. First of all, the matter of your judgement.'

'Ah, the ambush.' Ruth Mott looked back at Sawbridge. 'Would that be about the reason my survey in East Greenland was shut down?'

'I did wonder if we might touch on that—'

'No, please, let me, I was actually there. Mr Thornton, the court, reporters, everyone: I believe my survey in Qarrtsiluni was discredited in order to close me down, so that Sean's partner Joe Kingsmith could push ahead with his mining assay. They used the fact that I was in a relationship with my Inuit guide to press for me to leave.' She was breathing hard. 'Does that touch on it enough for you?'

'Oh, and the drinking,' said Sawbridge.

Sean felt ashamed.

'Sure,' Ruth Mott dug in to endure it. 'Plenty of it, at the time. But I still know that Joe Kingsmith of Midgard Lodge is the same Joe Kingsmith of Prism Exploration in East Greenland, and the same Joe Kingsmith of Prism Mining in the Central African Republic – before Ebola closed him down there. That was one of the things Tom and I talked about, overnight. The last time I saw him.'

'Mmm.' Sawbridge rubbed his chin. 'Thing is, that's neither here nor there, is it? Because Tom died when the ice-cave collapsed, very possibly because of a lake of meltwater on the ice cap feeding through and destabilising the glacier, as we have heard. The cause of this tragedy is not because of what happened to you, a long time ago, in another country. Or who does what in which developing nation, filling you with moral outrage. Though I can understand why, at some level, you might want to connect it all together.' Sawbridge looked around the courtroom. 'Perhaps you need to damage my client Mr Cawson's good reputation, because you need to make someone, *anyone*, responsible for your loss. But you are misguided and your reasoning is specious.'

He looked back at Ruth Mott with a pained compassionate smile.

'So there we are, a few bugbears unearthed – but for now, can we go back to your autopsy of the actual bear, in the hangar at the airfield at Longyearbyen? Am I right in thinking that, were it not for that random accident, of a polar bear being killed on that particular day, and requiring someone – anyone – with the credentials to do it, to perform the autopsy, you would not have met Mr Harding that day? Because neither of you were aware of the presence of the other.'

'Longyearbyen is still small.' She was white-faced. 'There was every chance we would have seen each other.'

'But you were not staying at the Polar Dream, were you? Where Mr Cawson's party had rooms? You were far downhill at the Radisson, where you were booked to have dinner with holiday guests and afterwards to talk to them about the Arctic and polar bears and eclipses and so on. Those hotels being some distance apart, you were not intending to eat at Amaruq that night – which was not only fully booked, but extremely expensive and an unlikely venue for a single diner on a modest lecturing fee, let's put it like that. Not to diminish the importance of highly qualified after-dinner speakers – it sounds like a very good tour company! And Mr Cawson's party certainly had no plans to go out bar-hopping later, so it's fair to say the odds were slim, of a chance meeting with Mr Harding.'

Sean watched Ruth Mott's face as Sawbridge let the black powder burn towards her. The room knew the explosion was coming. Go on, Ruth. Let rip. You're really upset, no one will hold it against you, and I will publicly forgive you. But she listened calmly and Sawbridge pressed on.

'The dead polar bear was the random agent that brought you into contact with Mr Harding again.'

'I told you: the bear was from East Greenland. Its lip tattoo proved it. What could be less random?' Ruth Mott made sure the press bench was paying attention. 'It travelled about eight hundred miles. So it either swam, which would be extraordinary, or it went the whole way around the North Pole clockwise, *or* the polar currents are already so disrupted by climate change that it came counter-clockwise. All sorts of marine species are found where they've never been known before; it's like all the ocean currents are scrambling, invasive species travelling in ship bilge water—'

'Bravo! Bravo!' Professor Kelly stood up at the back of the court, clapping. 'Exactly what I've been saying! When are people going to listen? Does no one understand England has a monsoon season now? Oh, another rainy June – NO! Wake *up*!' He sat down quickly before the clerk could get to him, and vigorously gestured to Ruth Mott to go on.

'So yes,' she said, her voice stronger now, 'yes, it might be random that a bear comes from East Greenland to Svalbard. It might be random that Joe Kingsmith wrecks his way around the world but I end up opposite him at dinner. And it *might* be random that before I got sacked in East Greenland I was studying reproductive anomalies in female bears, which is exactly what the eclipse bear in Svalbard was full of. Undeveloped blastocysts with evidence of pollution at the deepest cellular level. So, Mr Thornton, before you pull me off this witness stand because a dead bear has nothing to do with why Tom died, let me say that I believe she did, at a causal level. And another bear led the way to the ship finding his body.'

The journalists pattered away. Sawbridge waited for quiet again.

'Thank you, Dr Mott – a fascinating perspective on the facts. You've said to ask you anything, so I will. It's clear you and Mr Harding shared the kind of passionate feelings that, frankly, make me rather envious. A great love. A – primal bond?'

'Yes.'

'But turbulent, in the past?'

'Yes.'

'Did you and Mr Harding arrange that he would visit you, after the dinner?'

'Absolutely not. He persuaded a colleague to tell him my room. I'd talked to her about him. So she knew what he meant to me.'

Sawbridge sighed in sympathy.

'You said you, um, *talked* all night. Did Mr Harding get *any* sleep? I won't insult your intelligence, you'll know what is at the root of my question. Was he – perhaps – in a state of emotional exaltation but physical fatigue that next day, due to lack of sleep? We of course have no way of knowing, but you do.'

'To a man like Tom, a sleepless night would make no difference. He had great endurance, he was very strong.' She leaned forward. 'He said he felt reborn.'

'Marvellous. I can completely understand why you would want to believe it made no difference – because it would be unbearable, would it not?' Here Sawbridge gathered up Angela Harding and Granny Ruby in his compassionate glance. 'Quite *unbearable* to think that a night of passion had cost Tom vital energy when it came to the physical ordeal he was unwittingly about to face. To be just that crucial bit below par. To be … tired.'

Ruth stared at him in shock. So did Sean. To lead people to blame Ruth – he couldn't bear it. Sawbridge shook his head gently, as if he too, could hardly bear to think it. 'No further questions.' As he sat, she spoke again, but her voice was weak.

'He didn't trust Kingsmith.'

Sawbridge half-rose, as if to be polite to a lady. 'If I might respectfully suggest, Dr Mott, it was *you* who did not like Mr Kingsmith, but in your grief, to protect yourself from the possibility of culpability, no matter how innocently, in his death – you now project that fear posthumously onto Mr Harding. Who was, I remind you, quite happy to be in business with Mr Cawson, Mr Kingsmith—'

'He wasn't! He was full of doubt! And I believe something happened inside the glacier or before, I don't know what—'

'Dr Mott, you've led research teams in the Arctic on a number of occasions, been a senior scientist in your field – yes? Have you never doubted yourself? Never had a moment of wondering if you're doing the right thing, right time, right team? Never made a decision, then gone over your reasoning again before implementing it? A sort of safety routine?'

'I think things through very carefully, so that I trust myself. You can't lead a team if you're indecisive.'

'Or if you've lost your job.'

'No. Don't use that.' Sean said it impulsively, and the court turned to stare. Sawbridge held up his hand and nodded soothingly.

'My client is a very generous man to feel protective towards you, Dr Mott, but I'm afraid for his own sake I must persist with this line of questioning—'

'Nicholas, don't, you've said enough.' Sean was on his feet now, but Sawbridge refused to look, keeping his palm up as if stopping traffic, his eyes trained on Ruth Mott.

'Nothing you could say would be any worse.' She looked as if she were mortally wounded, but still standing. Sean wanted to go to her, but he too was frozen.

'Isn't the reason you're now an after-dinner speaker,' continued Sawbridge, 'rather than a respected working scientist, because you made a fatal error of judgement in your last position? Isn't it because of that business about the fatality with the sponsored bear? I didn't want to bring it up, but wasn't it to do with your responsibility for administering the wrong dosage of the tranquilliser? A case of being over-confident in your decisions, rather than having the humility to check, to question yourself, to *doubt*, on occasion?'

'Someone sabotaged me. I know I loaded the right amount.'

'Ah,' said Sawbridge. 'The mysterious *Someone*. But not a shred of evidence.'

'Someone on my team. Prism paid them, I was the only one fighting to protect the denning site, the rest of them had already taken the money!'

'So you blamed Mr Kingsmith's company for the closure of your study?'

'Rightly!'

'And then when you met him with my client, Mr Cawson, quite by happenstance, in Svalbard, you perhaps felt every wrong could be righted in one go, if you could only separate Tom from his purpose with them. You'd lost the man and the job you loved, but here was a second chance. No wonder you wanted to hang on to him for every minute you could.'

Sawbridge reverted to compassion.

'I think the coroner will take into account that – in Mr Harding's likely fatigued state due to lack of sleep following a highly intense reunion – we have found a strong contributory factor to his inability to save himself in this tragic accident. I thank you, Dr Mott. No further questions.'

I once met a woman who saved her own life by eating her husband and her children.

My husband and I were on a journey from Igdlulik to Ponds Inlet. On the way he had a dream in which it seemed that a friend of his was being eaten by his own kin. Two days after, we came to a spot where strange sounds hovered in the air. At first we could not make out what it was, but coming nearer it was like the ghost of words; as it were one trying to speak without a voice. And at last it said:

'I am one who can no longer live among human kind, for I have eaten my own kin.'

We could hear now that it was a woman. And we looked at each other, and spoke in a whisper, fearing what might happen to us now. Then searching round, we found a little shelter built of snow and a fragment of caribou skin. Close by was a thing standing up; we thought at first it was a human being, but saw it was only a rifle stuck in the snow. But all this time the voice was muttering. And going nearer again we found a human head, with the flesh gnawed away. And at last, entering into the shelter, we found the woman seated on the floor. Her face was turned towards us and we saw that blood was trickling from the corners of her eyes; so greatly had she wept.

'Kikaq (a gnawed bone),' she said, 'I have eaten my husband and my children!'

She was but skin and bone herself, and seemed to have no life in her. And she was almost naked, having eaten most of her clothing. My husband bent down over her, and she said:

'I have eaten him who was your comrade when he lived.'

And my husband answered: 'You had the will to live, and so you are still alive.'

Then we put up our tent close by, cutting off a piece of the forecurtain to make a shelter for the woman; for she was unclean and might not be in the same tent with us. And we gave her frozen caribou meat to eat, but when she had eaten a mouthful or so, she fell to trembling all over, and could eat no more.

She is still alive to this day and married to a great hunter, named Igtussarssua, and she is his favorite wife, though he had one before. But that is the most terrible thing I have known in all my life.

Across Arctic America: Narrative of the Fifth Thule Expedition (1927)
Knud Rasmussen

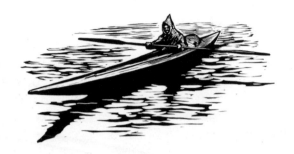

30

Sean bluntly refused Sawbridge's offer to have lunch. Ruth Mott would now believe that *she* might be culpable for Tom's death. It would blight the rest of her life.

'You underestimate the lady,' Sawbridge was ever affable. 'She strikes me as very resilient. And when it comes to reputations in a courtroom, it's a zero-sum game. Ours or theirs, never both. You're paying me to know this and act accordingly. So hear this: squeamishness in a client comes from one of two things. One, he's innocent but frightened no one will believe him. Or two, he's a coward who'll let someone hang in his place but please don't make him watch. Obviously, you're the former.' Sawbridge looked at his watch. 'You're confident he'll come?'

'Already landed.' Sean had received a text message from a new number, a Kingsmith move on arrival. Too many calls, otherwise.

Sean let Sawbridge peel off, then got himself a coffee and a ham-and-mustard sandwich and found a bench by a weir. Birdsong threaded through the sound of an open-air market and the water rushed fast and bubbling. As Sean ate, his mouth filled with wheaten mulch and long-dead meat. He forced himself to swallow then looked in the sandwich – it smelled normal, but it sickened him. The coffee was bitter and cloying. Could it be stress? Jenny Flanders came to mind. He didn't want to see her again but he knew he would.

Young people walked past him – pretty girls. For once he did not look carnally at their taut hips and flinging hair, but instead saw them as only just past childhood. Boys followed, young men unmarked by life. Early twenties, Sean guessed. For a moment he saw himself and Tom, and Gail and Ruth, laughing by the river all those years ago, just before they had become two couples.

He watched the foursome pausing to look down at the weir. They seemed held in a golden glow, they were sex and youth and promise and they had all the time in the world. They moved on but he still sat there, a middle-aged man with a paper cup and a sandwich, invisible on a city bench one weekday lunchtime.

Since Sean had saved Tom's bacon at the Lost Explorers' Society dinner, Tom Harding made a point of getting to know this stroppy waiter whose Arctic obsession outstripped even his own. Sean had gone to meet him at the King's Head that first time, and was amazed and touched, that this young man of similar age but in every other way from a different planet really and emphatically did want him to go to Greenland as his expedition partner. Sean could spot those who were privileged from birth – the Abbott's School and Oxford had taught him that – but there was nothing snobbish about Tom, and he was wildly impressed with Sean.

When Sean was finally forced to admit that he couldn't afford to go to Greenland, Tom immediately offered to pay. He refused.

'No charity, unless I'm the one giving it. But thanks.' Sean got up to go, but stopped at the sight of two lovely girls heading their way. One of them grabbed Tom and amorously embraced him, and Sean and the girl's friend looked away as Tom reciprocated enthusiastically. With their friends absorbed in each other, they smiled at one other awkwardly.

'Clearly they're back on again.' The girl rolled her eyes. 'I can't keep up.' She touched her face. 'What? Is it pasta sauce? Ruth cooked it in her room. It was horrible.'

'It was delicious. And cheaper than going out.' The girl called Ruth looked around, aglow with happiness. She was sitting on Tom's lap, his arm was around her waist and he was grinning stupidly. He looked up at Sean.

'You're going?'

'Oh,' said the other girl, 'are you?'

Sean suddenly decided he wasn't going anywhere. He pulled out a chair for her, and found out her name was Gail. Before he'd come back from the bar with the round he'd bought with his week's food money, he was in love. She was studying art, her parents lived in the country, she was unfashionable and didn't care, she followed Ruth around so that she could meet interesting people – like Sean ...

Ruth and Tom were wrapped up in each other so Gail and Sean talked, and ate crisps, and drank beer and he spent far more than he should because he refused to let her pay for anything, and it occurred to him that if he was going to be friends with Tom Harding – and this girl had sealed it for him – then he had better find a way to make more money, quickly.

But at a painful meeting the following week his bank manager refused him a loan or an overdraft. He had no family, or at least none he could ask. The trip to Greenland would cost five hundred pounds – plus the contribution to the Lost Explorers' Society annual funds and the membership. It was impossible, and he was a fool for thinking he could keep up with that sort of crowd. He went to Tom's college and left him a note explaining why he couldn't do it, and then one at Gail's college, saying he couldn't afford to go out with her, and he was very sorry.

But Tom had other ideas, and so did Gail. They ambushed Sean at the Crown and Sceptre, and presented a plan. A businessman with a reputation for supporting young people was coming to speak at the Oxford Union. They must go, and ask him for sponsorship.

The businessman was Joe Kingsmith, and the Union was packed with students eager to see this exotic American animal, the maverick entrepreneur who preached something called globalisation, and avoided paying tax by living in the air or out at sea on a yacht – or so rumour had it. Sitting at the back, Sean craned to see him.

Tall and heavy in the shoulders, his ridged bronze dome of a head giving him a gladiatorial look, Kingsmith offset his air of danger with an easy manner and elegant low-key clothes. Shunning the small platform at the front, he welcomed the audience from the floor of the

Union, as if it were his own space, then spoke of the need to remove all trade borders and regulations and release the energy of free enterprise. He mused on the family fortunes built on colonial exploitation, and how expansion and investment must now happen in a more just way, as he practised it. Security was essential, but so was a genuine profit for the less technologically sophisticated partner: it was only good business.

Kingsmith had no qualms about enumerating his own achievements – his work in Chad, his mines near N'Djamena, how he was bringing health and prosperity to the whole country. He told the audience not to be timidly nationalistic but think boldly and globally, to mistrust terms like government, and coup, belligerent or insurgent. Take Burkina Faso, for instance, where the most recent coup had been celebrated by the people.

The chamber was silent in astonishment. Kingsmith smiled. 'Oh, it's quite true,' he told them. Power was security, and security was power. They shouldn't feel squeamish to hear it said, or guilty for wanting it. Just for a second the American caught Sean's eye – and he felt a jolt of energy.

Kingsmith moved on, talking about catastrophe bonds and how they were going to be the big financial news of the future, but Sean was more interested in his dominance of the space, how people at the ends of the rows moved their legs out of his way as he strode towards them, the avid expressions on their faces as they looked at him. He felt the same expression shaping his own face.

And then suddenly Kingsmith was thanking them for the invitation, they were lucky kids to be here, he hoped they knew that – and he must leave for a meeting. The pink-cheeked president of the Union stood up, astonished. Awkwardly he explained that they'd booked him to speak for an hour and he was sure the audience had many questions to put to him, but it had only been fifteen minutes. Kingsmith looked at him kindly.

'Kid, you've misunderstood. I was curious to see this place. A lot of friends of mine have spoken here. I've said what I wanted, so good evening to you.' He walked out, raising his hand to salute the few timid boos that grew louder when he was safely out of the chamber.

Sean was on his feet at once, pulling Tom with him. They ran out in time to see Kingsmith fold himself into a cab, which they chased on foot as far as the Randolph Hotel, where he got out. Panting, they followed him into the lobby and begged him for five more minutes, they had a question. He laughed and told them to wait in the bar.

Sean and Tom collapsed at a table. A waiter arrived to tell them Mr Kingsmith invited them to order whatever they would like. Daringly, they ordered bottled foreign lager, the taste of adventure and sophistication. Sean looked around the Randolph Hotel. There were people who lived like this always. He wanted to be one of them.

'He must be a multi-millionaire.' Sean tried not to sound too admiring.

'At least.' Tom was excited as well. They had scooped a meeting with a big beast, and now they mustn't blow it. They practised what they were going to say when Kingsmith returned – which was sooner than they expected. Sean felt his heart pounding as Kingsmith came in and spotted them. They both stood up in automatic respect, and he grinned and motioned them back down.

'Nice of you to run so fast,' he said. 'You don't look like assassins, but I could still be wrong. What do you want?'

'Sponsorship to go to Greenland,' Sean said straight away. 'Not charity.'

Kingsmith laughed. He waved away their compliments and they got to the point: the Lost Explorers' Society, and the fees. He looked at Tom, then at Sean.

'But only you need it. Right?'

'How do you know?'

'You're wearing your best clothes.'

Sean felt humiliated. It was true. 'How can you tell?'

'You were dressed smarter than everyone else in your row, and you paid attention to everything I said. Don't worry, kid, I read a room fast. A lot can depend on it. And I like it when someone shows respect.' He looked at Tom, in jeans. 'Right?'

'I always wear jeans.' Tom looked confused. 'Unless it says black tie.'

Kingsmith turned back to Sean. 'You got black tie? They love it here.'

'I've never needed it.' Sean heard himself, defiant and upset.

Kingsmith smiled. 'I'm betting you will, and soon. Go on then, your Greenland vacation. What's in it for me?'

This, they were ready for. They told him about all the minerals hidden under the ice, the copper and rubies and diamonds and gold, the lithium, the uranium – the centuries-old attempts to find the fabled sea route from Europe, the ancient Chinese beads found on Inuit spears, how Pytheas the fourth-century Greek trader was the first to tell of the frozen seas to the north, how it wasn't Peary who first set foot on the North Pole but his Negro manservant Matthew Henson—

Kingsmith held up his hand to stop them. He looked at Tom. 'Why don't you lend him the money? Or give it? Isn't that easier than running after a stranger?'

'He won't take it.' Tom shook his head. 'Sean, come on, he's just playing with us. Let's go.'

'If he was going to say no he wouldn't still be talking to us.' Sean looked Kingsmith in the eye. 'Will you or will you not sponsor us to go on the Lost Explorers' Expedition to Greenland? We'll give you something in return, but you have to tell us what you want.'

Kingsmith burst out laughing. 'The chutzpah! *He's* making the deal!'

'I'm not a joke and I don't want charity.' Sean didn't smile. 'I'm reading Economics, I'm hard-working, I don't mind getting my hands dirty and I don't get tired.'

'And what's the most important thing you've learned so far?'

'Seize your chances.'

'What's your name?'

'Sean Cawson.'

'And what's your problem? Lack of money's only the symptom.'

Sean suddenly choked up. 'I just – need – to go to the Arctic.'

'You *need* to ...' Kingsmith looked at him with deeper interest. 'Why?'

For a second Sean was on that landing, looking across the void of stairwell where the light caught the peeling wall, gazing at the painting of the icebergs.

'Why not take charity?' Kingsmith held him in his gaze, and Sean felt the back of his eyes burning. He pushed the feeling down.

'I've had enough of it. I spent time in care. There was a painting of the Arctic there. It was where I went. When I needed to.' He looked at Kingsmith, defiant again. 'All right?'

'Good on you,' Kingsmith said. 'And good instinct to stay.' He looked at Tom. 'You're worrying about your friend but you don't need to. He'll be fine. And I can tell you're thinking, this guy doesn't know either of us from Adam, how can he say that—'

'That's right,' Tom said. 'I was.'

'Your friend reminds me of me.' Kingsmith turned back to Sean. 'Plus, you got me on a good night, I just had some nice news. So here's the deal: I don't know much about your fancy society, but I like how you two operate, so I'll take a chance. You boys go to Greenland for me, you have a good time, you tell me about it.'

He sat back and waited for effusive thanks. But Sean frowned.

'What's in it for you? That's no kind of deal.'

'Ah, he's sharp. OK, not much at first. But if what you say's remotely interesting, I might send you somewhere else you want to go. You love the Arctic? I'm pretty interested too. So go have a trip on me, and we'll take it from there.'

'Is this the give before the take?' Sean stared at him, and Kingsmith laughed. 'For sure! Come on, it's easy: I like to have scouts on a new frontier.' By some signal, a waiter came to his elbow and Kingsmith glanced up and signed the bill. He turned back to them. 'One-time offer: take it or leave it.'

'Take it.' Sean put out his hand. 'We'll take it, thank you.'

'Yes,' said Tom, a moment later. 'Thank you.'

Kingsmith shook hands with Sean, then Tom, and gave him a business card. 'Lawyer,' he said. 'Call him tomorrow afternoon, he'll advise.'

'On what?' Tom looked at the card suspiciously.

Kingsmith winked at Sean. 'Where to send the money.'

At the half-landing on the way up to Court No. 1, Sean passed Mrs Osman, motionless by the window. Over her asymmetric shoulders he saw a black Vauxhall saloon swing into a narrow space in the court car park. Then the welcome shape of Kingsmith unfolded from the driver's door, dusting imaginary specks off his jacket. He slammed it and looked up, as if he knew he was observed. Sean raised his hand in greeting and went down to him. Mrs Osman continued to the court.

Kingsmith gave him his familiar heavy clap on the shoulder. He was as well dressed as ever, a dark linen suit for the hot October weather, light leather brogues and an olive cashmere sweater over one arm. His head was tanned and smoothly shaved. 'Bearing up?'

'Sure. Thanks for coming.' Sean smiled the truth away. Kingsmith didn't like sickness or weakness, never succumbing himself. 'That's not the car I thought you'd drive.'

'Now I just drive what my PA books, it's easier. Come on. Let's get you through this so we can go have some fun tomorrow.'

Sean had to think for a moment what he meant. Tomorrow was the benefit dinner, for Tom. Fun was the last thing it would be, but it was good that Joe was upbeat.

In the courtroom, after a brief introduction to Sawbridge, Kingsmith made straight for Angela Harding and respectfully introduced himself. Sean and Sawbridge watched him take her hand in his two big ones and speak in a low sincere voice. Then he came back to Mrs Osman, who was speaking with her two aides sitting by the aisle. Fascinated, Sawbridge dropped all pretence of not listening.

'Mrs Osman?' Kingsmith had done some research. 'It's an honour to meet the lawyer who ensured justice for the Waterby girls. We heard about that case in the States. Beyond words. But at least you brought peace for their families.'

Mrs Osman's eyes were so dark, and the sockets so deep, that if she turned her head a certain way as she now did, she resembled some ancient blind seer.

'Peace? No. Justice, maybe. But it's poor coin for murder.'

Sean was surprised, first that Kingsmith knew anything about it, and then that Mrs Osman had anything to do with those young abductees, missing for two agonising years and then unearthed. He watched her move away to talk to Ruth Mott, who sat hunched and had clearly been crying. The lawyer murmured to her, they heard the word 'bathroom'. She walked out, painfully slow. Her back must hurt, Sean thought. Years of black document cases, and their darker contents. Kingsmith sat down heavily beside him.

'You've met Osman.' Sawbridge leaned forward with a grim smile.

284

'I heard she also arranged the killer's cellmate.' Kingsmith glanced around, but Osman had gone. 'And that justice was protracted.'

Sawbridge grimaced. 'Yes. We do hear that.'

Kingsmith took in Ruth Mott. 'And our good biologist?'

'Ah. Quite docile now, I think.' Sawbridge answered before Sean could.

As the chairs scraped and the afternoon session began, Sean looked over at Ruth Mott, no longer fierce and bright, but bowed by her broken heart.

Kingsmith took the Christian oath in his deep and pleasant baritone. He would have made an excellent actor, broad-shouldered and deep-chested, and now in that ageless state that money brings a man who keeps his fitness, dresses well, and whose tan will never fade. The court stared at this exotic animal with his powerful face. He projected the confrontational quality of a man used to the submission of others.

Kingsmith gave his home address as being in Zurich – Sean recognised the street as the same as one of the banks he used. Perhaps, like so much in Switzerland, the lie was part of a larger and absolving arrangement. He watched his mentor in skilful deferential mode, the coroner at ease at once. Sean felt likewise reassured. The cavalry had arrived, and he would take Ruth out for lunch when this was behind them. It was a shared loss, and he would find a way to support her in rebuilding her life.

Mr Thornton seemed rather charmed that Mr Kingsmith had made a very long journey to attend his court, and invited him to simply give his account of everything he felt was relevant to the tragic outcome of their trip to the ice-cave. He himself would interject as required, and counsel would please signal – and here Mr Thornton looked severely at Mrs Osman's late return from her bathroom break – if they wished to ask a pertinent question.

Kingsmith began. He described in glowing terms his long relationship with both Tom and Sean boy – and went on to sketch out their shared love of the Arctic, placing himself in a line of worthy hard-working miners going back to his father's humble beginnings. He stressed his own hard-scrabble entrepreneurial journey and glossed the global empire part, before returning to Sean and Tom's pursuit of him when he spoke at Oxford, back in the Jurassic age.

Kingsmith's smile was genuine. To everyone who didn't know, he wanted to say that those young men, with their dreams of discovery and heroism, were just irresistible. Before he knew it, he'd agreed to underwrite their Lost Explorers' Society, and that was how he knew them both. Over time, Sean better, Tom, less so.

Mrs Osman put her hand up.

'Why was that? Why did you know Tom ... less well?'

Kingsmith nodded thoughtfully, as if grateful for the question.

'Sean liked how I did things, he knew he could learn from me. And he has. Tom had his own ideas – but that's good too. I'm a maverick myself, so I value independence very highly. But we had philosophical differences. On a grand scale! Everything on the grand scale with Tom. But I'm the same.'

Sean noted Kingsmith didn't try his coroner-style charm on Mrs Osman, but was harder-edged. 'I sent them on a few trips, in return for building up my knowledge. They were my eyes and ears, all over the Arctic. I funded their passion, in return for information. Mostly just background colour. Sean stayed close. That's all.'

'Where did they go for you?'

'Greenland.' Kingsmith made sure people saw him look over to Ruth Mott, and nod to her. Sean knew he was signalling that he was ready for whatever she might try. Ruth looked away.

'A remote place of great interest,' observed Mrs Osman. 'At that time. When was that exactly? 1988? 1989?'

'I guess round then. But even though the Arctic isn't remote any more – even though it's open for business, it's still dangerous.' Kingsmith looked out. 'The people who set up the infrastructure take the biggest risks. The pioneers. That's me, that's Sean over there, that was Tom. And that's what happened at Midgard – the pioneers, taking the risks for everyone else, suffered a terrible loss. It could have been any of us, or all of us, or none of us. It was Tom. And I am so, so sorry.'

Sean was completely caught up in the performance. Once again, Kingsmith had the room in the palm of his hand. Like Tom had in Claridge's. What a force he and Kingsmith would have made, on the same side.

'Let me make something very clear,' Kingsmith went on. 'And this might be unpopular but I'm used to telling it like it is. I don't care how many movie stars and popsicles you get pushing a stuffed polar bear round the streets of whichever capital. I don't care how many idealistic young people chant Save the Arctic and chain themselves to how many corporate towers. Hear this: It's. Too. *Late.*

'Business is already there, making money and doing it safely. It's not the story that sells but it's the truth. Change is part of life, and Tom knew this one was unstoppable. But what he also knew was that it's all about the *how*. *How* you ship, to bring down the price of goods. How you extract the commodities that the world needs. How you fish, to feed more people. How you set up your comtech.'

'Comtech.' Mr Thornton peered at Kingsmith. 'Satellite technology.'

'Right. And while we're on it, ask why it's business gets the beating in the Arctic, not the military or tourism. Naval war games everywhere, cruise ships in the gaps. The place is heaving! So dry your tears, because the new Arctic has just unblocked a load of congestion on our crowded planet.'

'What mendacious and utter bollocks!' Professor Kelly stood up, turned to the press bench and pointed at Kingsmith. 'He is a dangerous man and we are sheep to the slaughter if we believe him!'

'Professor Kelly, I regret my decision to allow you to stay,' called out the coroner.

'Do not believe a word he says! Get your hands off me!' Professor Kelly beat away the clerk attempting to usher him out. A couple of journalists took the opportunity to photograph the exchange, and Mr Thornton also pointed them out to the clerks he had summoned by discreet means.

Sean saw Ruth Mott, pale-faced with fury, Osman keeping a light finger on her arm to hold her back. Professor Kelly could still be heard shouting as he was escorted down the stairs. Then there was silence, and Kingsmith took it.

'But about what happened in the ice-cave. I have a confession.' He gathered the room in his pause.

'I'm not proud to say it, but I was very frightened. I thought I'd be OK, until the ice walls started to get closer together the further in we went. When Sean and Tom went on ahead, I realised I was hanging back with the girls. Then I wasn't feeling good and, bless her, Radiance got the sense of it and she said we should go back. I'm not used to feeling scared, but that's what was happening. I started getting these weird flashes. Some kind of panic attack, if you believe in those. She and I started back for the entrance then Martine came right behind us, calling on us to wait. She said Sean and Tom were having a quick look in at the Great Hall and then they'd be right after us. The three of us had just gotten back to near the ladder when we heard this bad sound. We knew it was bad, there was this rumbling, like heavy furniture falling in the room next door.'

Kingsmith rubbed his head with both hands.

'When we tried to go back to see, the passage was blocked. There was no room to move and the three of us were all shouting and treading on each other in there, trying to yell to them through the ice – and then we all felt it give again under our feet and after that we ran for the ladder, because you can't help people if you're trapped too.' He looked at the coroner. 'Danny and Terry were already at the top to get us out because the storm was coming. They didn't even know about the collapse. They were very good, they checked inside the entrance, then they got us back down to the Lodge just before the blizzard hit.'

Kingsmith looked for Angela Harding in the silent courtroom. 'That was the right safety protocol, no matter what. If it had been me down there, trapped in the ice, they'd have done the exact same thing. As soon as the phones came on again, we raised the alarm, but that wasn't until the storm passed. I can only offer my most sincere condolences to all Tom's family.' He turned back to the coroner.

Mrs Osman put her hand up and rose. 'Mr Kingsmith,' she said in her hoarse voice. 'Can I go back to when you met Tom and Mr Cawson, when they were students at Oxford and you were already a very successful ... entrepreneur.' Kingsmith nodded.

'You took Mr Cawson on as your ... protégé. Is that right?'

'I mentored him. Still do, if he wants.'

'You mentioned differences, with Tom. Did you fall out, at any time?'

Kingsmith frowned slightly. 'As in, ever have a disagreement? Or a fight?'

'Either,' Osman said mildly. 'At any time, right up until ... I suppose ... the incident in the ice-cave.'

'I do wish you wouldn't call it that.' Sawbridge stood up fully. 'Your Honour, don't you think it gives a very unpleasant slant to things? Mrs Osman is no stranger to correct terminology, so I fail to understand why she doesn't use it. It was an *accident*.'

'Mr Sawbridge, I will tell you what I think in my summing up and not before. Mrs Osman, I am in no doubt there *was* an accident: please use that term for now.'

'Thank you,' Sawbridge emphasised, directing the remark to Mrs Osman.

'*Accident*,' she drawled, making it sound far worse. 'The *ac-cident* ... in the ice-cave. Were there any ... arguments? Before you went in?'

'Arguments?' Kingsmith looked bemused.

'Yes. Arguments.' Mrs Osman looked through her file, laboriously. Everyone waited. She looked up. 'Because Dr Mott received a call from Tom on the morning of the eclipse, from Midgard Lodge itself. Before his phone was cut off.'

Sean's eyes went to Ruth – she was right there waiting for him. She nodded. *That's right.* He looked away, his heart pounding. Tom had told her.

Quickly Sean leaned into Sawbridge and whispered. Sawbridge nodded vigorously and popped up again.

'Objection! My client insists that no phones were "cut off" by human action, and that it is a most pejorative claim we dispute in the strongest terms. My client reiterates that it is a feature of the location that regular cell phones will not work, and the signal for the iridium phones provided by Mr Cawson to the whole party, and with which Mr Harding was also personally familiar from other remote travel, were also being affected over the whole of the archipelago, by the solar eclipse. It's well documented. Mr Harding's phone was certainly not "cut off", but might well have been functioning erratically.' He stared at Mrs Osman. 'I hope that is quite clear.'

'But they did have a few seconds to speak ...' Mrs Osman pulled out a sheet from her file. 'Here is Dr Mott's phone record for that day, which shows it as 10.58 a.m., registering one minute. Dr Mott says it was less, but one minute is the basic unit of record by the phone company. She says Tom was agitated about something.'

'Mrs Osman, why did you not give this to me sooner?' Mr Thornton was losing patience.

'I apologise. I must have mis-filed it.' She handed the page to one of her aides, who took it to the front. As the coroner studied it, Sean felt his spine prickle.

'In Dr Mott's words—'

'Dr Mott is sitting in my courtroom, so if she does not mind, I will ask her to come back to the witness stand and tell me herself. Dr Mott? Are you willing?'

Ruth Mott nodded. 'Mr Kingsmith, would you mind? You don't need to leave the platform.'

'Of course.' Kingsmith stepped aside, his eyes fixed on Ruth Mott as she came up the aisle. She looked back defiantly, puffed up like a small threatened cat against the dog that could kill her. The coroner directed her where to stand. Now she ignored Kingsmith completely.

'I'll consider you remaining as sworn in. Please tell me what Tom said, in this very short phone call.'

'He said there was a cave full of guns. He said it was unbelievable.'

'Dr Mott, why have you not mentioned this before?'

She looked at Mrs Osman for a moment before she answered. 'I went through a bad depression when I lost my job. I'd been completely professionally discredited, I'd lost the man I loved, I was trying to put everything behind me and move on. But when his body was found – I knew I had to speak.'

'You've had ample opportunity,' said the coroner. 'I find it very—'

'I asked her not to,' Mrs Osman interrupted. Sawbridge made a loud sound of exasperation and looked around for support.

'Because?' Mr Thornton was now visibly annoyed.

Mrs Osman remained calm. 'Because I believed, had Mr Kingsmith known of this detail, there was a chance he might have found himself busy today. And I thought it useful for him to be here, as scheduled.'

The courtroom was silent, all eyes now on Kingsmith. He stared at Mrs Osman, and licked his lips once. Sean was suddenly put in mind of a Komodo dragon, tasting the air. Then Kingsmith smiled.

'Well, I'm delighted to meet you too, Mrs Osman. But let me tell you, the décor at Midgard Lodge is truly impressive. There's this majestic window, double storey, looking straight down Midgardfjorden. Stone fireplace on the back, same height. And then my collection of antique firearms on the walls.'

'No,' Ruth Mott said firmly. 'He said it was a cave. A cave full of weapons.'

Kingsmith looked at her sympathetically. 'That's absolutely the feeling of that part of the room. But the way you describe it makes me think it does strike the wrong note. It might feel threatening. Sean, maybe you want to look at that.' Kingsmith spoke as if he were happy to talk about interior design all day. 'Anything else?'

'Yes. Dr Mott, can you tell me anything more about this phone call?'

'He said they were about to leave. He didn't say where. Then his phone cut out.' She looked at Sean. 'For whatever reason.'

Sean remembered. Immediately after their confrontation in the boathouse, and before leaving on the skidoos, Tom had gone back into the Lodge. He'd said he needed to pee. But he hadn't. Sean closed his eyes. As soon as he'd seen Tom heading for the boat hangar, he sensed trouble and told Terry Bjornsen to block the Wi-Fi. But he hadn't done it in time.

'OK?' Sawbridge murmured it. Sean nodded, his eyes on Ruth Mott.

'Your Honour?' Mrs Osman spoke. 'I do have a few questions more for Mr Kingsmith.'

He bowed. 'Please.'

'Thank you. A point of curiosity really, but perhaps … of relevance. Why are you driving an armoured car?'

'A *what*?' Kingsmith laughed.

'Your Vauxhall Insignia. It's armour-plated.'

'What an extraordinary thing to suggest!'

'Not really,' she replied. 'When you're familiar with them, the sound of the heavy door closing is quite distinctive. Then, when I walked around it, I noted it does indeed feature inch-thick bullet-proof glass. I merely wondered.'

'Ma'am, with the greatest respect, you're mistaken.' Kingsmith smiled. 'But I'd be very happy to let you inspect it at your leisure, if you fancied a spin.'

'I don't, thank you. What I really want to ask is how you would characterise your role in the affairs of Midgard Lodge.'

'Surely.' Kingsmith switched tactics, as relaxed as if they were flirting in a bar. 'I'm valued as a very amiable sleeping partner. For a long time, Sean and I have been involved in business ventures together. It started with me inviting him in, but in recent years he's done a lot more hosting – by which I mean he's thrown the party and I've brought the bottle and sometimes some of the guests, if you follow me.'

'I'm afraid I don't.'

'OK. If there's an interesting financial opportunity, we like to help each other out. That's how you grow. One way or another, I've been investing for him since his student days, and it's no secret he's done pretty well for himself on the gains. And for some time now, I'm pleased to say the pupil's returned the favour and brought the old man in on a few deals.'

'So Midgard Lodge was a financial opportunity, in which Mr Cawson invited you to participate? Yes or no would be the most helpful answer.'

'Ah, Mrs Osman – you know how they so often limit our understanding.'

'Or seek to obfuscate it.'

'Business is always about relationships. They're delicate living things, way past the yes and no binary. Relationships are about politics, and politics is always about needs, resources and access. And before you pull me up for being evasive, I *am* answering the question fully – if you'll just stay with me a minute. When Midgard Lodge came up for sale in Svalbard, Sean saw a great business opportunity – but he's made plenty of money. This time he wanted more. Sorry, Sean boy, but let's be honest and help this inquest along. Plain and simple, he wanted glory. Anyone thinks he's a playboy in a suit, hasn't got him. In his heart, he's an explorer, and they're the world's greatest romantics. No amount of money makes up for a lack of adventure in life. Not for men like us.'

Sean felt an untimely surge of pride. *Men like us.*

'And then this chance of a lifetime comes up – it fits perfectly with his brand, and it's the part of the world that's closest to his heart. And now he's mature enough to want to give, not just get.'

Kingsmith came out from behind the witness stand, the better to connect, and the clerk moved out of his way. Sean thought of Kingsmith the first time he'd seen him at the Oxford Union, how people had physically reacted to him, instinctively drawing away. As though they were afraid.

'Protecting the Arctic is a job that needs doing and it goes hand in hand with trying to steward best business practice there. Sean's trying to do both – he knew he needed Tom's help.'

'Mr Kingsmith.' The coroner was less enamoured. 'You're not running for office, so please simply answer my questions. Do you think Mr Harding shared your view on development in the Arctic Ocean?'

'Yes, as his vision became more sophisticated.'

'That is a lie!' Ruth Mott said it to Kingsmith, then turned to Sean. 'What did you *say* to him? What lies did you tell him, to get him in? He knew, didn't he? He found something out – I *know* he did!'

'Dr Mott, please, if you have some evidence – other than your wishful thinking—' Sawbridge was also standing, 'you've had ample opportunity to bring it to the coroner's attention. We understand you're very upset, but while we sympathise—'

'Being upset does not make me a fool! Making mistakes in the past does not mean I'm going to miss this chance to do the right thing!' Ruth Mott also came out to the front of the stand, looking ready to punch the next person who spoke.

'Everyone sit down!' The coroner banged his palm on the table. He pointed at Mrs Osman: 'Not you.' And at Kingsmith, who was unperturbed: 'Or you.'

'There's a cover-up!' Ruth Mott turned to the coroner. 'I know it!'

Sean wanted to grab her by the shoulders and shake her, and yell in her face to shut up, none of this will bring Tom back so just let it go, we all have to move on without him, we all have to live with our mistakes. Tom is dead and we're going to make a huge fucking donation in his name tomorrow night and put it into what he believed in. Tom forced the issue and look what happened. It didn't have to happen!

Ruth looked right back at him as surely if he had actually yelled it out loud instead of in his head. Then, trembling and white-faced, she walked off the platform and between the staring rows of people.

'Dr Mott!' called the coroner, but she did not stop, and as she went to push the double doors it looked as though they were opened from the outside. Sean caught a flash of a tall figure in a red jacket.

'Let her go.' Sawbridge put a restraining arm on Sean's, but he broke free.

'Mr Cawson!' called the coroner. 'Mr Cawson!'

Outside Court No. 1 the lobby was empty. Then Sean saw her, huddled in the seat on the first-floor landing, her face turned away. Sean looked around for whoever had opened the door for her, but they were alone. There was no one in a red jacket, and the only movement was Ruth Mott's shoulders, shaking. She knew he was there.

'Something else happened.' She did not look up. 'I absolutely know it.'

Sean could not help himself, he went to her.

'Ruth. We both lost him.'

To his surprise, instead of shoving him away, she held out her hand. He took it and felt the bones and the muscles and the warmth of her skin tighten around his own. He crouched down beside her, then he put his arms around her. Her grief went through him like a shock wave.

'Ruth,' he heard himself say, in a tender tone he'd not used in so long. She heard it and turned and clung to him, and through her sobs he felt the heat of her wet face against his neck, and held her closer. He felt her breasts pressing against him, and the curve of her ribs under one hand. He let go abruptly.

'Sean, you're freaking me out.' Ruth stood up and wiped her eyes on her sleeve. 'I can't breathe in here. I have to get out.' She ran down the stairs.

Sean stayed where he was until her footsteps were gone. He wanted air too. A thread of freshness was coming from somewhere and he turned to find the source. It came from a door on the staircase landing, opening onto the black iron fire escape. It was slightly ajar. He became aware of someone repeating his name.

'Sean!' Sawbridge stood higher up, outside the double doors of the court. 'Thornton's about to lose it. Are we bailing for the day?'

'No I'm there.' Sean went back in, but as he did, suddenly he understood. The fire escape led down to the car park. Mrs Osman's dark hooded eyes had a new brightness as she met his gaze. Her bathroom break had been her chance to go out onto the fire escape, and down to the car park. That was the only way she could have examined Kingsmith's car. Smiling faintly, she turned away.

If we only had a little pemmican to eat when the tent is pitched, we should not mind being fatigued, for pemmican is easily cooked, and then one can lie down and rest. But dog's flesh must be boiled for a long time to make it eatable at all, and it is hard to keep awake until it is done. We let it stew for about an hour and a quarter – we cannot wait any longer, and for the last five or ten minutes we are wakeful enough, digging and poking at the meat with a sail needle, to see if it is tender. As soon as we think it is cooked, soup and meat are divided as fairly as possible; the soup is what we value most, for there is not much meat, and what there is, is tough as leather. I have considerable difficulty in eating it, for my teeth are still loose from the scurvy, and to my great annoyance I cannot even pick the bones clean.

Lost in the Arctic: Being the story of the 'Alabama' Expedition 1909–12 (1913)
Captain Ejnar Mikkelsen

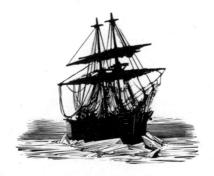

31

At the end of Kingsmith's cross-examination at 16.30 on the Wednesday afternoon, Mr Thornton announced that, in the light of the new evidence – the phone record and subsequent testimonies – he needed more time to consider all factors. He knew an event connected with Tom's legacy was being held the following evening, so he had *hoped* (and here a look specifically to Mrs Osman) to deliver his conclusion before that time. Instead it would be Friday morning.

'Better, actually,' Sawbridge said, packing his papers as the courtroom dispersed. 'Gives you a chance to recover before your big night. Chin up, it might be very therapeutic for you.'

Sean nodded and smiled, but he was dreading it. After these three days, his starring role would be a very particular form of torture. Smiling, pressing the flesh, raked over by five hundred pairs of eyes as he eulogised Tom. For once, he loathed the thought of the spotlight. At least in black tie he would blend in and disappear. And at least Angela and the Harding family had declined his invitation.

'You'll have Martine by your side,' Sawbridge said wistfully. 'She's rather wonderful.'

Sean smiled, but if Martine had suddenly needed to go away on business, he would have been glad. He wanted telly and wine and to bury himself in comfort. He wanted to disappear.

'Told you this was a bugger,' Sawbridge said, 'but you've done very well. Always tell my clients, book yourself a really good holiday afterwards. Push the boat out. These things are like throwing a bloody great rock in a pond – ripples long after the whole thing's past. Got to physically get away, mental and physical space. Move on.'

'Good idea.' Sean thought of the blazing chandeliers of the Carrington, the colossal floral arrangements, the swarms of dull people he would have to charm and connect and fan to life. 'Are you sure you won't come tomorrow? We can easily find you a place.'

'Good grief no, completely wrong signal, having me along. Make you look nervous! Never travel with your KC – unless you did it.' Sawbridge glanced up and his chortle died in his throat. He switched to sober respect incarnate. 'Mrs Harding.' He withdrew.

'Excuse me, Sean,' Angela touched his arm. 'You're probably very busy, but at six o'clock we're going to light candles in the cathedral for Tom, if you'd like to come?' She lowered her voice. 'I asked Ruth and a few other people. I – I just thought I'd ask you too.' She walked away quickly, before he could answer.

Relieved to have a reason not to go back to London straight away, Sean said goodbye to Kingsmith in the lobby – he would see him at the Carrington tomorrow evening. Sawbridge was visiting friends in Kent, and staying in Canterbury until the inquest was over. Back in his room in the White Bear, Sean checked his mail and messages. It was mercifully quiet, all his managers were good. Danny Long had nothing to report from Midgard, and Rupert Parch sent a cheery line confirming he would see him tomorrow evening, and that his master also sent his best wishes. He added an emoticon: a smiley face version of Munch's *Scream*.

Martine had left a voice message: everything was perfect and in place for tomorrow, it was going to be a triumph. She knew things must be OK or he would have called her, so she was out at a dinner tonight if he was still away, or cancelling it to be by his side if he needed her. Something in her tone hoped he wouldn't.

Sean texted back all was well but he had to stay another night. He'd call her tomorrow. He clicked on the x key. It looked strange. He made it a capital, and sent it. He emailed Jenny Flanders to ask if she had any time tomorrow before five. Then he put on his last clean shirt and went to the cathedral.

Angela Harding hadn't said where in the vast structure they would be. It was almost dark outside so the stained glass was subdued, but now the stone contours were alive in the candlelight. Once again, he followed the sound of singing deeper into the nave. The chapel where he had signed the book was dark and quiet, and the singing came from below. He found them in the chapel of Thomas Becket.

Tom's mother gladdened at the sight of him. 'Oh you came.' She embraced him as she had done all those years ago, when he used to wolf food at her table, and Granny Ruby rapped Tom's knuckles for dropping scraps for Roxy. She was there too, holding hands with Ruth Mott, who looked surprised to see him.

'Sean! I'm – it's good you came.'

'Thank you.' He kept his distance this time, standing with people he didn't recognise. But one knew him.

'All right?' It was John Burnham, the publican from the Feathers. They nodded awkwardly to each other. Sean was embarrassed at the thought of Sawbridge's superior attitude to the man.

'Here.' Angela Harding gave them each an unlit candle and moved on. They stood in silence, until Sean remembered Flip-flops.

'Do – do you have a daughter called Beth?'

'Oh, I know, she's been in there, hasn't she? I said, don't you make trouble—'

'She hasn't. She's extremely bright. I've got one too, a bit older.'

John Burnham's forbidding expression disappeared, and the trials of teenage daughters transformed them from wary mourners to commiserating fathers. Sean found himself speaking of Rosie as if she were still his loving daughter, until the deacon interrupted with her lit taper. She arranged them in a semi-circle, then in a high singsong voice asked for blessing on the friends and family of Tom Harding at this difficult time, before leading them in the Lord's Prayer.

Wanting to do the right thing, Sean murmured a few words, but it felt hypocritical so he tailed off into silence. Surreptitiously, he looked up to see what other people were doing, and caught Ruth doing the same. For a second they shared a complicit look, intercepted by the disapproving deacon. Ruth snorted with a giggle, which Angela Harding interpreted as tears, and reached out to hug her. This toppled Ruth into real grief, and they wept together.

Sean's eyes stayed dry. He could smell beer on John Burnham's clothes and it was a friendly smell. Tom's spirit wasn't in some cold crypt, solemn and spiritual as this was – it was in the diamond whirl of sunny Arctic air, or the clink of pints. It was rammed next to Sean at a gig, roaring along with the crowd, Ruth and Gail on their shoulders. It was racing on a sled in Greenland, and making the dogs howl in song when they bellowed their way through Bowie's 'Heroes'. *That* was the hymn he wanted to sing for Tom, he wanted to hear it blasting through the cathedral, and howl like a dog for the friend he'd lost.

He would never see Tom again. It hit him.

He felt Ruth looking at him again, and then the strange sensation in his face: his mouth was shaking, his eyes were burning, and something was running down his cheeks. Ruth left Angela and came to him. Without a word she put her arms around Sean and held him. He went rigid for a moment and then a great gasp came out of his mouth, and sobs began to tear out of his very core. He didn't know if the deacon was still speaking but he felt hands touching him, patting his back, rubbing his arm; he didn't know who it was and he was too ashamed to look. When he regained control, he apologised to whoever was there but he couldn't look up. He pulled away and hurried out of the crypt, back to the White Bear and went straight up to his room. He wasn't hungry, he didn't want a drink. He kicked off his shoes and crawled into bed. He curled himself into a ball, shaking.

Only in the morning, waking fully clothed under the covers he didn't remember pulling over himself, did he realise he'd slept the whole night through.

It is impossible to go through all the challenges faced by or limitations placed on the freedom of movement of ships. What makes the ensuing limitations or attempted restrictions on the freedom of movement so problematic is that they are undertaken multilaterally, by involving competent international organisations, as well as unilaterally or bilaterally. Such limitations are not easy to harmonise since they have different legal bases.

Furthermore, it is their cumulative impact on the freedom of navigation/right of innocent passage/transit passage which should be cause for concern as regards the legal framework established by the United Nations Convention on the Law of the Sea.

The legal situation in respect of international straits raises particular problems, given the enhanced status of international navigation.

Whether ships carrying weapons of mass destruction which are not targeted against a particular State may be interdicted on the high seas by warships of another State without the consent of the flag State concerned is a matter of controversy. The exclusive jurisdictional relationship between a flag State and one of its vessels on the high seas is well-rooted in customary international law.

Judge Rüdiger Wolfrum
President of the International Tribunal for the Law of the Sea
8 January 2008

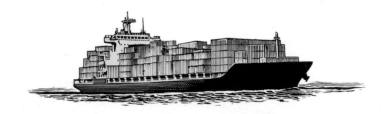

32

'I've been seeing Tom,' Sean said to Jenny Flanders, before he'd even sat down. After his full night's sleep, he had considered cancelling, but it felt right to keep the appointment. The end was in sight and this was part of the process of closure. She'd done some tidying since his last visit – the windows were sparkling clean and he could actually see the Victoria and Albert Museum in the distance. The rugs were brighter, and the cardboard boxes were gone – he felt relieved, as if a difficult decision had been made. So she was staying. She was all in beige again and he wondered if she had several copies of the outfit.

'No flowers today?' Some indistinct jade thing sat where the rude tulips had sprawled. 'I bought some afterwards, the same kind.'

She looked. 'Oh, the parrot tulips. They're seasonal,' she said. 'Very brief.'

'You've got a good memory.'

She smiled but did not speak. Suddenly he was anxious again. He'd come prepared to talk, but now he changed his mind. He kept his eyes on the jade thing. Bad feelings fluttered inside him like moths.

'You're not my friend, are you? I'm just paying you to listen to me.'

'That's right. But I still want to help you.'

'Then help me.' Sean felt himself slipping again, he heard himself talking, he hadn't even realised he had begun, but Jenny Flanders sat there with her pale eyes on him, nodding as he told her about the walrus wife in a film he'd seen who stayed to watch her mate be butchered on the ice, and how he would never have this kind of love with Martine, how he wasn't sure he even *liked* Martine, how Midgard Lodge was a dangerous place, with a maelstrom in the fjord now, new since the calving that brought out Tom's body, and how it wasn't true he was all crushed and purple, Tom still felt alive, he still couldn't quite believe he was dead, he didn't know what it was going to take if the funeral hadn't done it—

Sean had the sense of tipping out a great bag of rubbish on her sitting room floor. A great huge mess for her to sift through with her pals Jung or Freud or whoever she thought made sense of things. But Jenny Flanders just sat quietly. The rumble of traffic drifted in from the Cromwell Road. His fingers started burning. Soon it would be time to go to the Carrington.

'Why do you say Midgard Lodge is dangerous?'

'The Arctic is dangerous.' He went to the window. Outside, the plane tree leaves were still green, and people wore shirtsleeves and light dresses. 'It's all wrong. It's nearly Halloween but it's like summer. Any second we'll start hearing White Christmas, and we're never going to see another one of those at this latitude.' He came away from the window. 'No one wants to face the truth.'

'You said you've been seeing Tom.' There was a stillness to her, as if she were a statue, or a paralysed oracle. For some reason, Sean thought of Ursula Osman: agile and dusty and penetrating.

'Do other people with PTSD ... have what I have? Do they ... see things?'

'Sometimes.'

'And how do you treat them?'

'We start like this. Talking. It's a painful process.'

Sean stared out. He knew Ruth Mott was a friend again, despite what he had told Sawbridge about her. In the crypt, she had held him as only a true friend could. He was flooded with conviction he must make some reparation to her. He would ask her – humbly, not as a rich patron – if he could fund her to start her research again.

'You're smiling.' Her face reflected it.

'I was just thinking ... maybe I've got some things wrong.' Sean felt slightly dizzy at the thought. 'Midgard was supposed to be a good thing, but Tom died there. And it feels like ... it's getting out of my control – but I'm the CEO.' He felt his heart thumping, like it had when he saw the bear. 'Can you give me something to take, for anxiety?'

'You would have to see a medical doctor. I'm just a PhD, but I can refer.'

Sean felt the kayak swinging in the current. He put both hands down on the armchair to steady himself. He did not remember coming back from the window. He felt the bear's eyes on him, intelligent and intimate.

'I saw this bear. On the glacier. He was calculating how he could get to me, he wanted to eat me.' He put his hand on his chest and felt his heartbeat under his ribs. 'I imagine it. And at night I hear my blood in my ears. When Sawbridge first told me about you and suggested I might have it, PTSD, I thought he was joking. Do other people get that pumping sound? It's like bass coming through the wall. The vibration makes you feel sick.'

'Do you feel sick now?'

'Not physically. But what happened with Tom did something bad to me too.' The words fly round the room on their own. *What happened with Tom.*

Jenny Flanders re-crossed her legs, and he saw her inner thighs, pale and plump. He looked away. 'Nothing can bring him back. It's all over tomorrow morning. It's either climate change that made the cave fall in, in which case the whole world's to blame, or it was Ruth Mott keeping him up all night so that he was too tired to save himself. I got a full night's sleep and I survived. That's what it can come down to, a night's sleep. I was able to hang on and get out. But Tom slipped. He couldn't hang on.'

Jenny Flanders looked at him with the same kind expression. Sean realised his right hand was clamped in his left armpit, and his fingers were burning. He pulled it out. His eyes fell on the jade Buddha.

'You're not a Buddhist, are you?' he said again. 'It's just decoration.'

'That seems rather important to you.'

'It's like you're pretending to be someone you're not.'

'Me?'

Sean stared at the jade. The beautiful blue-green colour of the melt-water lakes, on the Midgard glacier. The seeping water, undermining everything. The colour of danger.

He got up. Jenny Flanders glanced at her watch.

'We still have some time.'

'No. We don't.'

'May I ask why you suddenly feel you have to go?'

He looked at her. 'Instinct.'

Only when he had pulled the big black front door shut behind him, did he breathe more deeply. One more day and it was over, and he and Martine – he winced at what he'd said about her in there – they could go somewhere, into nature, far from people. He wasn't sure if he meant it, that he didn't like her – or that it was even necessary to like the person you were with, all the time. He was exhausted, that was what it was, he needed to rest, and they could do that together, and then see.

Standing at her first-floor window, Jenny Flanders watched him go, then dialled a number. Two miles away in a small, unfavoured Whitehall office, Rupert Parch answered, and listened with interest.

In Svalbard on Christmas Day in 1921, trapper Georg Nilsen went out to visit the German research station at Kvadehuken. When he failed to arrive, two of the station members went out searching for him, but they too disappeared, their bodies not found until June 1922. Later that summer the German station master took his own life.

In 1965, the remains of a skeleton and a rifle were found – a cartridge jammed in its chamber. People believe that it was Georg Nilsen and his gun, and that he probably died when he met a polar bear, took aim and fired, but the bullet stuck. They speculate how he must have felt, as the bear came toward him, and killed him instead. They are careful to keep their weapons in full working order, but accidents still occur.

The jammed rifle is now in the Svalbard Museum.

As told to the author, Svalbard 2013

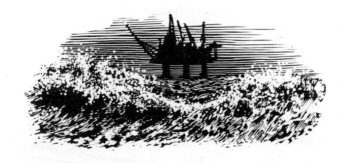

33

Sean's taxi pulled up under the illuminated portico of the Carrington. The smell of the flowers grew thicker as he went to find Martine in the ballroom. Everything was black and white with accents of gold, conservative elegance to reassure the donors. He looked at the big board of placement on the easel by the door, then decided he did not care who sat where. He felt in his pocket for the speech cards and then remembered he had left them on the dresser. It didn't matter, he didn't need notes. His deepest feelings about Tom were not a performance for this crowd, or the coroner. He'd present the award, say something truthful. Long, short, awkward, eloquent – it didn't bloody matter. Tom was dead.

Sean looked about him irritably. Martine was supposed to be here to meet him, or he would not have come this early. He checked his phone – still switched off after his troubling appointment with Jenny Flanders. He turned it back on, that electronic nipple he constantly sucked from.

'Sean – there's a problem with Midgard. Kingsmith's in a state.' Martine was at his side, her face strained. She was in a dress he hadn't seen before, a column of heavy lime-green silk which draped her small high breasts and dropped in a low V back, showing off her toned musculature and – he admired it dispassionately – boyish arse.

'What's the problem?'

'I don't know, he practically threw me out – he's got no respect for you if he talks to me like that. One minute we're having mint tea and planning a diving trip on *Brisingamen*, the next he gets a call from Danny Long and kicks me out.'

'Out of where?'

'His suite. Sean, I texted you to say I'd be there; it's huge, much better to get ready in. You're not jealous, are you? Are you calling him?'

Sean didn't answer, because his phone was on now and he scrolled down the list of calls – nothing from Danny Long, or Midgard, or Terry Bjornsen. Or Kingsmith.

'Shit.' Martine smoothed her dress, then waved across the room. 'Darius! I'm so glad you're first!' She touched Sean's arm before she left him. 'My investors have a stake in Midgard too, so whatever's going on, I need to know. But no drama.' Then she clicked into gear, a lithe green flame moving across the room to warm the wallets of the early birds.

Sean waited for the lift to the tenth-floor suites. He looked at the man in the copper-burnished mirror as he ascended. Good-looking, calm, entitled. Kingsmith did not have crises. He occasionally assisted in them and took his profit. But no one made money constantly, there had to be some reversals. Even for Kingsmith. More than likely, Martine's hostess stress had made her melodramatic. But Danny Long's phone went straight to message again.

He paused outside the door of Kingsmith's suite. At first there was silence, then he heard the muffled rise and fall of his voice. Sean knew at once by its timbre: Kingsmith was agitated. Not wanting to be caught eavesdropping, he squared his shoulders and pressed the buzzer. Immediately there was silence within. Kingsmith would be padding to the door to look through the spyhole. Then he opened the door, almost completely dressed but for the tie and shoes. He smiled broadly at Sean.

'Hey! Sean boy, you're through the fire. Come in, have a drink. How's it looking down there?'

'Battle-ready. They've started arriving.'

'What'll it be?' As Kingsmith went to the bar, Sean saw the laptop open on the console table. Kingsmith pushed the cover down as he passed, but not before Sean glimpsed the flashing green dots of the AIS shipping location screen.

Kingsmith held up a heavy crystal tumbler with a finger of topaz liquid. 'You don't like Scotch, but this is beyond that description. I bought some tweed from the island it comes from – that's all they do. Tweed and whisky.'

'Just water,' Sean said.

'Come on. The worst is behind you. You've been a star.'

'Martine said you got a call from Danny and there's a problem at Midgard. His phone's going straight to voicemail. So is Terry's. And the main office.'

'It's their weekend off. The weekend they only get every ten days – you want them there twenty-four seven, three-six-five?' Kingsmith grinned. 'Lucky they'll never have a union.' He stretched. 'Sometimes it's good for them all to kick back together. It's bonding; no visitors, nothing to do – so a whale breaches or a bear stops by; one time they miss it.'

'Joe. Is there a problem?'

'OK, OK. You know Danny, conscientious to a fault. He picked up a signal that he thought meant trouble, so he let me know.'

'You? But I've already told him—'

'Yes, me, Sean, because you know fuck-all about sailing, but I live on the ocean, remember? And by the way, have you made sure your pal in Oslo tips us off when something's going on up there, because the Sysselmann's office always forgets. It's like they don't trust us or something. Keep on that, OK?' Kingsmith was talking a lot, as genial as if he were a new contact.

'Who were you talking to before I buzzed? You sounded agitated.'

Kingsmith took another sip of his Scotch.

'Sean, I know women are your thing, or at least they were, but you are sounding like a jealous lover. Excuse my French, but I'm going to put it down to stress from that fucking inquest. Midgard might be the centre of your world, but believe me, it's not mine. So cut it out.' He smiled. 'Come on. Take the edge off with something.'

'I said just water.' Sean rubbed his forehead. Then he took out his phone and pressed the key for Danny Long. It went straight to voicemail again. 'Danny: it's Sean Cawson, your CEO. Call me immediately.' He hit the red button and looked at Kingsmith, ignoring the annoyance in his eyes. 'Joe, we both know he's always supposed to answer. His phone is never supposed to be off. You just spoke to him.'

'That wasn't him! And I am telling you, Sean, so listen to me: everything is cool. You really do need that vacation, so I've let Martine bully me into lending you *Brisingamen* in the Seychelles. Fully crewed. How does that sound?'

'It sounds like you've told them not to talk to me.'

Kingsmith broke their stare.

'You'll give yourself a nervous breakdown, which is what I'm trying to spare you after the week you've had. It's not a big deal, and we do not want to make it one, but there's a cargo ship with engine trouble. I didn't tell you straight off because I knew you'd freak. But if you insist, here, have it. It's no big deal.'

Sean forced himself to speak calmly. 'If a cargo ship is in trouble near Midgard Lodge then we have to render aid. It's part of our deal with Oslo.'

'*Our* deal? Way back when, right here in this room, you told me you were the only person to set it up and handle it, remember? Critically important it all went through you, and you alone. But don't worry: the vessel is not so near, and she hasn't requested assistance. She's doing OK.'

'Engine trouble in the Arctic, in October, how can that be OK?'

'I knew this would be too much for you right now, that's why I tried to shield you from it. You've had so much stress you've lost all perspective. For everyone's sake, step back and let me handle it.'

Kingsmith passed his hand over his bald head, and Sean heard the faint rasp. It was the one tell of Kingsmith's that he'd ever picked up on. He'd been too busy to shave – which meant an emergency. Out of the corner of his eye, Sean glimpsed another laptop on the bathroom counter.

'I need to pee.' He went in and clicked the lock before Kingsmith could stop him. He touched the mouse pad and the AIS screen popped to life, the green dots of ships bright on the black, but the central one unmoving. He clicked the mouse to enlarge the view of the Barents Sea – the irregular yellow line showed the contour of Wijdefjorden. Before he could further enlarge it the screen was turned off at source.

Sean flushed anyway.

Kingsmith tapped on the door. 'Sean. I've cut you some slack, but it's getting boring.' He paused. 'Come on out now.'

The instant he unlocked the door Kingsmith slammed it into him and took the laptop. He looked at Sean in the mirror.

'Don't do that again.' He went back out into the suite. 'And get out here. We are going to talk about what's been happening and I am going to tell you what you are going to do.'

Sean sat down, winded. Terry Bjornsen, Danny Long, all of them, were taking their instructions directly from Kingsmith. He'd never been their boss.

Kingsmith snapped his fingers in front of his face. 'More importantly,' he said, and Sean smelled the Scotch on his breath, 'you are not going to panic. You're going to stay calm and you're going to trust me, because if you don't, if you let your ego ride you any more – oh, we will come to that too – you will bring down more trouble than you knew one man could wreak in this world.' He clicked the laptop back on and turned it to face Sean. 'What do you see?'

'Wijdefjorden, just outside it. And right there, a ship, not moving.'

'She is, very slowly. She's only got a bit of engine trouble and they're fixing it as we speak, but if they haven't sorted it by the time she's into Icelandic waters and if she still needs it – then she'll get all the help she needs.'

'Why Iceland, when we could render aid now?'

Kingsmith smiled. 'Along with setting up that generous endowment in her name, for the Sino-Icelandic poetry translation prize, Radiance also bought a port. So your ship can go there.'

'*My* ship?'

'Sean boy, have I taught you nothing? First rule of business is good housekeeping. But you just see the dividends; you stopped looking at the delivery vehicles a long time ago. What was it you said? That's right: "*You understand them, so I don't have to.*"' Kingsmith chuckled. 'Out of the mouths of babes.'

Sean went cold. It was completely true. Kingsmith had been investing for him for twenty years. He'd grown his entire business from seed capital created in this way. He was financially grafted to Kingsmith's root stock.

'What have you put me into?'

'You don't want to know. Or rather, why start caring now, at this late hour?' Kingsmith's smile had faded. 'Don't feel too bad, most people are the same. Give them enough profit, and they'll skip the details. Unless they're very strategic too.'

An image of Radiance came to Sean, on the plane, three years ago. Her red toes wiggling as she trounced her online chess partner. The realisation clubbed him.

'You and Radiance – that was you she was playing chess with, on the plane. While you were in the bedroom. I didn't introduce you at all.'

'Sean, you kill me! Of course you didn't. But you just assumed you did, and it was funny. We were going to tell you, but somehow we missed the moment. And it made life easier, you know? Plus everyone underestimates her. She's a very clever girl. Speaks perfect English, good French and Russian, gets by in Arabic – but she puts on the bad grammar to let people feel superior.'

Sean got up. 'I don't own any ships. I've never signed anything.' But as he said it, he could not be sure.

'No, not wholly – but you share an interest with one of my other protégés. You've even had a private meeting with him, earlier this year, at Midgard. I'm sure Danny has some photographs of you two shaking hands.' Kingsmith watched him. 'I did try to stop you going, but you insisted ...'

'Benoit.'

'Benny boy, another eager protégé. You see? You are into Africa after all.'

Sean could barely breathe.

'You've used me. You're using Midgard – what are you using it for?'

'Now, Sean, don't be like Tom, going off half-cocked with half the facts. You of all people know how dangerous that can be.' Kingsmith looked him deep in the eye. 'Which is why you're not going to bother Danny or Terry or the Sysselmann because the—' Kingsmith stopped himself. 'Because the ship herself hasn't yet done that. And I don't think she's going to. I think she's going to be OK.'

'What's her name?'

'The Doesn't Fucking Matter.'

'What's she carrying?'

'Useful things.' He winked. 'So we want her to get where she's going.'

'You're supplying Radiance's businesses in Africa.'

'Sean boy! I'm starting to believe there's hope. Yes, *we* are. And can you guess what's the on-board treat?'

Sean could hardly bear to say it. 'You're taking arms across the Arctic and my name's on it.'

'Of course not; that would be illegal. Just home improvement supplies. Biodegradable 3D printers, 4D, if they can afford it; changes use over time – means elegant and ecologically approved deniability. Robotics are so impressive. Plus supplies, of course: raw materials, chemicals for all the full effects – no half-measures with Radiance and her pals.'

'Does Martine—' He couldn't bear to think of that.

'As if I'd do that to you! Anyway, she's a short-range thinker; she'd slip up as soon as it stopped being about her. Look at the glass half-full, Sean boy, see how our clever Radiance and her friends are investing to raise the standard of living for a whole country, once all the chaos, panic and disorder is cleared up. Even your secret friend Mrs Larssen needs a helping hand sometimes, and haven't you been a helpful errand boy to her?'

Kingsmith poured a Scotch and left it by him, then topped up his water from a carafe.

'And since we're having a frank chat, watch out for Philip Stowe – I find him slippery. Though I admit that having you as our go-between has made everyone's life a bit easier these last three years. So I'd say you'll be getting your Safety in the Home medal.' He went to the mirror and began to do his tie.

'Ah come on, lighten up. We're just clearing the air – and long overdue it is, too. Once you get over the shock, you'll see the funny side. You've been a great boy scout – without you, I'd have missed out on the TransPolar Route. I'm grateful!'

Sean sat rigid, trying to believe it. His money, his Midgard, tied into Kingsmith's arms trafficking. And it was true, he had brought Kingsmith into the very heart of the Arctic, he'd begged for his help in setting up Midgard's security. Or so he thought. In reality, he'd created an Arctic base for Kingsmith's mercenaries, tacitly approved by Philip Stowe. It could not be.

At ease, he'd said when Danny Long had introduced him to those men in the dorm room. The barracks – the standing force of men in Midgard's name – *his* name – and all the while he had refused to see it. It was like saying Defence Expo instead of Arms Fair, or alt-right instead of fascist. Kingsmith nodded to him in the mirror.

'Let's get you down off of that meat hook. You've done a good thing, you'll come to see that. You've created a service station on the newest trade route on the planet! International waters too, so no political shackles. Tom was all about the whales and the Inuit and the climate, but who knows what's going to happen? We won't be alive to see it.'

'My daughter will.'

'She'll be fine.' Kingsmith turned. 'How's that? Taken me years to get it right. I think I look pretty damn handsome. By the way, your British defence universities are the best in the world. But with all our business investment, so they should be.' He watched Sean sympathetically. 'How else do you think I know Philip Stowe? Tennis parties?' He sighed. 'Sean boy, stop with the suffering. Midgard is still a truly special place on earth, just not what you think. It's more; the reality is *better*. Don't lose heart – it's a foot in the Arctic door for British business. Follow Uncle Joe's advice and don't worry about one little ship in the night. Think about your knighthood.'

'Fuck the knighthood!' Sean stared at Kingsmith. It wasn't possible he'd misplaced his trust so badly. 'Did you – did you never believe in anything we were trying to do?'

'Hmm. How to say this nicely? It. Didn't. Matter. The world doesn't understand carrot, only stick. Midgard Lodge is a beautiful, organic, fairly traded exquisitely cooked, fucking carrot.' Kingsmith tied his shoes and finished his drink.

'But what is also true, is that you and Tom really did have this big romantic thing going on for the Arctic, and I loved that. You were so right to bring him in, you totally seduced the Pedersens. They even took less money, because you two so utterly believed in what you were selling. Midgard Lodge meets so many needs for so many people; I take my hat off to you.'

'What's happening with that ship. Pull it up again.'

Kingsmith smacked himself on the forehead.

'Sean, you've not understood a word I've said. You know how elegantly you dealt with that problem in the cave? I thought you might be a rightful successor, one day. Poor Tom, falling like that. Nothing you could have done.'

'What do you mean?' Sean stood up. 'What problem in the cave?'

Kingsmith shrugged. 'Your skilful leverage of force majeure. No need to tremble, come on, it's over. Back to the situation in hand – this is just another opportunity to practise. Life isn't black or white, it's in the grey, and if you weren't so fucking overwrought, I'd kick you up a grade and let you handle this one yourself. But as you *are* ... I'm telling you to stand down. Better to lose that ship than make a mess of the scale you'll create.'

They both became aware of someone knocking on the door. Kingsmith strode over – and then as he looked through the spyhole, his back relaxed, no longer gathered to strike. He beamed as he opened it.

'Martine! You look criminally gorgeous. Was I a bit short earlier? Forget about it, it's all sorted now. And may I say, Sean is one lucky bastard.'

She smiled thinly, then looked past him.

'Sean, you have to come! I cannot do this without you there. It's heaving, everyone wants to talk to you.'

Kingsmith stepped aside, making sure Martine saw him admire her. He gripped Sean's shoulder as he went out to join her, and smiled.

'Front of house. Very important.'

Sean went down in the lift with Martine, listening to her rattling off the people who'd come and the money they'd already raised. He looked at the immaculate man in the black tie, and the beautiful woman in the green backless dress.

The doors opened and the party hit him.

I was trapped. The hole was too small to let me get through, my beard would not let me retire into my grave again. I could see no way out. But what a way to die – my body twisted in an unnatural position, my beard frozen to the sled above, and the storm beating my face without mercy. My eyes and nose were soon filled with snow and I had no way of getting my hands out to wipe my face. The intense cold was penetrating my head, my face was beginning to freeze and would soon lose all feeling.

With all my strength I pulled my head back. At first the beard would not come free, but I went on pulling and my whiskers and some of my skin were torn off, and finally I got loose. I withdrew into my hole and stretched out once more. For a moment I was insanely grateful to be back in my grave, away from the cold and the tortuous position. But after a few seconds I was ready to laugh at my own stupidity. I was even worse off than before! While I had moved about more snow had made its way into the hole and I could hardly move, and the bear skin had settled under my back where I could not possibly get at it.

I gave up once more and let the hours pass without making another move. But I recovered some of my strength while I rested and my morale improved. I was alive after all. I had not eaten for hours, but my digestion felt all right. I got a new idea!

I had often seen dog's dung in the sled track and had noticed that it would freeze solid as a rock. Would not the cold have the same effect on human discharge? Repulsive as the thought was, I decided to try the experiment. I moved my bowels and from the excrement I managed to form a chisel-like instrument which I left to freeze. This time I was patient, I did not want to risk breaking my new tool by using it too soon. While I waited, the hole I had made filled up with fresh snow. It was soft and easy to remove, but I had to pull it down into my grave which was slowly filling up. At last I decided to try my chisel and it worked! Very gently and slowly I worked at the hole. As I dug I could feel the blood trickling down my face from scars where the beard had been torn away. Finally I thought the hole was large enough.

Vagrant Viking: My Life and Adventures (1953)
Peter Freuchen

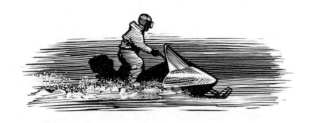

34

Pre-dinner cocktails were in the mirrored and filigreed Chinese Room. Sean's plan was to flash a smile with Martine then disappear somewhere he could check on the Svalbard shipping situation, but he found himself the target of pension chiefs, insurance barons and private bankers all wishing to offer their condolences about Tom – and re-imprint their faces as they did so.

He went to stand by the big photograph of Tom, hoisted on a gold easel by the bar as if at auction. The magnitude of what had just happened up there on the tenth floor was too great to take in. Part of him desperately wanted to believe Kingsmith, that maybe the ship had a bit of mechanical trouble, trouble that could be fixed enough to get it into Icelandic waters. That kind of thing happened all the time at sea. There were maritime insurance bosses in the room right now who wouldn't be remotely surprised to hear of losses or accidents unreported – it kept the prices down.

And how could he check what was really happening, when he didn't even know the ship's name? But of course that was not true. Sean put himself onto smile-and-nod autopilot, splitting his mind off to rack up his options. If the ship had not turned off its AIS locator then it could be found – there were not so many vessels in that area that it would take very long. Then, he could call the coastguard and raise the alarm by saying ... What? There's a ship in trouble in Svalbard waters, I believe it's trafficking arms across the TransPolar

Route and by the way I'm a part-owner. That's right, Sean Cawson of Midgard Lodge. Yes, the one your Assistant Defence Minister Mrs Larssen thinks of as a friend. Would I rather go to prison in the UK or Norway?

He exchanged small talk without hearing a word, his shirt sticking to his back. Soon they would all have to go in to dinner. If he disappeared now, Martine would definitely come looking for him. He was making the speech and presenting the award. Perhaps it was a grim joke Kingsmith was playing on him, telling him he was involved, simply to frighten him off raising the alarm. Or ... perhaps by the time he'd investigated which ship it was, the problem would be fixed, and he'd only make trouble. Jeopardise everything he'd worked for.

It was certainly true he was exhausted by the inquest. Maybe he should just focus on the dinner, and look into it afterwards. He'd trusted Kingsmith for years, what was one more night? And hadn't he just been to see Jenny Flanders this afternoon – it felt like years ago – to tell her he'd been hallucinating? Before he'd run out without knowing why. He looked up at Tom's handsome face, smiling back down at him.

'Is that him in Nepal? He climbed Everest and Annapurna, didn't he? Wow!'

Sean turned to see a pretty young waitress beside him, a glass of juice on a tray. She cleared her throat. 'Sorry to ramble! I was told to look after you.'

Across the room Sean saw Martine, the centre of attention of a grinning group, each member soon to be several thousand pounds lighter. Grateful for her thoughtfulness, he drank it. He watched her shine brighter with every man's attention. He turned to flirt with the waitress, but she'd already gone.

The juice was refreshing and primed him for a vodka tonic, which he drank in three pulls, to steady his nerves. *The world works in the now.* And here he was, in the thick of a buzzing social event, the Chinese Room full to capacity with smiling faces and laughing voices. Martine's green flame burned in another part of the room. Jenny Flanders was right: he did not trust himself. The week had shot his judgement – no wonder he'd had a run-in with Kingsmith. If the ship was really in danger, the crew would raise the alarm. But still, he had to know.

Sean slipped out into the great lobby and tried all the numbers again: Danny Long, Terry Bjornsen, Lodge reception. All went to voicemail. He tried getting onto the AIS system online from his phone but he needed a laptop. A false alarm would make trouble, but if there really was a terrible situation and he did nothing ... He pulled up the Sysselmann's emergency number on his phone, but did not press the call button. Suddenly his vision was blurry as a snow dome. He shook his head to clear it.

He wouldn't raise the alarm until he had spoken to Radiance. They had their own relationship independent of Kingsmith. They clicked – he got her, he liked her – he would just come out with it all, and she would laugh and put him straight – Kingsmith was a bad joker, right! That's what he needed to hear her say. Sean blinked away the black flashes in front of his eyes, trying to focus on the scroll of names. Then the phone was taken out of his hand and Kingsmith sat down heavily beside him. 'Don't even worry.' He laid his arm over Sean's shoulder as he pocketed the phone. 'I was looking for you to tell you it's all sorted.' He clapped Sean on the shoulder in his old familiar way. 'Relax already.'

Sean wanted to push him off, but his body wouldn't do it.

'You're lying.' His voice was thick in his ears.

'A lie down? Good idea. You're probably feeling a bit strange. But first, look at all the people who want to meet you!'

Sean saw the lime green flash of Martine's dress and tried to get up.

'Easy now.' Kingsmith kept him down and she approached, trailing a group of young men in old-fashioned black tie, with short side-parted combed-back hair. A few wore tweed Alpine plus-four trousers and roll-neck sweaters. They were in their early and mid-twenties. They all smiled at Sean.

'The Lost Explorers' Society bought a table and they can't wait to meet you.'

Sean stared as one by one the young men came forward and introduced themselves to him, effusive in support of the event, of Tom, of finding Arctic careers now it was all opening up. They surrounded him, eager and loud. Their features blurred and a tumble of noises came out of their mouths. His brain felt like some heavy cold weight was sliding around inside.

'Sir? Are you all right?' one of them asked.

'Boys,' Martine stepped in, 'it's been a tough week. Go have a drink. We'll see you later.'

All Sean could feel was the burning in his fingers. Kingsmith leaned down.

'PTSD,' he said in Sean's ear. 'Hallucinations, delusions. The stress of an inquest could definitely trigger it.' He dropped his voice even more. 'So can guilt. That's what Jenny Flanders says.'

At that name Sean twisted round and slipped. Kingsmith hoisted him up. 'Martine,' he said, 'our boy's had one too many – and I don't blame him. You better do the Tom eulogy. It's too much for him.'

Martine crouched down in front of him. Sean saw the concern – and irritation – in her eyes. She slid a golden arm around him. 'Oh, darling.'

Sean's mind clung to consciousness. Joe had his phone. Martine must not go. He reached for her hand and grabbed her dress instead. She pulled back and he felt it rip.

'You're right,' she said to Kingsmith. 'Take him. I'm really sorry.'

'Don't you worry about a thing,' he said. 'It's been tough on you too, princess, and it won't be the first time he's crashed with me. I'll take care of him.'

The green shimmer disappeared, then Sean felt himself hoisted up.

'When you're so tired,' Kingsmith said in Sean's ear as he hauled him towards the lifts, 'sometimes even a juice can put you over the edge. Lucky I'm here.'

The impeccable staff took care not to notice the over-refreshed guest, being assisted by his older and very solicitous pal. Sean felt the rising motion and shut his eyes against the gold and mirrors. The doors opened with a long hiss and he staggered along the deep mossy carpet, one wrist tight in Kingsmith's grip, the older man's sinewy arm around his torso. Whatever he had been given was coming on even stronger now.

'You just sleep it off, Sean boy,' Kingsmith gritted in his ear, 'where I can keep an eye on you and make sure you don't do anything stupid and dangerous – like touch the fucking phone when I told you not to.'

He held him against the wall while he used his key card. 'And I thought Tom was the problem.' He opened the door, quickly checked up and down the empty corridor, then flung Sean in with great force. The door clicked shut behind them.

The carpet slammed into Sean's face and body but did not hurt. He saw Kingsmith's black patent dress shoes very close to his face, then one of them lifted up.

He felt the blow in his stomach and heard the gasp – but still there was no pain. He heard the order to get up, he was struggling to do that anyway—

From his knees to the floor again, then the blows – he kept his brain awake counting them – one two three—

Instinct rolled Sean into a ball, coughing. His shirt was tearing – he was being hauled to his feet, he still couldn't feel his legs but somehow he was flying backwards, landing on something soft—

Kingsmith was in his face, he bent over Sean as he half sat, half sprawled on the sofa. He punched him twice in the face, and the picture of the icebergs filled Sean's mind. Great big icebergs, the glassy green foot—

He felt his body jerking under the blows, he kept his imagination on the icebergs, the pink light on the strange shapes—

'Tired – and emotional.' Kingsmith stopped and stood back, breathing hard.

Sean returned to consciousness with the shock of water flung in his face. He coughed. He felt himself grabbed up, his hands flailed for something to hold on to. He smelled the Scotch, heard the familiar voice.

'You know what happened, Sean boy?' Kingsmith held him by his lapels so that he could punch him again. 'You needed some air. You got in a fight outside, some poor fucking taxi driver I had to pay off not to make a scandal. You – were very – *stupid!* Lucky for you I was *there.*'

A ping came from the laptop, and Kingsmith paused his assault and went to check. He sipped his Scotch, then brought the rest of the glass back and forced it into Sean's mouth. 'What a fucking waste, but you just couldn't stop, could you?' He slapped Sean around the face. 'You're a lazy – greedy – little – fucker, and that's why I'm having to do this, you hear me? Everything I've done for you, but you've got – no – fucking – *loyalty.*'

Sean felt his body jerk with different impacts, but the drug muffled the pain.

They were all as children, yet they had served us well. They had, at times, tried our tempers and taxed our patience; but after all they had been faithful and efficient. Moreover, it must not be forgotten that I had known every member of the tribe for nearly a quarter of a century, until I had come to regard them with a kindly and personal interest, which any man must feel with regard to the members of any inferior race who had been accustomed to respect and depend upon him during the greater part of his adult life. We left them all supplied with the simple necessities of Arctic life better than they had ever been before, while those who had participated in the sledge journey and the winter and spring work on the northern shore of Grant Land were really so enriched by our gifts that they assumed the importance and standing of Arctic millionaires.

The North Pole (1910)
Robert E. Peary

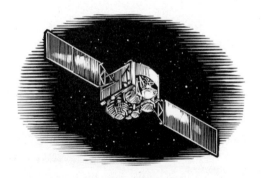

35

Half an hour before the sun rose over London, long after the Grand Ballroom of the Carrington had been restored to cleanliness and order and Tom Harding's photograph taken home by an ardent waitress, Sean woke breathless with pain. He rolled over to touch Martine – who was not there – and he gasped as his face pressed against some cold hard thing. He could hear a strange ragged rumbling sound, and he realised he was lying on the floor. Very slowly he opened his swollen eyes.

He was on the carpet in the gap between a sofa and a coffee table. So many parts of his body hurt as he slowly turned his head, but instinct told him not to make a sound. A furlong of carpet led to the dark cave of a room, the source of the rumbling sound. A man's snore. He deciphered heavy gold drapes. Rugs. Huge vases of flowers. The silver oblong of a laptop on the table. This was Kingsmith's suite, and something bad had happened.

His tongue explored slippery clots on the inside of his sore cheeks – he let one fall out onto the carpet. Dark bloody jelly, from where his own teeth had cut into his mouth. He couldn't think why he was lying here and the pounding in his brain made him lay his head back down. Nausea swirled in his guts. Through the glass of the coffee table he could see the crystal hobnails of a tumbler of water. As he moved slowly to try to reach it, he saw something else. Attached to the underside of the table frame was a round silver button. A circle of matt metal with a shiny central depression. Swallowing the gasp of pain, Sean twisted his head to check that Kingsmith was not stirring. Then he reached up and pulled the button off the frame.

Held on by ineffective double-sided tape, it dropped to the carpet. Sean lunged to retrieve it and lie still, just as he felt the shift in the floor as, from the bedroom beyond, a heavy form got out of bed and padded into another room. He heard Kingsmith urinating, but not flushing. He clicked the silver button repeatedly then closed his hand over it and lay perfectly still as he felt the footsteps come closer. The red of his eyelids turned black and he knew Kingsmith was standing over him. Then he felt the sofa being pulled back, exposing him. The door buzzer rang, and Kingsmith muttered. Sean felt his footsteps move away, then Kingsmith called out he didn't need anything.

Sean clicked the silver button again and again before he felt Kingsmith's tread returning. He still didn't know what had happened but he kept his eyes shut.

'Sean, I know you're awake. So stupid: you did this to yourself.'

The door buzzer rang again, and this time Kingsmith swore. As Sean felt him move away he staggered to his feet, ignoring the pain.

'Help me!' he shouted hoarsely as the door opened. 'Don't go!'

Kingsmith spun around, but the butler had seen him. Sean caught his shocked expression in the moment before Kingsmith tried to close the door.

'We're fine.'

'Are you sure, sir?' The butler was young and slight, but he put his foot in the door against Kingsmith's pressure, long enough for Sean to crash the older man aside and break out.

Sean lunged into the corridor, where mirrors reflected a bloodied man in black tie. Other butlers hurried down the corridor towards the room, panic in their averted eyes. Behind him he could hear Kingsmith calling to him to come back – *Sean boy!* – but he stumbled on, his vision still blurry and his head splitting. He hit his fist at every door buzzer, he knew he needed witnesses – but no one came out and no one stopped him. A frightened-looking maid jumped back as she came out of the staff staircase and Sean barged through and grabbed hold of the brass rail, the only thing he could focus on, and started running down the black and white stairs until there were no more and he found himself in a lobby that smelled of disinfectant and food, where more faces stared at him.

He was on the service floor, doors in all directions. Through one pair he could hear noise and bustle, he went in and it was the kitchen, bustling with the breakfast orders. Nobody stopped him; instead, they opened doors for him, passing him through their space as fast as they could, until Sean found himself out in the cold air by the huge waste bins. Someone was gripping his arm then a gate was opening and hands were pushing him through it – and Sean found himself on his knees on the grey and grimy Mayfair pavement, at dawn.

Automatically he reached for his phone that was not there. He got to his feet and managed to walk to the kerb, to the corner. His head felt like an axe was jammed through his skull, every pulse of his blood hurt the back of his eyes – he went to the corner and stared out.

Kingsmith sitting down beside him. Taking his phone.

He heard the surge of Park Lane. A cab went by with its yellow light on, but when he stuck out his hand it accelerated past him. The next cab switched its light off, and the next. He put his hand up to his face, and his fingers came away with blood on them. The corner of his mouth was bleeding again. He looked down and saw the blood on his shirt front. Why had Kingsmith taken his phone? Why was he frightened of him?

The corridor, the stream of butlers – Sean started walking towards Park Lane, just because he knew the route. The way home. He had to go home, he knew that, and if he got into the park he could walk.

Horns blared as he stepped into the traffic, he held up his arm and crossed over to the central grass reservation of Park Lane, and then stared up towards Marble Arch, where the red buses loomed. He waited until two of them went past, then stumbled across the south-bound lane, with more screeching horns. The green of the park was ahead, he could feel the cool of it. He stared at the trees. He walked unsteadily along the black metal railings until he found a gate. He was just about to go into the park when he saw them, in the distance. The cavalry horses, being exercised.

Even now, bleeding and blurry, the horses held him. He hung on to the railing, focusing on the animals gathering on the curve. He was in time, they were starting to trot – he felt pain in his face as he smiled, they were going to canter and he was right there—

He felt them in his feet, he heard one of the riders shouting at him to stay back, and then they were upon him, he felt the rhythm of their feet in his body, he saw the light on their necks and the darker sweat patches, the flowing black manes and tails – their sweet warm animal smell cut through whatever was in his head—

Sean, are you at home? I've got bad news—

The horses passed by and then there was just the vast expanse of Hyde Park before him, and the roar of morning traffic behind him. Sean kept hold of the railings.

Sean boy, they've found Tom—

Tom's inquest. Tom's inquest, the last day in Canterbury, starting this morning. And there, across Park Lane, the Carrington hotel, and Joe Kingsmith – and the ship, the ship he remembered it now—

He spat in his hands and pushed back his hair, pulled his lapels up to hide the worst of the blood stains, and drew himself up straight. Then he ran back to Park Lane and in the most autocratic way he could, raised his arm at the next taxi with its light on, and jumped in before the driver could object.

'Canterbury,' he said into the intercom.

'Canterbury? You need a hospital, mate.' The driver frowned at him in the mirror. 'I'll take you.'

'No. I have to get to Canterbury for the summing up.' Sean fumbled at his wrist and took off his watch. He wiped some blood off it and passed it through the window. 'I have to get there. You can have this if you take me.' Horns blared as the driver pulled across into the slip road at the top of the park, and stopped to examine it. He looked back at Sean in the mirror.

'This feels real.'

Sean winced as his smile split his lip again. 'I know.'

'It's a Cosmograph. My son's dream.' The cabbie held it up so the light caught on the ice-blue face. 'Sure now? Can't change your mind halfway.'

'I won't.'

Sean sat back and closed his eyes. He thought his nose might be broken, but he didn't want to check in case he started bleeding. He worked backwards, to take his mind off the lurching and bumping of the ride. The white twisting stairs with the shiny handrails, the staring staff, the open door out to big wheelie bins – the Carrington hotel. Kingsmith's carpet. The laptop on the table. *The ship.* He clicked the intercom.

'I need the news. I have to hear the news, Radio Four—'

The cabbie muttered something but changed the channel. Sean listened. Voices arguing, but nothing about any ship. He sat back, paralysed by the fear of what he was about to do.

At 8 a.m. the driver turned the news up without being asked.

'Just in case I'm an accessory, mate,' he called back. He held up the watch. 'Still got a deal, though.' In the back, Sean listened equally attentively. He was rewarded, or punished, with the last item, an as yet unconfirmed report of a capsized cargo ship off the coast of Svalbard, travelling late in the season on the still-contentious TransPolar Route. Reports just coming in suggested fuel oil was already leaking into the water, threatening the pristine Arctic archipelago of Svalbard. The presenter hesitated, then with great excitement told of the latest report, that there had been a firefight between rival rescue teams. They would of course bring more details when they had them. They moved on to the environmental threat, the risks of shipping, and three, two, one, segued to the stagnant situation in Suez, before the sports news.

Sean stared out unseeing. A firefight between rival rescue teams. One would surely be Midgard. The other – probably Russian. Kingsmith left the Russians alone, even he knew his limitations. But if he was trafficking arms through Russian-contested territory – and the TransPolar Route ran right across the Lomonosov Ridge – then he might well prefer to lose the cargo than face that music. No wonder he wanted to get the ship to Icelandic waters. Or – Sean felt sick at the possibility – let it go down, rather than be exposed.

He wanted to weep at his own stupidity. But it wasn't just his: he was the trusting go-between, but Philip Stowe and Mrs Larssen imagined they'd bought themselves a guard-dog at Midgard – they were duped too. At least the Midgard clients were simply greedy and vain, delighted to feel they were worth a standing security detail of presidential calibre.

All he'd seen was the money multiplying from everything he did with Kingsmith, more than he could keep track of – and so he didn't.

If Kingsmith told him something was good, it invariably was – financially. He'd had the freedom to do whatever he wanted with it, and what had he chosen?

Any and everything to claim his place at the top table, to feel secure. It was not enough to be married to a woman he had loved and whose background gave him status, not enough to be able to dishonourably indulge himself with the stream of beautiful women passing through his clubs. Not enough to be rich, to break bread with and profit massively from the appetites of the 1 per cent he catered to. Because nothing was ever enough.

You always were a greedy little bastard—

Kingsmith was right. And so was Tom, who had never really trusted Kingsmith, even that first night at the Randolph Hotel. His own frozen friend, ever ready to take on injustice and cruelty whenever he found it. But Sean had valued money and position more highly.

He caught the cabbie's eye in the mirror. They were now in the slow approach to Canterbury, where a state school gate was crowded with parents depositing their children, and the traffic crawled. Men and women were kissing their children goodbye. His vision was less blurry now, and he saw the pictures on the cabbie's dashboard – a young couple with two small children. Son and grandkids, he guessed. They were on the ring road outside the old city walls. Almost there. He braced himself for what was coming.

Emergency kit
*During the 1940s and 1950s ... the Canadian government, in order
to establish sovereignty in the Arctic, essentially forced the Inuit into
settlements, in some cases moving entire populations hundreds of
kilometres from their homes. There was one old man who refused to
go. Fearful for his life, his family took away all of his tools and
weapons, thinking this would oblige him to leave the land. Instead,
in the midst of a winter storm, he stepped out of their igloo,
defecated, and honed the feces into a frozen blade, which he
sharpened with a spray of saliva. With this knife, forged by the cold
from human waste, he killed a dog. Using its rib cage as a sled and
its hide to harness another dog, he disappeared into the darkness.*

As told by Olayak Narqitarvik to anthropologist Wade Davis in Arctic
   Bay, Canada
The Wayfinders: Why Ancient Wisdom Matters in the Modern World
   (2009)
Wade Davis

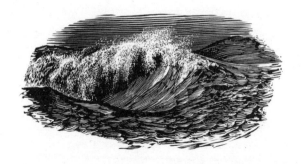

36

The cabbie switched on the intercom.

'Say where.'

Sean looked out as they passed the street the court was on, and saw the white outside broadcast vans and a small crowd. 'Two more blocks.'

The cabbie went on, then pulled over. He had the watch on his wrist now.

'Can't change your mind.'

'I haven't.' Sean looked at the photograph on the dashboard. 'Is that your son? The one who loves watches?'

'Yeah.' A world of pride in that one syllable.

'Tell him enjoy it. And get a better dream.'

Sean got out and the cab pulled away almost as he slammed the door. He stood on the street, stunned by the sudden pain. The interior of the cab was limbo, it was unreal, but now he was here, the court was two blocks away. He didn't have to go, he could go to hospital instead. He felt the bruising and rawness and pulsing of what he was sure was his broken nose. He doubled over and was sick, traffic hooting at the debauched sight, at this decent family hour.

He didn't have to go through with it, he could call Martine – now he thought of her, in her green dress – the benefit – but he had never memorised her mobile number. He could go into any police station, any hospital – he found himself walking down the street to the grim-looking pub, the Feathers, where he and Sawbridge had gone a thousand years ago. He could stop here, for a moment.

The front door was shut but there was a side gate for deliveries, and before he could lose his nerve he stepped through into the brick court-yard. A radio was playing inside the building. He went closer. He could see into the kitchen, were John Burnham was at the stove frying bacon, and Flip-flops, his daughter Beth, was sitting at the yellow table eating cereal and checking her phone.

'What the—' John Burnham spun round, fists ready as Sean came in. Then he recognised him. 'Who did this?' Before Sean could answer, he went outside and looked around. Then he locked the gate to the street and came back.

'There's a ship sinking off the coast of Svalbard,' Beth said. 'It's on the news. Is that to do with you?'

'You wait a minute, miss,' said her father. He turned to Sean. 'What the fuck's going on? Why are you here?'

'I – came here because – you were a friend of Tom's. And I'm testi-fying again. I don't want to make trouble for you …'

John Burnham stared at him. He sighed as he sat down. 'A friend of Tom's is a friend of mine.'

Sean felt his lip and saw the blood on his fingers. 'Do you need to warn anyone I'm here? I'm not too pretty.'

'Don't worry.' His daughter put a mug in front of Sean. 'It's a pub. We've seen worse. Milk?' She added it anyway.

Sean wanted to smile, but it would split his lip again. 'You're lucky,' he said to Burnham, who looked at his daughter. She pulled a face at him.

'When she's not gurning, or kicking off.' But there was love in his eyes. 'What's yours again? Rosie?'

'Yes. Did I tell you?'

'In the crypt, mate. Smells and bells.'

Now Sean remembered. The hands on his shoulders, the people around him. Talking to John about their daughters. That feeling that tore out of his chest, in great gasps.

'If you want to get there, I'll go with you.'

'And can I take your photograph? Can I write about it? Dad you know this is far more important than school, so don't even try.' Beth looked at Sean. 'It's the summing up now, isn't it?'

'Conclusion,' he said. 'Be accurate.'

'Conclusion. Thank you.' She took his picture with her phone. 'Seize your chances, that's what you said in your interview. Do you want to clean up? Or is it better all bloodstained? Bloodstained. Can I interview you?'

'Afterwards.' Sean closed his eyes.

At first the journalists and waiting crowd just saw the stocky figure of John Burnham striding down the street in his white trainers and jeans, beefy arms loose, Spurs supporter shirt tight over his barrel chest and belly. His slip of a daughter hurried alongside. It was only when they passed the first of the outside broadcast vans that anyone noticed the state of the man behind them, and who it was. First they stared, then they shouted.

'Mr Cawson! Sean! Sean, what happened? Sean, do you know anything about this ship? Sean, over here – can we have a word?'

John Burnham shoved their cameras and microphones back at them and Beth blocked their lenses with her schoolbag. A small crowd of young people clustered together in the street. Some had placards saying *Save the Arctic*. When they saw Sean, they ran towards him, their faces distorted with anger.

'Arctic poisoner!' shouted a girl, and someone else screamed 'Save the Arctic!' but John Burnham was well practised in crowd control. He opened his big arms wide and took up position on the steps, holding them back so that Sean could get into the court, but one girl darted through and grabbed Sean's arm.

'Dad, what have you done?' cried Rosie – and then she saw the state of him.

Sean threw his arm round her and John Burnham understood. He blocked the rest and Sean pulled his daughter into the lobby. They stared at each other.

'Dad.' Rosie's eyes were full of tears. 'What have you done?'

'I'm going to make it right.'

'You can't!' she cried. 'There's no way—'

'Yes. There is.'

'Of course there is,' Sawbridge came forward, 'and I must say we're all very glad to see you. My god, London's getting so rough, I hope you reported it. Quite the panic, everyone looking for you.' He flashed a quick smile. 'You must be Rosie.'

'I want to speak to my father.' She was trembling.

'Of course, but we have a rather urgent matter in hand – Sean, a private word?'

'A ship is going down in the Arctic!' cried Rosie. 'What's more urgent than that!' Then she saw Martine running forward and her face hardened. Dressed for work and with evidence of crying, Martine ignored Rosie and grabbed Sean.

'I've been going crazy wondering where you are! Joe said you ran away – no one knew where you were – why didn't you call me?'

'No phone,' Sean said. 'That hurts where you're holding me.'

'Joe's been trying to find you – even Rupert's been calling the whole time.'

'Parch? Did he know about the ship?' Sean drew back. 'Do you?'

'Me? Of course not! I heard on the news, but it's got nothing to do with us. Has it?'

'Absolutely nothing.' Sawbridge stepped between Sean and Martine, and included Rosie in his caring authoritative look. He lowered his voice. 'Were they migrants, do you think?'

'*Migrants?* What are you talking about?'

'Chaps who attacked you. Or was it only one? Very brave to tackle you, but of course drugs do that. I've heard they hang around the best hotels, picking off the wealthy and well-refreshed. We really must give the police greater power—'

'Dad! Talk to me!'

'Your father's got a crisis to deal with.' Martine tried to be kind. 'You can see him later, I promise.'

'Don't tell me when I can see my father!'

'Ah, splendid, it's free.' Sawbridge threw open the door to the small meeting room they had used before, but before he could guide Sean in, Mr Thornton appeared.

The coroner stopped at the sight of him. 'Good grief, Mr Cawson. What on earth happened?'

'I have to testify again.' Sean felt the blood seep from his lip.

'He can't, Your Honour,' put in Sawbridge, 'you can see he's not fit to—'

'He needs to go to hospital at once,' Martine agreed.

'Shut up!' Rosie looked as if she were about to punch her. 'If that's what my dad wants—'

Sawbridge blocked Sean's way. 'It's PTSD, this poor man—'

'Mr Cawson will testify,' the coroner told his clerk. 'Any more? No? Good.' They went on.

'Please, dear chap,' Sawbridge implored Sean. 'It's been beyond abominable for you, but I beg you, don't waste it all now. We are so close. It's so nearly all over. Think of Tom's family, and what's kindest for them.'

'I am.' But Sean stepped inside. Martine followed, her phone in her hand.

'It's Rupert, he won't stop ringing me until I let him speak to you to prove you're alive.' She gave him her phone.

Sean took it. 'What.'

'Man alive, am I glad to hear you!' Parch sounded like he was outside somewhere windy. 'What the fuck happened? Martine says you were mugged outside the Carrington? London's like Mogadishu these days. Are you OK?' His voice seemed to move inside. 'Course you're not. Matey, you're beyond heroic, getting yourself back there, but it just proves you're off the scale. No one expects you to say another word, you need the best TLC money can buy. A car's on its way—'

'No.' Sean turned away from Sawbridge and Martine's intent gaze. He felt Rosie take his hand, and he squeezed it gently.

'*Yes*, matey,' said Parch. 'Because you've got PTSD, which rhymes with, get out of jail free. Do you understand what I'm saying?'

Sean glanced at Sawbridge, his debonair expression forgotten. He felt his daughter's hand in his. Warm and alive.

'Tell me, so I do.'

'OK, listen: all the goodwill you have so brilliantly earned, truly you have, and all the rewards for which you are so truly deserving, are still yours if you'll only—'

'I won't. Goodbye.' Sean pressed the red button and returned Martine her phone. She stared at him in horror.

'Dear me.' Sawbridge shook his head. 'Sean, even if you senselessly throw yourself on Tom's publicity pyre, nothing will bring him back.

It's not heroic, it's pure self-indulgence. You're deeply unwell, you're injured – you need help.'

'What's happened with that ship?' Sean slammed his hand down on the table so hard Sawbridge jumped. Martine's eyes filled with angry tears.

'No one knows! I don't know, Nicholas doesn't know, it's only just been on the news! The *Zheng He* has nothing to do with us, and if it does then I've got fifteen per cent equity in a disaster and what are my investors going to say?'

'The *Zheng He*. You knew its name.' He almost laughed. 'Was it sabotage? Look how upset Joe got with me, when I suggested going public.'

'They said the name on the bloody radio! Sean, you're crazy. Surely you're not saying Joe did this to you? OK, you're done – I'm calling an ambulance—'

'Leave him alone!' Rosie stepped in front of her father.

'Security!' called Martine. 'We need help in here!'

'Rosie, stop it,' Sean said to her, as two stewards arrived.

'She needs to leave,' Martine told them.

'Don't touch my child.' Sean turned to Rosie. 'Now you can sit in court or—'

'Don't tell *me* what to do,' she cried. 'You've made this fucking mess.'

The stewards stood back to let her pass.

Just under two thousand miles away to the north, the stricken *Zheng He* lay on her side in the Barents Sea, off the coast of Svalbard. Helicopters from Longyearbyen, Barentsburg, Midgard Lodge threshed the freezing air above and harnessed news cameramen zoomed in as close as possible on the black seep spreading out across the water.

The closest vessel was the Sysselmann's new coastguard boat, and others bearing the Norwegian flag blocked the Russian tug and the two RIBs from Midgard Lodge, one of which was now disabled and roped to the other. A high wind stopped the sound of the conflicting tannoy shouts being intelligible to the news crews in the air, but it was clear that it was not a united rescue effort. The *Zheng He* reared up as if she would right herself – and then, very slowly, tipped up on her stern and began pointing her bow to the sky.

Outside, in the street directly below the windows of Court No. 1, a roar went up – and it was clear that the crowd of demonstrators had swelled. 'She's sinking! She's sinking!' And the boos started.

'There's nothing I can do about the noise,' Mr Thornton told his courtroom. 'And may I remind you all, that in this room we are strictly concerned with the events concerning the tragic death of Mr Thomas Walter Harding in Svalbard three years ago – and not this morning's news. As of 9 a.m. I was ready to deliver my conclusion, but between then and now, we have had an extraordinary request which I must grant. Mr Cawson has asked to make additional testimony, so thank you for your patience.'

'Dear chap,' murmured Sawbridge, 'I *implore* you. Let me handle it, it will all be all right. You're about to cross the finish line, it's all over—'

Sean stood. 'I'm ready.'

In the time it took for Sean Cawson to walk up the aisle and take the secular oath, the Sysselmann's vessels moved back, the Midgard boats and the Russian tug pushed even further away, guarded by every boat the coastguard had. Helicopters hung overhead, pulverising the air. Slowly, the bow of the *Zheng He* began to rise, so that at first it appeared that her 400-metre length was rising up out of the sea like a metal iceberg, the water cascading like skirts from her sides. She balanced upright on her stern for one long moment, and then as gracefully as she had risen, with news cameras her witnesses, she sank into the frigid deep of the Barents Sea.

And now from the far-away western horizon a fiery serpent writhed itself up over the sky, shining brighter and brighter as it came. It split into three, all brilliantly glittering. Then the colours changed. The serpent to the south turned almost ruby-red, with spots of yellow; the one in the middle, yellow; and the one to the north, greenish-white. Sheafs of rays swept along the sides of the serpents, driven through the ether-like waves before a storm-wind. They sway backwards and forward, now strong, now fainter again. The serpents reached and passed the zenith. Though I was thinly dressed and shivering with cold, I could not tear myself away till the spectacle was over, and only a faintly-glowing fiery serpent near the western horizon showed where it had begun.

Tuesday, 28 November 1893
Farthest North: The Norwegian Polar Expedition 1893–1896 (1897)
Fridtjof Nansen

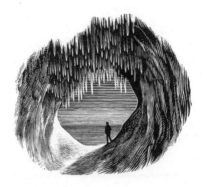

37

In Court No. 1, Mr Allan Thornton studied the man on the stand.

'I have to say, I'm very concerned by your physical state. Are you both mentally and physically fit enough to testify?'

'Of course he's not, look at him!' Sawbridge called out.

'I am.'

Ruth Mott nodded, her eyes never leaving Sean. Beside her, Angela Harding and the family were like stone. On the press bench, the keys tapped like rain. And then moments later, a great boo rose up from the street.

'Ignore it,' said the coroner. 'Go on.'

'Everything happened as I said,' Sean continued. 'But I left certain things out. When we went up for the eclipse, Tom discovered that we – my other partners and I – had a wider agenda for Midgard Lodge than he knew about. Ruth was right, he did find weapons.'

'*Yes!*' she said, and he saw in her eyes she was willing him on.

'I tried to explain they were for the good – because I was allowing Midgard to be used as a base to help Norway gather intelligence on Russia—'

'Intelligence gathering?' The coroner leaned forward.

'Not personally. But I enabled it.' Sean avoided Martine's burning glare. Sawbridge had his hand over his mouth. Mrs Osman sat calmly as her two aides made rapid notes. The only person in the room he felt connected to was Ruth. Her clear gaze steadied his freefall. *Don't stop now.* He nodded to her.

'I agreed to use the cover of our in-house security to host a small private militia, which I arranged through Joe Kingsmith and which would be available to the Norwegian government should they need it. Tom was furious. He was going to publicly denounce it and withdraw his name.'

He saw Martine whisper in Sawbridge's ear and Sawbridge push her back, intently focused on his client's self-destruction. Mrs Osman put up her hand.

'Absolutely not – Mr Cawson, please go on.'

'Ruth Mott met Joe Kingsmith when we all went to the restaurant in Longyearbyen. Greenland came up, and his business interests – his mining, and they got in an argument. Next day, Tom saw the strong room and he thought the worst.'

'Meaning?'

'He thought I'd deceived him. But we didn't get to that because we never got to talk properly. We went to the ice-cave and ...' Sean stopped and wiped a hand over his forehead.

'Mr Cawson, your face is bleeding. You need medical—'

'Afterwards.' Sean touched his lip where it had opened again. The clerk passed him a few tissues and he took them. 'I found out last night about the *Zheng He* being in trouble near Midgard Lodge.' He stopped on the brink.

You always were a greedy little bastard.

'I believe it's carrying arms.'

'Darling, stop! You're not well!' Martine stared at him in disbelief.

'Shut up.' Ruth Mott looked at her with such fury that Martine sat back out of her eyeline. Mrs Osman put her hand up again and the coroner allowed her to stand.

'Mr Cawson, this is very courageous of you. But are you telling us that the ship ... the *Zheng He* ...' and Mrs Osman looked at her phone, 'which has just been confirmed ... as sunk, was connected with Midgard Lodge?'

'I believe my backer Joe Kingsmith was using it to transport weapons to the Central African Republic and South Sudan, via the port of Bissau.'

'PTSD, you know,' Sawbridge said, to anyone who'd listen. 'Terrible cross.'

'I believe it loads in the Chinese port of Dalian.' Sean looked over to the press bench. He felt a grim satisfaction at meeting their eyes. Let them have at him.

'Dalian is where our other partner, Radiance Young, owns a wharf, and I believe Joe Kingsmith uses it in the supply of weapons and their components, including 3D printers, to several end users. One is Radiance and I believe another is a man from the Central African Republic called Benoit. I believe Joe Kingsmith's main business is private militias, supporting Chinese corporations as they expand in certain African countries where he has interests. The Central African Republic for one, South Sudan another. I believe he might have been involved in Guinea Bissau when I first met him, in 1988. Because of my own greed and stupidity, I've been his unwitting assistant since that time.' Sean forced himself on. 'I think *Zheng He* was carrying chemical weapons.'

The press bench was so stunned that for several seconds they did nothing – and then their fingers clattered and raced. Some got their phones out and started making calls. One journalist – Sean's old enemy – raised his hands and clapped slowly.

'I haven't finished.' Sean gripped the stand, the riptide of adrenaline making him dizzy. 'I thought Tom was naïve and he thought I was corrupt. We were both right, but now I realise I was naïve as well. We were so angry with each other that we missed the signs in the cave. I said I helped him, but it was the other way round. It always was.'

Sean and Tom hear the groan and creak in the ice before they feel the sliding planes around them. With one long ripping sound the floor of ice splits apart, the two sides peel away from each other, and from above stalactites plummet and shatter against the sides of the chasm as they fall. Sean is on one side, Tom the other. A great chunk of ice drops, wedging across the top of the break.

'Quickly,' Tom whispers, shining his head torch on it. 'Crawl over now, while you still can.' Sean stares as the bridging block slowly begins to slip.

'Don't look down, look at me,' Tom calls to him. 'Over here—' He reaches out and they grab each other in the hand-to-forearm boat grip. Tom pulls Sean across. They haul themselves back towards the passageway – but everything has changed.

'You're still a lying shit,' Tom pants to him as they go, 'don't think you're not. Nothing's changed when we get out.'

Sean stopped speaking. His hands were freezing. His legs shook and he could feel the surge of the drug breaking down in his brain. Then he saw Gail's face at the back of the courtroom. She was looking at him steadily, as if she had come to his execution and would not look away. He would die properly then. No half-measures.

'We started to go back,' he said, 'and we knew we had to be quick because there was water coming in from somewhere, it was flowing, and I couldn't believe it because Tom started asking me about the Lodge again, and what else I was hiding, and what was Kingsmith hiding, he wasn't letting go of it even when we might both die – that was what he was like.'

The odd sound was Ruth Mott clapping, standing up, her face wet with tears, nodding at him. *Keep going.*

'We were both so angry with each other, even in this situation, but we kept going on, Tom kept saying *"Fram"* like we used to, *Forward,* like he wasn't frightened at all. He said we were going to get out, *he* was going to get out because he wanted to get back to Ruth.'

He saw her put her arms around herself and close her eyes.

'We felt one of the plastic grip tiles and we knew we were closer to getting out and then everything goes sideways, the whole thing collapses again and Tom's shouting where he's wedged so he doesn't drop, and I've found a rope in the wall, I grab hold of it with my left hand and I reach for him with the other.'

'Here, Tom,' Sean reaches out his right hand, but not quite far enough. His wavering head-torch beam is on Tom's face. 'But first promise not to say anything. Give me your word. When I explain it to you—'

'Give me your fucking hand!'

'I will, just promise me—'

Tom falls. Sean's beam arcs down into blackness. He calls out. Again, again, louder. There is no reply.

Sean fixed his gaze on the back wall of the courtroom, unable to meet a single pair of eyes. His right hand was tingling. Not from frostbite, he knew that now. From what he had not done. He felt about to burst into flames. 'I killed Tom. Not deliberately. But I did.'

In the silence in the courtroom Granny Ruby slowly got to her feet. 'Shame on you,' she said, and her voice was small but as piercing as her eyes. Outside, the booing started again. A mob sound.

'Silence! Everyone!' The coroner stood and addressed Sean. 'Mr Cawson, you are telling the court, you are telling me, that you delayed rendering aid to Mr Harding, in order to attempt to elicit his promise not to say what he had witnessed at Midgard Lodge?'

'Yes.' Sean closed his eyes a moment. 'Tom would not have got involved if he'd known the true scope of what we were doing. And had I known the extent of Joe Kingsmith's other activities, I would not have accepted his investment.'

'Irrelevant, irrelevant, irrelevant!' Sawbridge had had enough and was on his feet as well. 'Your Honour, I move that it is impossible to know if my client could or could not have saved Mr Harding's life, despite his desire to throw himself on his sword, and that because of my client's post-traumatic stress disorder—'

'Mr Sawbridge, sit down—'

'—he is incapable of distinguishing truth from paranoia and is completely delusional. He is suffering from a psychotic disturbance!'

'Must I have you removed?' Mr Thornton shouted it, and Sawbridge sat down. Mrs Osman raised her hand and the coroner permitted her to stand.

'Mr Cawson,' she said quietly. 'I admire your courage. And I am legally bound to tell you that, if you answer my questions, those answers might cause this inquest to be moved, in the public interest, to a criminal trial.'

'I understand. I accept.'

'Are you financially involved with the ship the *Zheng He*, now sunk off the coast of Svalbard, and which you believe is carrying chemical weapons across the TransPolar Route?'

'Yes.'

'You also said you are complicit in allowing Midgard Lodge to be used for intelligence gathering by Norway on Russian activity in the Svalbard archipelago. Are you willing to expand on this?'

'Yes. It was with the approval of Philip Stowe, the British Defence Secretary, and Skadi Larssen, Assistant Minister for Defence, in Oslo. She said Norway was very concerned about Russian expansionism, she said many countries were. We met at the arms fair in London in November, three or four years ago. I brought Kingsmith in on it, but he and Stowe also know each other. I believe I was the go-between.'

He wondered how he could still be standing there, alive. Mrs Osman held his eyes, and he felt her support.

'Do you also have a theory about the cause of this shipping disaster?'

Mr Thornton appeared to have forgotten what was relevant and what was not, and leaned forward for the answer. Sean nodded.

'I believe it ran into trouble in a storm, but, Joe preferred to let it sink rather than report it in distress and have the cargo exposed. He wanted me to think it would cause a massive diplomatic incident. But it was to protect himself.'

The tapping of the press bench went out almost live, online. Outside on the street a hundred smart phones picked it up and the chant rose, loud and angry in the courtroom.

Eco-cide! Eco-cide!

Sean felt the liberation of self-destruction. There was nothing more to hide.

'My meeting with Philip Stowe was arranged by Rupert Parch, his private secretary. He implied I'd get a knighthood for my trouble. At one time, I wanted it.' He found Gail's face at the back. 'I wanted stupid, empty things.'

'Sean!' called Martine. 'You're delirious! Look at me!' She twisted round to see what he was looking at, and saw Gail. 'Did you ask her to come?'

'No.' Sean looked at Martine as if seeing her for the first time.

'You've got no business here,' she called out to Gail.

'Miss Delaroche, you will please leave the court,' said Mr Thornton. 'Now.'

'Fine. But there's something I need to do first.' Martine stood up and turned to Osman. 'You wanted this to happen. You're evil.' She flung the contents of her water glass in the barrister's face and strode towards Gail. 'And you did too, didn't you? You've always wanted to destroy us.' Martine's face tightened. 'Answer me!'

Gail didn't look at her, but nodded to the stewards who held the doors open. As they took a step forward, Martine's eyes burned hatred at Gail – then she stormed out before the stewards could touch her.

Everyone's eyes returned to the extraordinary spectacle of Mrs Osman carefully slicking down her wet hair and standing up straight. The hunch was gone, and her face, though still unusual in its stark bone-structure, was rather beautiful. Nor was she as old as Sean first thought. Meeting her eyes, he saw the amusement in them, before she turned back to the coroner.

'Your Honour, I believe we have heard enough to request a verdict of unlawful killing, and that it is without question in the wider public interest that this inquest be moved to a criminal court.' She looked around. 'I don't expect Mr Kingsmith is available today? No, I rather thought not.'

Sawbridge, slightly recovered, did a half push-up.

'Your Honour, might I cross-examine my own client? As everything is so highly irregular?'

'Please.'

Sawbridge waited until Mrs Osman sat.

'Now, Sean,' he said gently, 'you've been having psychiatric treatment for PTSD, haven't you? You've suffered hallucinations. Remember? In that restaurant? And panic attacks on the Underground—'

'I never told you that.' But he had told Jenny Flanders.

'Memory lapses, confusion – fact is, you're *not* a competent witness. I think His Honour and even my learned friend Mrs Osman can see that. Survivor's guilt is one of the most pernicious burdens facing our returning armed forces. Who here hasn't put a note in the bucket for Help for Heroes? In his own way, Sean Cawson has served his country and paid the price. Shouldn't we respect his sacrifice? Let's remember both Sean and Tom shared a lifetime's obsession for the Arctic and both knew the risks. That was part of the appeal! Yes, they had political differences; yes, they argued, but at the end of the day even heroes can die, and that's what's so hard for Sean to accept. That's why he's trying to make himself responsible for everything that ever went wrong. Survivor's guilt.'

Sean looked to Mrs Osman.

'I stand by everything I said.'

In the silence, the coroner drew a deep breath.

'The court will recess for fifteen minutes.' As he walked out, the courtroom burst into noise.

Sean couldn't hear anything as he walked down the aisle; he felt half dead but it was not unpleasant. The stares no longer bothered him. Gail stood up as he reached her. They regarded each other in silence. He saw the delicate lines around her eyes, her mouth, he saw her neck, her breasts, the small knots of gold in her earlobes – he saw the girl inside the woman.

'You haven't changed.'

'You have. Well done, Sean.' Her smile broke his heart. Before he could answer, Sawbridge took him by the arm.

'Terribly sorry, but the moment is critical – Sean, you must come now.'

'Wait,' he said. She nodded.

He stood with Sawbridge in the small room. The angry chanting floated up. *Eco-cide! Save the Arctic!* He forced open the window, peering down into the street where police had arrived to manage the situation.

'Something far more urgent here, old chap.' Sawbridge held up his phone. 'Let's see: don't believe anything until it's been officially denied twice – we're way past that. Denials flying in all directions, official rebuttal of all your "specious claims" from Stowe's office – already online so you know it's serious. Yep, google-translated in every country in which you've got us into the deepest diplomatic excrement. Ah, here we are, British trade talks with the Sino-Arctic Alliance suspended – aren't you clever? Just from one, stupid, undisciplined, outburst. All this fuss. I'm your counsel, did you even think how it would reflect on me?'

Sawbridge wound up with a quick, pained grin. 'Never mind, worse things happen at sea, don't they just.' He glanced at his phone screen, flashing with incoming emails. 'And completely par for the course, the Sysselmann's office in Svalbard has questioned the legality of your ownership. Midgard personnel in altercation with Russian search and rescue from the Arktik Dacha – all Greek to me, but maybe means something to you? – yes, and here we go, links to more outrage – you're trending, Sean! All the fame you can handle. Nobody's cared for years about the flouting of the Svalbard Treaty until you show them up as a bunch of hypocrites. You didn't mean to, I know; you were just playing geopolitics with your Lego, and now you're in all this trouble.' Sawbridge squinted at the screen. 'Aha. Someone I think you know.'

He turned his phone to Sean, where a YouTube clip played: a furious Skadi Larssen denying everything in Norwegian, with English subtitles. He winked. 'Honey trap, was it? Must say, I'd probably fall for it too—'

Sean knocked the phone from his hand. A tiny angry Skadi spun on the floor. Sawbridge picked his phone up and examined it sadly.

'I'll add it to the bill. Be a good chap and pay me before the deluge of all your other costs comes in, won't you? Much obliged.' He peered into the crazed screen. 'More emails, oh dear, so many from our mutual friend Rupert Parch – you seem to have greatly upset him. But he really shouldn't cc me.' Sawbridge brushed a few invisible specks from his jacket. 'Shall we agree that I'm not the best representation for you going forward? Excellent.' He looked at his watch. 'Tell you what, we'll stop the clock yesterday. Do excuse me, and the very best of luck with everything.'

*

Sean sat alone in the small cell of a room, with the flat-pack furniture and the damp-curled carpet tiles, and the blue upholstered chairs. The soreness and damage to his face and body felt more insistent, but it was nothing compared to the pain in his heart. Outside, the chants were louder – the crowd had grown. He looked at the blank space on his wrist. He hoped the cabbie's son would be happy. He felt grateful to John Burnham and his fiery daughter.

And to Rosie – he felt a flush of love at the thought of his daughter who had come back to him, violently angry though she still was. He burst out of the room in search of her, straight into Mr Thornton, Mrs Osman, Ruth Mott and the Harding family, heading back in for the summing up. He halted, waiting for the abuse to fall on him – but instead Ruth Mott put her hand on his arm. Angela Harding looked him in the eye. 'Thank you, Sean,' she said quietly, and walked on with her mother-in-law. Sean followed behind, with Ruth.

'It's not true, you know,' she said. 'You did help Tom. When you spoke for him, when he was too drunk, when you stopped Redmond from hurting him more in Greenland. When you told him not to care what people thought, to do what he wanted with his life. He told me those stories so many times. Sean, he loved you.'

Granny Ruby turned. 'And you loved him. We saw that.'

They went in. Mr Thornton entered a silent courtroom full of standing people. The Harding group went to one side, but Sean, now alone, walked to his empty row. No Martine, no Sawbridge. Gail remained at the back, Rosie now by her side.

Mr Thornton was brief. Despite Mr Cawson's astonishing and, he agreed, most courageous testimony, he had not changed his opinion.

If there were evidence that Mr Cawson had wilfully let Mr Harding die, there would be a case for unlawful killing. But it was his belief that, although Mr Cawson made a morally unwise attempt to coerce Mr Harding into a promise under extreme circumstances, he had neither wished his death nor sought it in any way.

It was also Mr Thornton's belief that Mr Harding, whilst he might not have become involved in the Midgard Lodge purchase bid had he been in possession of all the facts, was nevertheless experienced in Arctic travel, and knew its risks. He had entered the ice-cave of his own volition.

He was therefore of the considered opinion that Tom Harding lost his life due to the proven collapse of the Midgardbreen ice-cave system, most probably due to the pervasive action of meltwater on the ice cap above. This was arguably an effect of climate change but even if so, and he believed it was, that was not in itself a direct cause of Mr Harding's death.

He also stated for the record that Mr Harding's body was believed irretrievably lost in the ice-cave on the date of the accident, until it was revealed by further action of the glacier, in the calving witnessed by the passengers of the cruise ship *Vanir* – at which point it was recovered.

But – and Mr Thornton looked at Sean as he said this – given Mr Cawson's new testimony, and the wider events in the world, namely today's sinking of the cargo ship the *Zheng He* off the coast of Svalbard, he believed a further investigation into the activities and partners of Midgard Lodge was warranted.

He waited until the sound of cheering and applause from the street died down and then looked to the press bench.

'Are you transmitting this live?'

They all nodded. At the back, Beth Burnham also raised her hand to be counted.

'Whilst I therefore return a narrative conclusion to this inquest, that the cause of death of Mr Thomas Walter Harding be recorded as Nature Unknown, I also recommend that the entire body of evidence I have collected in this process be moved on to criminal investigation, as requested by Mrs Ursula Osman, KC.'

Ruby Harding rose to her feet applauding, joined by a number of people in the court, the sound drowned out by the roar from the crowd in the street below.

Mr Thornton and his clerk left in a sweep of robes, the courtroom burst with noise and movement, but Sean stood where he was. Someone came up to take his photograph with a phone but Gail pushed the phone aside.

'Leave my husband alone.'

That phrase brought Sean back. He looked at her.

'Slip of the tongue,' she said. 'Need a lift? I've got my car at the back.'

He felt as slow as a dream, the Rohypnol spiking again. 'Where's Rosie gone?'

'Outside. She knows some of those people.'

'Gail ...' He saw the lines around her eyes, he wanted to touch them. 'Would you bring the car round there? I have to do something first.'

When she'd gone, the clerks and security guards allowed Sean a moment alone in the courtroom to collect himself. He stood in the empty space, the mints spilled on the floor, the disordered chairs, his own toxic sweat. He sat down and put his face in hands that no longer burned. It was over.

The crowd were chanting for him. The ugly sound swelled as they saw him coming through the lobby but Sean stepped straight out onto the steps.

An egg broke against his shoulder, then another one. People jeered and booed and he wondered why the police weren't there – but they were. There were just so many protestors – hundreds more had arrived, some with placards and masks, others whose fresh young faces opened and closed in angry shouts he couldn't quite hear. For a moment it all swam in brightness and he felt the drug still in his system. Even the young could look ugly, if they were angry enough. He picked out the word Arctic in their chants and screams.

'Arctic,' he repeated, trying to bring himself back from the dangerous haze on the edge of everything. 'The Arctic,' he said. He heard another word. 'Ecocide.'

Arc-tic! Eco-cide! A heavy paper cup hit him, and the coffee smelled good.

He recognised a red jacket and a friendly face in the crowd – of course it was Tom, Sean was pleased to see him. He waved. Young and handsome, Tom waved back, holding something up. Something brown and pointed. Sean recognised it. The shit chisel. He held up his own imaginary one, and thinking he was addressing them, the crowd shouted louder.

'Let him speak!' Armed with a megaphone, Rosie furiously elbowed her way out of the crowd and joined her father on the steps. 'Just shut the fuck up for a minute,' she said through it, his warrior daughter and human shield. Sean gazed at her in wonder as she handed him the megaphone. 'Quick,' she said under her breath, 'if you're going to.'

'You're right to be angry,' Sean called out to them. 'I've been stupid and greedy and blind, I've betrayed and lost my best friend, and I've destroyed everything I've touched. And the *Zheng He* has sunk—'

He waited for the noise to die down, 'But I am going to cooperate in every way I can to make sure this cannot happen again, and I'm going to do it in a criminal court. And I want as many of you there as will fit in, I want you in the room because Tom can't be there. And I don't want there to be a conservation bequest in his name. I want there to be no need for one.'

To his surprise, there was a smattering of applause. He looked at the crowd of young people holding up their phones recording his shame. But standing there with his daughter who had returned to him, and his wife – she still was – coming for him, he felt the opposite. As if some burden he hadn't known he carried was lifting.

He saw a mineral white BMW coming up the street, slowly parting the crowd. It took a moment to recognise the woman at the wheel as Gail. He went down the steps, Rosie by his side, flashes going off in his face. He heard the door locks click open, and he climbed in.

'I'm staying.' Rosie had tears in her eyes as she smiled. 'You did good, Dad.' Before she could close the door on him, he grabbed her hand and kissed it. She thumped the car twice on the roof and Gail clicked the locks as photographers tried to block them for more pictures. She drove slowly into them and they jumped back, cursing. Sean looked at her in amazement. She shrugged.

He moved around in the seat and fiddled with the controls. Something occurred to him. Some tall bastard had sat here with his long legs. Gail's lips twitched, as she understood what he was processing. She had had a lover. A tall one. Maybe she still did. Sean was harpooned by jealousy.

She pulled out onto the ring road and they drove in busy silence for a while.

'Rosie called me Dad again.'

'I heard.'

Neither was aware of the black Vauxhall Insignia following two cars behind.

'Where shall I take you?'

'Home.'

'I'm not going to bloody London—'

'Nor am I.'

She looked at him a moment. 'Sean – you can't just come back like that.'

'No. I know.' He waited a moment. 'Is the tall bastard still around?'

Gail did laugh now, but she didn't answer. They drove on in silence for several miles. He recognised the roads. He looked at his watch, or the space where it had been.

'Do you mind if we have the news?'

She turned it on. The environmental disaster of the *Zheng He* was now the top story and the Ministry of Defence had issued a denial of the shocking allegations at the inquest of respected environmentalist Tom Harding—

Sean looked out at the familiar fields, the hedges, the fences, as the news presenter explained about the environmental integrity of Svalbard, the suspension of British businessman Sean Cawson's troubled Arctic venture ...

There was the Acorn, the beautiful country pub where they hadn't been in years, he would like to go there again—

... investigations to be carried out over a suspected breach of the Svalbard Treaty ... trade relations ... historic allies ...

Sean didn't care that the Russian ambassador had already made a formal complaint in London, he didn't care if he never walked into a smart party again, if all the grand doors in grand houses owned by grand people slammed in his face – because what mattered was that his daughter had grown up while he wasn't looking but that now she had come back to him. What mattered was that he was with Gail again and the band around his chest, that he hadn't even known was there, was gone and he could breathe again. He recognised the roads, and the trees, and the fields as they sped home in her new car. And that tall bastard would never sit in his place, because he was going to make her happy again, and come back from the ice and finally deserve her love.

*

In another, chauffeur-driven car, Martine and Sawbridge sped back to London in silence, listening to the same news, caring very much about the formal complaint by the Russian ambassador, and the mention of Midgard Lodge. In an office overlooking Whitehall, whilst checking three other screens and writing an email on a fourth, so did Rupert Parch, his eyes not remotely merry, and his disposition far from playful.

Cruising at 36,000 feet, Joe Kingsmith cut into a blue steak, three phones and two laptops open beside his plate. Occasionally he swept them all with a glance. Nothing.

In Canterbury, the Feathers pub was doing uncharacteristically brisk business for the hour, as activists and journalists crammed in, and John Burnham had put the football flat-screen on to watch the breaking news about the ship. In the hubbub, Ruth Mott and Rosie Cawson sat together, both tearstained, and drinking pints. Ruth had her arm around Rosie, and Rosie had her phone out, listening and nodding while Ruth spoke.

Sean sat back as Gail drove. In his wing-mirror he saw a black saloon approaching fast, indicating to overtake. Gail glanced up in the rear-view mirror and saw it too. How extraordinary that he felt no pain about Martine. She had abandoned him in court, but he felt nothing, not even anger. Yet to leave Gail had been agony only trumped by lust. Sean saw as the black car overtook that it was a Vauxhall Insignia. Its brake lights glared red, it suddenly skewed to the side and Gail hauled on the wheel – but it skewed again, forcing them the other way – their speed too fast and the road too narrow to miss the long drystone wall. The impact hurled the BMW into the air.

*

Ah, sighed Anaralunguaq, *and we used to think Nature was the greatest and most wonderful of all! Yet here we are among mountains and great gulfs and precipices, all made by the work of human hands.*

The BMW crashed down on its roof, activating its on-board emergency satellite communication. Two hundred miles above the road accident it reported, that information was beamed back down to earth, and the relevant civic authorities.

Nature is great; Sila, as we call it at home; nature, the world, the universe, all that is Sila; which our wise men declared they could hold in poise. And I could never believe it, but I see it now. Nature is great, but are not men greater?

Four hundred metres down the road, where the drystone wall ended and the road curved around, the driver of a Dutch-registered eighteen-wheeler had stopped for a break in a layby. As the oncoming Vauxhall flashed its lights, two men inside opened the rear doors and dropped the hinged ramp. The Vauxhall drove in and braked hard. They pulled up the ramp and closed the doors. The lorry drove away.

The wheels of the BMW spun slowly to a halt. Nothing moved but the wind.

One of Kingsmith's phones flashed. Still chewing, he slid it towards him. A blank text from a UK number. He deleted it then signalled the steward for more wine.

*

In the press, on social media, in Chatham House, in bars, in cafés, even in Highgrove House (where the King was hosting an interdisciplinary debate on the role of monarchy and the wilderness) speculation raged over the connection between the sinking of the *Zheng He* and the death of environmentalist Tom Harding.

Those tiny beings we can see down there far below, hurrying this way and that. They live among these stone walls; on a great plain of stone made with hands. Stone and stone and stone – there is no game to be seen anywhere, and yet they manage to live and find their daily food.

On the floor of the Barents Sea, the steel hull of the *Zheng He* settled into the swirling sediment. Her oil, and other substances lighter than water, continued to leak out into the darkness, towards the troubled gyres of the seven seas.

Have they then learned of the animals, since they can dig down under the earth like marmots, hang in the air like spiders, fly like birds and dive under water like the fishes; seemingly masters of all that struggled against ourselves?

Inside the inverted vehicle, a human voice speaks from the onboard computer, assuring the driver that BMW have been informed of the collision and location, and that assistance is on its way. A rap ringtone interrupts, coming through the car's digital system.

Gail manages to reach up and press the button on the steering wheel.

'Hi,' She's hoarse, and gasping. The remote voice coming from somewhere in the car continues to reassure the passengers.

'Mum?' says Rosie's voice. 'Dad, can you hear me? What's that noise? I've got major anxiety about my dysfunctional parents – but I just want you to know I love you both.'

Sean reaches out to hold Gail's shoulder. The blown airbags make it difficult. He clenches back a gasp of pain. 'We love you too.'

'Rosie,' Gail calls out. 'Remember, deep breaths.'

I see more things than my mind can grasp; and the only way to save oneself from madness is to suppose that we have all died suddenly before we knew, and that this is part of another life.

The mineral white BMW blocks the road, emergency lights flashing. Motorists have stopped to help, traffic is starting to back up. Inside it, Sean and Gail have found each other's hand. Sirens wail. They hold on.

AUTHOR'S NOTE

Since the fourteenth century, men have sought a northern maritime trade route between Europe and what was once known as Cathay; the Far East. Countless sums and lives have been spent in its pursuit.

The end of the Arctic summer sea ice means that finally, the long-sought TransPolar trade route directly over the North Pole is now open; through the 1.1 million square miles of the international waters of the Arctic Ocean – covered with permanent ice for all of human history, until now.

Distance savings compared with traditional trade routes using the Suez or Panama canals, can be as high as 35 per cent. And with possible closures to both these historic routes due to political instability, traffic across the TransPolar Route increases every day.

A VERY PARTIAL BIBLIOGRAPHY

Bones, Stian and Petia Mankova (eds.), *Norway and Russia in the Arctic: conference proceedings from the international conference 'Norway and Russia in the Arctic', Longyearbyen, 25–28 August 2009* (University of Tromsø, 2010)

Byock, Jesse L. (tr.), *The Saga of the Volsungs: The Norse Epic of Sigurd the Dragon Slayer* (Penguin, 1990)

Chapman, F. Spencer, *Northern Lights: The Official Account of the British Arctic Air-Route Expedition 1930–1931* (Chatto & Windus, 1932)

Davis, Wade, *The Wayfinders: Why Ancient Wisdom Matters in the Modern World* (House of Anansi Press, 2009)

Gearheard, Shari Fox *et al.*, *The Meaning of Ice: People and Sea Ice in Three Arctic Communities* (International Polar Institute Press; University Press of New England, 2013)

Emmerson, Charles, *The Future History of the Arctic* (PublicAffairs, 2010)

Freuchen, Peter, *Arctic Adventure: My Life in the Frozen North* (William Heinemann Ltd, 1936)

Freuchen, Peter (tr. Johan Hambro), *Vagrant Viking: My Life and Adventures* (J. Messner, 1953)

Henson, Matthew, *A Negro Explorer at the North Pole: The Autobiography of Matthew Henson* (F. Stokes, 1912)

Horwitz, Joshua, *War of the Whales: A True Story* (Simon &

Schuster, 2014)

Klein, Naomi, *This Changes Everything: Capitalism vs. the Climate* (Penguin, 2014)

Lindsay, Martin, *Sledge: The British Trans-Greenland Expedition 1934* (Cassell & Co., 1935)

Lopez, Barry Holstun, *Arctic Dreams: Imagination and Desire in a Northern Landscape* (Scribner, 1986)

Malaurie, Jean (tr. Gwendolen Freeman), *The Last Kings of Thule: A Year Among the Polar Eskimos of Greenland* (George Allen & Unwin Ltd, 1956)

McFate, Sean, *The Modern Mercenary: Private Armies and What They Mean for World Order* (Oxford University Press, 2014)

McGhee, Robert, *The Last Imaginary Place: A Human History of the Arctic World* (University of Chicago Press, 2007)

Mikkelsen, Captain Ejnar, *Lost in the Arctic: Being the story of the 'Alabama' Expedition 1909–12* (William Heinemann Ltd, 1913)

Nansen, Dr. Fridtjof, *Farthest North: The Norwegian Polar Expedition 1893–1896* (Archibald Constable & Co., 1897)

Ovsyanikov, Nikita, *Polar Bears: Living with the White Bear* (Swan Hill Press, 1996)

Peary, Robert E., *The North Pole* (Hodder & Stoughton, 1910)

Rasmussen, Knud, *Across Arctic America: Narrative of the Fifth Thule Expedition* (G. P. Putnam's Sons, 1927)

Scoresby, William, *An Account of the Arctic Regions: With a History and Description of the Northern Whale-Fishery* (Archibald Constable & Co., 1820)

Scott, Jeremy, *Dancing on Ice: A 1930s Arctic Adventure* (Old Street Publishing, 2008)

Singer, P. W., *Corporate Warriors: The Rise of the Privatized Military Industry* (Cornell University Press, 2003)

Smiley, Jane (ed.), *The Sagas of the Icelanders* (Penguin, 2001)

Stirling, Ian, *Polar Bears: The Natural History of a Threatened Species* (Bloomsbury, 2012)

Wadhams, Peter, *A Farewell to Ice: A Report from the Arctic* (Allen Lane, 2016)

Wheeler, Sara, *The Magnetic North: Notes from the Arctic Circle* (North Point Press, 2009)

Wormdal, Bård, *The Satellite War* (CreateSpace Independent

Publishing Platform, 2011)

Worsley, Frank Arthur and Grettir Algarsson, *Under Sail in the Frozen North: The Log of the 1926 British Arctic Expedition* (Stanley Paul & Co., 1927)

ACKNOWLEDGEMENTS

This book was written with the support of a great many people. It is now my pleasure to thank: At 4th Estate Books, David Roth-Ey and Helen Garnons-Williams; Michelle Kane, Matt Clacher and Paul Erdpresser; Lottie Fyfe, Anne O'Brien and Tom Killingbeck; Jo Walker for the beautiful cover, and Chris Wormell for the woodcuts inside.

Thank you to my agents Simon Trewin and Dorian Karchmar, and to the Royal Society of Literature for the Brookleaze Grant, which I used towards research travel to Svalbard. When I got there Frigg and Frank Jorgensen showed me generous hospitality, gave me connections and rifle training; Arild Lyssand gave me invaluable research information throughout my process; my warmest thanks to all of them. Thanks in Svalbard also to Jason Roberts, Tom Foreman and Mark Sabbatini for Arctic guidance in many forms, and to Captain Daniel Rizzotti, Mikael Arman, Dima Litvinov and Arne Sorensen for hospitality aboard the Greenpeace ship *Esperanza*.

This book has benefited from the collected wisdom of the following authorities in their fields, and all errors and omissions in the text are mine alone. It is my pleasure to thank: Dr Peter Wadhams and the Scott Polar Research Institute in Cambridge; Rear Admiral John Kingwell and Mrs Alison Kingwell; Mr Michael Kingston, insurance representative at the International Maritime Organisation on the finalisation of the Polar Code; Mr Alan Kessel, Canadian Deputy High Commissioner in London; Mr Charles Emmerson, Senior

Research Fellow, Chatham House; Professor Klaus Dodds, Professor of Geopolitics at Royal Holloway College, University of London; Judge Rüdiger Wolfrum, member of the International Tribunal for the Law of the Sea; Mr Robin Hepburn; Mr Rod Downie of the World Wildlife Fund and Mr Geoff York of Polar Bears International; and my thanks again to polar scientists Dr Tom Smith, Dr Jon Aars, Dr Lily Peacock, Dr Christian Sonne and Dr Kristin Lairdre. I must also thank those individuals who, on condition of anonymity, confirmed the plausibility of one story element; also that truth is indeed stranger than fiction.

For permission to use her real performance as a cameo in this novel, I thank Polaris and Mercury prize-winner Tanya Tagaq, and for further insight into Inuit culture of Nunavut, I thank Mataalii Okalik. I also thank Peter Freuchen's grandson Peter Ittinuar, and his great-grand-daughter, Natalie Ittinuar, for their support.

Though he will not now read this book as he hoped, I owe thanks to Peter Cawson, one of the unsung heroes of the Polarati. In return for tea and fruitcake on Thursday afternoons in his funny little shop in St Leonards-on-Sea, he dug out rare old Arctic books and told me stories. Thank you to Beannie Nicholson for baking the best, and thank you too, Natascha Lampert, and Nick Foulkes.

For inspiration and support, I thank Clare Reihill, Jay Griffiths, Cal Moriarty, Clare Carlin, Anna Orenstein, Paul Dornan, Isabelle Grey, Liz Jensen, Ruth Gravelle, Natasha Bishopp, Maggie Doherty, Tessa Boase and Hattie Ellis. For patience and love during the writing process I thank all my family but particularly my mother and my daughter India Rose.

Lastly, I thank my husband Adrian Peacock, who ran base-camp and dangerous rescue missions like a true hero.